A CONSUMER'S GUIDE TO OVER THE COUNTER MEDICINES

A CONSUMER'S GUIDE TO OVER THE COUNTER MEDICINES

Dr Barrington Cooper, Dr Laurence Gerlis
and Elizabeth Jeannet

- All commonly used over-the-counter medicines included ●
- All widely available herbal remedies included ●
- A comprehensive survey of homoeopathic preparations ●
- Three-part arrangement for easy access ●
- Easy-to-follow table of drug interactions ●
- Invaluable table of effects of vitamin overdoseage ●
- Key medical terms explained ●

BCA

LONDON · NEW YORK · SYDNEY · TORONTO

Edited, designed, and produced by Curtis Garratt Limited
The Old Vicarage, Horton cum Studley, Oxford OX9 1BT

This edition published 1992 by BCA
By arrangement with Octopus Illustrated Publishing
Michelin House, 81 Fulham Road, London SW3 6RB
part of Reed International Books

A catalogue record for this book is available from the British Library

CN 4972

Printed in Great Britain

IMPORTANT
As the introduction explains, *A Consumer's Guide to Over-the-counter Medicines* is designed to be a self-treatment book **only for minor conditions**. It would be used, therefore, before consulting a physician to gain information about medicines which are available, without a prescription, from pharmacies, health food shops, and so on. On the other hand, the *Guide* is **not intended** to be a substitute for the advice of a prescribing physician nor for the instructions on the medicine's package. Similarly, it is advisable to consult a herbal or homoeopathic practitioner if you intend to use alternative therapies.

Every effort has been made to ensure that the information contained in the book is as accurate and up-to-date as possible at the time of going to press but medical and pharmaceutical knowledge continues to progress, and the use of a particular medicine may be different for every patient. **Always** consult your medical practitioner if any symptoms from which you are suffering persist or worsen.

The authors, editors, consultants, and publishers of this book can not be held liable for any errors or omissions, nor for any consequences of using it.

CONTENTS

Introduction

In 1990, our book, *A Consumer's Guide to Prescription Medicines*, was published for the first time. This has been a very successful publication and its companion volume, *A Consumer's Guide to Over-the-Counter Medicines*, follows on naturally from it. The aims and objectives of the two books are entirely different, however.

The purpose of the first book is to supply additional information to those patients who have consulted a doctor and who want to know more about the actions and side effects of prescription medicines. It was always meant to be used in conjunction with medical advice. In contrast, *A Consumer's Guide to Over-the-Counter Medicines* is designed to be a self-treatment book for minor conditions, and it would be used, therefore, before consulting a physician. If it is carried out properly, well-informed self-medication may make it unnecessary to see a doctor but we do advise everyone using this book to seek medical advice if the symptoms worsen or persist.

We have included in this book preparations which can be bought at a pharmacy or at a health food shop without a prescription. Although we work as orthodox practitioners, we are aware that a number of patients use herbal and homoeopathic remedies, so we have included a section on alternative therapies.

According to the *British Medical Journal* (1991, Vol. 302, pp 612-13), there is a boom in over-the-counter (OTC) medicines. Sales of these preparations account for 13 per cent of the European medicines market and 30 per cent of that in the United States. At the time of writing, the British public spends £600 million a year on OTC preparations.

You may be surprised to see that some extremely powerful medications are available as OTC products. Insulin and all of the accessories available for diabetic patients, for example, can be bought from pharmacies without a prescription. Similarly, anti-anginal nitrates and vasodilators can be purchased. Antifungals, antimalarials, anti-worm agents, antacids, bronchodilators, steroid creams, antihistamines, and anaesthetic gels can all be obtained without a prescription. Thus, the well-informed patient has available an armamentarium of drugs and herbs which can be used as first-line therapies for a wide range of illnesses. The purpose of this book is to provide that information.

This book contains a listing of a number of homoeopathic and herbal preparations with a note of their uses and indications. This information is made available to the reader to enable the understanding of alternative medicine, but we can not endorse the fine detail for these products because the mechanisms of action are not entirely clear and vary from person to person.

Thus, this book is intended to enable the reader to best use the medicines to which he or she has open access. These can be used to treat minor conditions which occur at home, recognizing the need for people to do what they can for themselves.

Potentially serious conditions, such as pain in the head, chest, abdomen, eye, or ear, which worsen or persist beyond forty-eight hours need medical attention, particularly if they occur as a result of injury. Where possible, a diagnosis should be made before treatment of any condition with any type of therapy.

No one should underestimate the value of the advice which may be obtained from the pharmacist or other ancillary practitioner.

The ethos of alternative medicine precedes modern therapy, and many current treatments are derived from earlier natural remedies. For these reasons, we include both conventional and alternative therapies in this book.

Dr Barrington Cooper
Dr Laurence Gerlis
21 Devonshire Place
London W1

1991

How to use this book

A Consumer's Guide to Over-the-Counter Medicines is organized into two major parts, the first of which is divided into a series of sections. Each section of the first part of the book is concerned with the various disorders of one part of the body. Thus, anyone suffering with an eye or ear condition should consult the relevant section. Treatments for skin infections should be

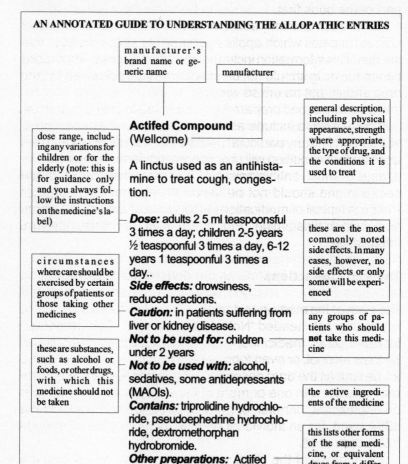

AN ANNOTATED GUIDE TO UNDERSTANDING THE ALLOPATHIC ENTRIES

manufacturer's brand name or generic name

manufacturer

Actifed Compound
(Wellcome)

A linctus used as an antihistamine to treat cough, congestion.

general description, including physical appearance, strength where appropriate, the type of drug, and the conditions it is used to treat

dose range, including any variations for children or for the elderly (note: this is for guidance only and you always follow the instructions on the medicine's label)

Dose: adults 2 5 ml teaspoonsful 3 times a day; children 2-5 years ½ teaspoonful 3 times a day, 6-12 years 1 teaspoonful 3 times a day..

Side effects: drowsiness, reduced reactions.

these are the most commonly noted side effects. In many cases, however, no side effects or only some will be experienced

circumstances where care should be exercised by certain groups of patients or those taking other medicines

Caution: in patients suffering from liver or kidney disease.

Not to be used for: children under 2 years

any groups of patients who should **not** take this medicine

these are substances, such as alcohol or foods, or other drugs, with which this medicine should not be taken

Not to be used with: alcohol, sedatives, some antidepressants (MAOIs).

Contains: triprolidine hydrochloride, pseudoephedrine hydrochloride, dextromethorphan hydrobromide.

the active ingredients of the medicine

Other preparations: Actifed Expectorant, Actifed Tablets,

this lists other forms of the same medicine, or equivalent drugs from a different manufacturer sought under the section on skin disorders, as well as among the antiseptics and antifungals.

All the preparations included in this book are also listed in the Index so that you may check on a drug that has been recommended to you. And, to allow even easier access to any given preparation, the second part of the book lists every drug included in the first part in strict alphabetical order. Diseases are listed in the Index, too, and you may find it easier to consult this part of the book first.

Within each section, some preparations are listed together with extra detail which applies generally to all the drugs in that section. This information includes side effects, contra-indications (when the drug should not be used), and interactions (what the drug should not be mixed with).

We have grouped preparations according to their general use and have tried to include as many preparations as possible. If you cannot find any particular preparation, the other productions used for that condition will give general guidance for usage. For example, most antihistamines listed here will cause some sedation and should not be used with alcohol. The entry for Piriton is typical of medications in this section and if you cannot find your antihistamine, Piriton will give you some general information.

Table of interactions

For each of the medicines described in detail in this book, there is a paragraph headed 'Not to be used with'. This paragraph includes other medicines, groups of medicines, substances such as alcohol, or even foods which should not be taken at the same time as the drug described. This is because the medicine may interact with one or more of the substances mentioned in an unpleasant, harmful, or potentially dangerous way. On the other hand, for an individual patient, there may be no serious interaction at all.

The purpose of the chart set out below is to depict, using a simple and familiar technique, whether or not major 'families' of medicines have been found to interact with one another in any way. It does not attempt to show the degree of interaction. To work out whether or not a medicine you have been prescribed is likely to interact with any other substance, just pick out the family to which it belongs in the vertical column, and trace it horizontally across the chart. Where a ' ● ' occurs, trace down the chart and you will find the name of the substance with which it may interact.

For detailed information concerning interactions, you should, of course, refer to the 'Not to be used with' paragraph for the particular medicine you have been prescribed.

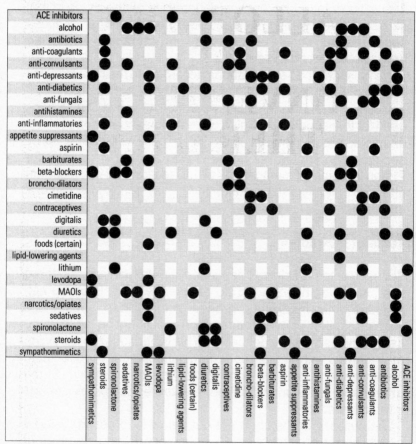

PART 1

ALLOPATHIC OR CONVENTIONAL THERAPIES

Eye conditions

The main eye disorders are infections, inflammations, cataract, and glaucoma. Because of the sensitive nature of the eyes, most of these should be treated by a doctor using a prescription medicine. A few eye preparations are available over the counter, and many of these can be used in the early stages of eye infections to irrigate and disinfect the eye. The Optrex range of products is useful in this respect as are Brolene eye drops. Eye Dew and Murine reduce reddening of the eye.

Eppy is used for the treatment of glaucoma and is available over the counter. Most of the other preparations below contain disinfectants or artificial tears for those people whose lachrymal glands are reduced in activity. Fluorescein and Rose Bengal are special dyes used to diagnose eye ulcers and degenerative cells respectively.

It is worth remembering that contact lens solutions, protein removers, and disinfectants are also over-the-counter medicines which need product licences from the manufacturer.

Redness of the eye, pain in the eye, altered vision, painful reaction to light, and pus in the eye are all symptoms which require medical attention relatively quickly. Self-treatment should not be prolonged beyond twenty-four hours unless there is definite improvement in the condition.

There is no accepted treatment, other than surgery, for cataract. Eye infections are most commonly due to bacteria and may improve after twenty-four hours use of one of the irrigations listed here. Thereafter, antibiotic treatment may be necessary after a consultation with a doctor. Some viruses affect the eye and can cause permanent damage and a medical opinion and the use of antiviral drugs will resolve the virus. Red eyes may be due simply to irritation caused by cigarettes, but prolonged reddening may be caused by infections or even iritis. This latter condition is due to local inflammation and needs to be treated by a doctor with steroids. Acute glaucoma (increased eye pressure) can also result in red eyes but chronic glaucoma can worsen without warning and cause visual loss.

Brolene Eye Drops
(Fisons)

These contain propamidine isethionate 0.1%, benzalkonium chloride 0.1%. An ointment is also available. These substances disinfect the eye and reduce redness. They may cause some local stinging and should not be used if redness of the eye persists or worsens. Allergies often in the eyes, particularly hay fever, cosmetic and dust allergies.

Eppy
(SNP)

Drops used as a sympathomimetic to treat glaucoma.

Dose: 1 drop into the eye 1-2 times a day.
Side effects: pain in the eye, headache, skin reactions, melanosis, red eye, rarely systemic effects.
Caution:
Not to be used for: patients suffering from absence of the lens, narrow angle glaucoma.
Not to be used with:
Contains: adrenaline.
Other preparations:

Eye Dew see Brolene Eye Drops and Optrex

Fluorescein
(SNP)

Drops used as a dye for staining purposes to enable abrasions or foreign bodies in the eye to be found.

Dose: 1 or more drops into the eye as needed.
Side effects:

Caution:
Not to be used for:
Not to be used with:
Contains: sodium fluorescein.
Other preparations:

Hypotears
(Iolab)

Drops used to moisten dry eyes.

Dose: 1-2 drops every 3-4 hours or as needed.
Side effects:
Caution:
Not to be used for: patients who wear soft contact lenses.
Not to be used with:
Contains: polyethylene glycol, polyvinyl alcohol.
Other preparations:

Isopto Alkaline
(Alcon)

Drops used to lubricate the eyes.

Dose: 1-2 drops into the eye 3 times a day.
Side effects:
Caution:
Not to be used for: patients who wear soft contact lenses.
Not to be used with:
Contains: hypromellose.
Other preparations:

Isopto Frin
(Alcon)

Drops used to lubricate the eyes when no infection is present.

Dose: 1-2 drops into the eye 3 times a day.
Side effects:
Caution: in infants and in patients suffering from narrow angle glaucoma.
Not to be used for: patients who wear soft contact lenses.
Not to be used with:
Contains: phenylephrine hydrochloride.
Other preparations:

Isopto Plain
(Alcon)

Drops used to moisten dry eyes.

Dose: 1-2 drops into the eye 3 times a day.
Side effects:
Caution:
Not to be used for: patients who wear soft contact lenses.
Not to be used with:
Contains: hypromellose.
Other preparations:

Lacri-Lube
(Allergan)

An ointment used for lubricating the eyes and protecting the cornea.

Dose: apply into the eye as needed.
Side effects:
Caution:
Not to be used for:
Not to be used with:
Contains: liquid paraffin, wool fat.

Other preparations:

Liquifilm Tears
(Allergan)

Drops used to lubricate dry eyes.

Dose: 1 drop into the eye as needed.
Side effects:
Caution:
Not to be used for: patients who wear soft contact lenses.
Not to be used with:
Contains: polyvinyl alcohol.
Other preparations:

Minims Saline
(SNP)
Drops used to irrigate the eyes.

Dose: use as needed.
Side effects:
Caution:
Not to be used for: patients who wear soft contact lenses.
Not to be used with:
Contains: sodium chloride.
Other preparations:

Murine see **Brolene** and **Optrex**

Normasol
(Seton-Prebbles)

A solution in a sachet used for washing out eyes, burns, wounds.

Dose: use as needed.
Side effects:
Caution:
Not to be used for:
Not to be used with:
Contains: sodium chloride.
Other preparations:

Optrex eye preparations
Optrex eye preparations contain dilute solutons of witch hazel.
This reduces eye reddening, and the solution acts to irrigate the
eye. Some people are particularly sensitive to witch hazel and the
treatment should not be continued if symptoms persist or worsen.
Local sensitivity will present as stinging in or around the eye.

Opulets Saline
(Alcon)

Drops used to irrigate the eyes.

Dose: use as needed.
Side effects:
Caution:
Not to be used for:
Not to be used with:
Contains: sodium chloride.
Other preparations:

Otrivine-Anistin
(Zyma)

Drops used as a sympathomimetic, antihistamine treatment for
allergic conjunctivitis and other eye inflammations.

Dose: adults 1-2 drops into the eye 2-4 times a day; children over 2 years 1 drop 2-4 times a day.

Side effects: temporary smarting, headache, sleeplessness, drowsiness, rapid heart rate, congestion.

Caution: in patients suffering from high blood pressure, enlarged prostate, coronary disease, diabetes.

Not to be used for: patients suffering from glaucoma or who wear soft contact lenses.

Not to be used with: MAOIS.

Contains: xylometazoline hydrochloride.

Other preparations:

Phenylephrine
(SNP)

Drops used as a sympathomimetic pupil dilator.

Dose: 1 drop into the eye as needed.

Side effects:

Caution:

Not to be used for: patients suffering from narrow angle glaucoma, high blood pressure, coronary disease, overactive thyroid.

Not to be used with: ß-blockers.

Contains: phenylephrine.

Other preparations:

Rose Bengal
(SNP)

Drops used as a dye to stain the eye for finding degenerated cells in dry eye syndrome.

Dose: 1-2 drops in the eye as needed.

Side effects: severe smarting

Caution:

Not to be used for: children.

Not to be used with:
Contains: rose Bengal.
Other preparations:

Sno Tears
(SNP)

Drops used to lubricate the eyes.

Dose: 1 or more drops into the eye as needed.
Side effects:
Caution:
Not to be used for: patients who wear soft contact lenses.
Not to be used with:
Contains: polyvinyl alcohol.
Other preparations:

Tears Naturale
(Alcon)

Drops used to lubricate dry eyes.

Dose: use as needed.
Side effects:
Caution:
Not to be used for: patients who wear soft contact lenses.
Not to be used with:
Contains: dextran, hypromellose.
Other preparations:

Topiclens
(S & N)

A solution in a sachet used to wash out the eyes, wounds, or
burns.

Dose: use as needed.
Side effects:
Caution: throw away any remaining solution.
Not to be used for:
Not to be used with:
Contains: sodium chloride.
Other preparations:

Ear conditions

The ear, like the eye, is a delicate organ. Infections in the outer and middle ear are common, and usually respond to prescribed antibiotics. Because infections may involve rupture of the eardrum, they are best seen by a doctor. Most of the preparations below are used for clearing ear wax although Auralgicin and some others are useful for mild external ear infections.

Ear wax itself is a simple condition but, even so, patients with perforated eardrums need to be careful when putting anything into the ears. For the same reason, syringing the ears must be carried out under medical supervision.

Wax blocking the ears may cause deafness, and wax-removing drops may improve the situation. Deafness may be due to infections behind the ear drum, however, and, in children, a chronic state of glue ear may develop. Hearing does deteriorate with age and, in addition, many people complain of noises in the ear (tinnitus). This can be due to wax or infections or to Ménière's disease which should be treated by a doctor. Vertigo or dizziness is also a symptom of ear disease because the balance mechanism is located near to the ear. Circulatory problems can also cause dizziness and many drugs, such as aspirin, can cause buzzing in the ears. Certain antibiotics can affect the ears particularly in patients with impaired kidney function.

Audax
(Napp Consumer)

Drops used as an analgesic to relieve pain associated with acute inflammation of the outer or middle ear.
Dose: fill the ear with the liquid and plug it.
Side effects:
Caution:
Not to be used for:
Not to be used with:
Contains: choline salicylate.
Other preparations:

Auralgicin
(Fisons)

A liquid used as an antibacterial treatment for inflammation of the middle ear.

Dose: fill the ear with the liquid every hour and plug until the pain is relieved, and then treat every 3 hours for 24 hours.
Side effects:
Caution:
Not to be used for:
Not to be used with:
Contains: ephedrine hydrochloride, benzocaine, chlorbutol, potassium hydroxyquinolone sulphate, phenazone, glycerin.
Other preparations:

Auraltone
(Fisons)

Drops used as an analgesic, local anaesthetic treatment for acute inflammation of the eardrum or inner ear.

Dose: fill the ear with the drops and plug lightly, repeating every

hour if needed.
Side effects: skin eruptions.
Caution:
Not to be used for:
Not to be used with:
Contains: phenazone, benzocaine.
Other preparations:

Cerumol
(LAB)

Drops used as a wax softener to remove wax from the ears.

Dose: 5 drops into the ear twice a day for 3 days may enable syringing to be avoided.
Side effects:
Caution:
Not to be used for: inflammation of the outer ear, dermatitis, eczema.
Not to be used with:
Contains: paradichlorobenzene, chlorbutol, arachis oil.
Other preparations:

Dioctyl Ear Drops
(Medo)

Drops used as a wax softener to remove wax from the ears.

Dose: 4 drops into the ear twice a day and plug with cotton wool.
Side effects:
Caution:
Not to be used for: patients suffering from perforated eardrum.
Not to be used with:
Contains: sodium docusate, polyethylene glycol.
Other preparations:

Exterol
(Dermal)

Drops used as a wax softener to remove wax from the ears.

Dose: hold 5-1 drops in the ear 1-2 times a day for 3-4 days.
Side effects: slight fizzing.
Caution:
Not to be used for: patients suffering from perforated eardrum.
Not to be used with:
Contains: urea hydrogen peroxide, glycerin.
Other preparations:

Molcer
(Wallace)

Drops used as a wax softener to soften ear wax.

Dose: fill the ear with the drops and plug with cotton wool; leave for 2 nights and then clean out.
Side effects:
Caution:
Not to be used for: patients suffering from perforated eardrum.
Not to be used with:
Contains: sodium docusate.
Other preparations:

Soliwax
(Martindale)

A red capsule used as a wax softener to soften and remove hardened ear wax and to clean the canal.

Dose: insert the contents of 1 capsule into the ear, plug, and leave overnight, then syringing if necessary.
Side effects:

Caution:
Not to be used for: patients suffering from perforated eardrum.
Not to be used with:
Contains: sodium docusate.
Other preparations:

Waxsol
(Norgine)

Drops used as a wax softener to remove wax from the ears.

Dose: fill the ear with the solution for 2 nights before they are to be syringed.
Side effects: temporary irritation.
Caution:
Not to be used for: patients suffering from inflammation of the ear or perforated eardrum.
Not to be used with:
Contains: sodium docusate.
Other preparations:

Diseases of the mouth

Many of the mouth conditions people complain of can be treated with antiseptic mouth washes and lozenges. These comprise most of the preparations available over the counter although there are some other interesting drugs which can be bought without a prescription.

Bioral is a formulation of an anti-ulcer drug which can be used for treating mouth ulcers. Local anaesthetics are available, including Merocaine, AAA Spray, and xylocaine gel, ointment, or spray. Aezodent is a dental anaesthetic and Bonjela (choline salicylate, cetalkonium chloride, menthol, alcohol, and glycerin) is useful for painful mouth conditions including ulcers and teething.

Antifungal preparations, such as Naxogin and Difflam, are available for thrush infections, and Daktarin Oral Gel perform a similar function. Blisteze lip salve is to be recommended for chapped or painful lips.

Artificial saliva products, such as Glandosane, are also available for those with reduced salivary gland action. Persistent problems should be seen by a doctor or dentist.

Vitamin deficiencies may cause soreness in or around the mouth, and dental conditions will often present as soreness or pain in the mouth. Thrush (fungal) infections are common in the mouth, particularly in patients taking powerful antibiotics (*see* Antifungal preparations). Ulcers which do not heal may need medical assessment. Bad breath can be caused by stomach or chest conditions or sinusitis; similarly, loss of taste can be caused by sinus infections. A sensation of water in the mouth (waterbrash) is caused by stomach acidity (*see* Stomach preparations). Many virus infections, including measles, can cause spots in the mouth. White patches in the mouth can be due to fungus or leukoplakia — the latter should be seen by a doctor. Cold sores are caused by a herpes infection on the mouth and they usually respond to prescribed antiviral agents. Stones in the mouth can result from salivary glands and occasionally these stones can block the gland and cause swelling. Gum infections (gingivitis) may respond to antiseptic mouthwashes, but, if persistent, it should be seen by a dentist. Spots on the tongue may be alarming, but often these are normal taste buds!

AAA Spray
(Rorer)

An aerosol used as an antibacterial and local anaesthetic to treat sore throat, minor infections of the nose and throat.

Dose: 2 sprays every 2-3 hours up to a maximum of 16 sprays in 24 hours; children over 6 years half adult dose.
Side effects:
Caution:
Not to be used for: children under 6 years.
Not to be used with:
Contains: benzocaine, cetalkonium chloride.
Other preparations:

Anaflex
(Geistlich)

A white lozenge supplied at a strength of 30 mg and used as an antibacterial and antifungal treatment for thrush and other bacterial infections of the mouth and throat.

Dose: adults 6-10 lozenges a day; children over 6 years half adult dose.
Side effects:
Caution:
Not to be used for: children under 6 years.
Not to be used with:
Contains: polynoxylin.
Other preparations: Anaflex Cream, Anaflex Paste, Anaflex Powder.

Betadine Gargle and Mouthwash
(Napp)

A solution used as an antiseptic to treat inflammation of the

mouth and pharynx brought on by thrush and other bacterial infections.
Dose: wash out the mouth or gargle with the diluted or undiluted solution every 2-4 hours.
Side effects: rarely local irritation and sensitivity.
Caution:
Not to be used for:
Not to be used with:
Contains: povidone-iodine.
Other preparations:

Bioral
(Winthrop)

A gel used as a cell-surface protector to treat mouth ulcers.

Dose: apply after meals and at bed time.
Side effects:
Caution:
Not to be used for:
Not to be used with:
Contains: carbenoxolone sodium.
Other preparations:

Bocasan
(Oral-B)

A sachet of white granules used as a disinfectant to treat gingivitis and mouth infections.

Dose: dissolve a sachet of granules in warm water and rinse out the mouth 3 times a day after meals.
Side effects:
Caution:
Not to be used for: patients suffering from kidney disease.
Not to be used with:

Contains: sodium perborate monohydrate, sodium hydrogen tartrate.
Other preparations:

Bonjela

Bonjela is a mouth ointment which contains choline salicylate (related to aspirin), chloride, menthol, alcohol, and glycerin. It is useful for mouth ulcers and teething problems. Small quantities should be applied every four hours because large quantities may deliver too much aspirin, especially to children.

Bradosol
(Ciba)

A white lozenge supplied at a strength of 0.5 mg and used as a disinfectant to treat infections of the mouth and throat.

Dose: 1 lozenge to be sucked every 2-3 hours.
Side effects: rarely local irritation and sensitivity.
Caution:
Not to be used for:
Not to be used with:
Contains: domiphen bromide.
Other preparations: Bradosol Plus.

Chloraseptic
(Richardson-Vick)

A solution supplied with a spray and used as a disinfectant to treat sore throat, mouth ulcers, minor mouth and gum infections.

Dose: adults 5 sprays every 2 hours as needed or gargle or rinse mouth with solution diluted with equal amount of water; children 6-12 years 3 sprays every 2 hours as needed or rinse

out the mouth.
Side effects: rarely local irritation and sensitivity.
Caution:
Not to be used for: children under 6 years.
Not to be used with:
Contains: phenol, sodium phenolate.
Other preparations:

Corsodyl
(ICI)

A solution used as an antibacterial treatment for gingivitis, mouth ulcers, thrush, and for mouth hygiene.

Dose: rinse with 2 5 ml teaspoonful for 1 minute twice a day.
Side effects: local irritation, stained tongue or teeth, may affect taste.
Caution:
Not to be used for:
Not to be used with:
Contains: chlorhexidine gluconate.
Other preparations: Corsodyl Gel.

Difflam Oral Rinse
(3M Riker)

A solution used as an analgesic and anti-inflammatory treatment for painful inflammations of the throat and mouth.

Dose: rinse or gargle with 3 5 ml teaspoonful every 90 minutes-3 hours..
Side effects: numb mouth.
Caution:
Not to be used for: children.
Not to be used with:
Contains: benzydamine hydrochloride.

Other preparations: Difflam Spray.

Eludril
(Pierre Fabre)
A solution used as an antibacterial treatment for throat and mouth infections, gingivitis, ulcers.

Dose: dilute 2 5 ml teaspoonsful with half a glass of warm water and gargle or rinse the mouth 3-4 times a day.
Side effects:
Caution:
Not to be used for: children under 6 years.
Not to be used with:
Contains: chlorhexidine digluconate, chlorbutol, chloroform.
Other preparations: Eludril Spray.

Glandosane
(Fresenius)

An aerosol used to provide artificial saliva for dry mouth and throat.

Dose: spray into the mouth and throat for 1-2 seconds as needed.
Side effects:
Caution:
Not to be used for:
Not to be used with:
Contains: carboxymethylcellulose sodium, sorbitol, potassium chloride, sodium chloride, magnesium chloride, calcium chloride, dipotassium hydrogen phosphate.
Other preparations:

Labosept
(LAB)

A red hexagonal-shaped pastille supplied at a strength of 0.25 mg and used as an antiseptic treatment for mouth and throat infections.

Dose: 1 pastille every 4 hours.
Side effects:
Caution:
Not to be used for:
Not to be used with:
Contains: dequalinium chloride.
Other preparations:

Medilave
(Martindale)

A gel used as an antiseptic and local anaesthetic to treat abrasions or ulcers in the mouth, teething.

Dose: apply to the affected area without rubbing in 3-4 times a day.
Side effects:
Caution:
Not to be used for: infants under 6 months.
Not to be used with:
Contains: benzocaine, cetylpyridinium.
Other preparations:

Merocaine
(Merrell Dow)

A green lozenge supplied at a strength of 1.4 mg and used as an antiseptic and local anaesthetic to treat painful infections of the throat and mouth, and as an additional treatment for tonsillitis and pharyngitis.

Dose: 1 lozenge allowed to dissolve in the mouth every 2 hours up to a maximum of 8 lozenges in 24 hours.
Side effects:
Caution:
Not to be used for: children.
Not to be used with:
Contains: cetylpyridinium chloride, benzocaine.
Other preparations:

Merocet
(Merrell Dow)

A solution used as an antiseptic to treat infections of the throat and mouth.

Dose: rinse the mouth or gargle with the solution diluted or undiluted every 3 hours or as needed.
Side effects:
Caution:
Not to be used for: children under 6 years.
Not to be used with:
Contains: cetylpyridinium chloride.
Other preparations:

Naxogin 500
(Farmitalia CE)

A white scored tablet supplied at a strength of 500 mg and used as an antiprotozoal treatment for acute ulcerative gingivitis.

Dose: 1 tablet twice a day for 2 days.
Side effects: stomach upset.
Caution: in pregnant women.
Not to be used for: children, nursing mothers, or for patients

siffereing from kidney weakness or brain disease.
Not to be used with: alcohol.
Contains: nimorazole.
Other preparations:

Orabase
(Squibb)

An ointment used as a mucoprotectant to protect lesions in the mouth.

Dose: apply to the affected area without rubbing in.
Side effects:
Caution:
Not to be used for:
Not to be used with:
Contains: carmellose sodium, pectin, gelatin.
Other preparations:

Oralcer
(Vitabiotics)

A green pellet used as an antibacterial, antifungal treatment for mouth ulcers.

Dose: adults allow 6-8 pellets to dissolve slowly near the ulcer on the first day, reducing to 4-6 pellets on the second day; children 3-4 pellets a day.
Side effects: local irritation.
Caution: do not use for extended periods.
Not to be used for: patients suffering from kidney or liver disease, overactive thyroid, intolerance to iodine.
Not to be used with:
Contains: clioquinol, ascorbic acid.
Other preparations:

Oraldene
(Warner-Lambert)

A solution used as an antiseptic rinse to treat thrush, gingivitis, ulcers, bad breath, stomatitis.

Dose: rinse out the mouth or gargle with 3 5 ml teaspoonsful 2-3 times a day.
Side effects: local irritation.
Caution:
Not to be used for:
Not to be used with:
Contains: hexetidine.
Other preparations:

Pyralvex
(Norgine)

A liquid used as an anti-inflammatory treatment for mouth inflammations.

Dose: apply to the affected area 3-4 times a day.
Side effects: local irritation.
Caution:
Not to be used for: children under 6 years.
Not to be used with:
Contains: anthraquinone glycosides, salicylic acid.
Other preparations:

Teejel
(Napp Consumer)

A gel used as an antiseptic, analgesic treatment for mouth ulcers, stomatitis, gingivitis, glossitis, teething, uncomfortable dentures.

Dose: rub gently into the affected area every 3-4 hours.
Side effects:
Caution:
Not to be used for: infants under 4 months.
Not to be used with:
Contains: choline salicylate, cetalkonium chloride.
Other preparations:

Tyrozets
(MSD)

A pink lozenge used as an antibiotic and local anaesthetic to treat mild mouth and throat disorders.

Dose: allow 1 lozenge to dissolve in the mouth every 3 hours to a maximum of 8 lozenges in 24 hours.
Side effects: additional infection, blackening or soreness of mouth and tongue.
Caution:
Not to be used for:
Not to be used with:
Contains: tyrothricin, benzocaine.
Other preparations:

Xylocaine

Xylocaine gel, ointment, and spray contain a local anaesthetic which can be used to suppress pain from local mouth disorders. It only masks the pain, however, and should not be used for more than a few days.

Skin disorders

Because many skin conditions are relatively minor, there is a number of skin preparations available over the counter. Many of these are antiseptics for cleaning infected or sore skin areas. Others are acne lotions, treatments for psoriasis, and treatments for warts. Skin softeners can be used for dry skin conditions. Skin infections can also be treated (*see* section below on Antiseptics) including fungal disorders. Dandruff is an irritating problem that responds to some of the preparations outlined below.

Mild steroid ointments (Dermacort, Efcortelan) contain hydrocortisone and can be used for mild eczema or dermatitis. E45 cream is a useful general skin softener containing white soft paraffin, lanolin, and light liquid paraffin. Calamine lotion is useful for skin itch, and witch hazel for itchy or irritating skin problems. Acriflex is useful for burns to the skin, and After Bite can be used to treat insect bites. The Uvistat range of products are useful for sensitive skin that burns in the sun; Hirudoid can be used for inflammatory conditions or the treatment of bruises. Chilblains may respond to Vitathone which is available as tablets or as an ointment.

Persistent skin problems, which do not respond to any of these treatments after fourteen days, should be seen by a doctor. In particular, bleeding or itchy moles, or moles which change colour, should be seen sooner rather than later because these signs may indicate malignant change. Any skin ulcer which does not heal should also be taken seriously.

Skin rashes are a common side effect to medications, particularly if there is allergy involved. These can progress to more serious urticaria. Local allergy or contact dermatitis often occurs with metals, such as jewellery, or with cosmetics. These will often respond to steroid creams. Antihistamine tablets may be used with local creams to treat allergic or itchy conditions.

Acetoxyl
(Stiefel)

A gel used as an antibacterial and skin softener to treat acne.

Dose: wash and dry the affected area and apply the gel once a day.
Side effects: irritation, peeling.
Caution: keep out of the eyes, nose, and mouth; children should use the weaker gel.
Not to be used for:
Not to be used with:
Contains: benzoyl peroxide.
Other preparations:

Acnegel
(Stiefel)

A gel used as an antibacterial and skin softener to treat acne.

Dose: wash and dry the affected area and apply the gel once a day.
Side effects: irritation, peeling.
Caution: keep out of the eyes, nose, and mouth.
Not to be used for:
Not to be used with:
Contains: benzoyl peroxide.
Other preparations: Acnegel Forte.

Acnidazil
(Janssen)

A cream used as an antibacterial and skin softener to treat acne.

Dose: wash and dry the affected area and apply the cream once a day for the first week, then twice a day for the next 4-8 weeks.

Side effects: irritation, peeling.
Caution: keep out of the eyes, nose, and mouth.
Not to be used for:
Not to be used with:
Contains: miconazole nitrate, benzoyl peroxide.
Other preparations:

Acriflex

Acriflex is a cream containing chlorhexidine gluconate as a disinfectant. It may be useful to soothe burns and to prevent secondary infection.

Alphosyl
(Stafford Miller)

A cream used as an anti-psoriatic to treat psoriasis.

Dose: massage thoroughly into the affected area 2-4 times a day.
Side effects: irritation, sensitivity to light.
Caution:
Not to be used for: patients suffering from acute psoriasis.
Not to be used with:
Contains: coal tar extract, allantoin.
Other preparations: Alphosyl Lotion, Alphosyl Shampoo.

Anthisan
(Fisons)

Anthisan is a topical antihistamine cream containing mepyramine maleate 2%. It is used for the treatment of allergic skin reactions and allergies.

Balneum with Tar
(Merck)

A bath oil used as an emolient and antipsoriatic to treat eczema, itchy or thickening skin disorders, psoriasis.

Dose: adults add 4 5 ml teaspoonsful to the bath water; children over 2 years add 2 teaspoonsful and use for a maximum of 6 weeks.
Side effects:
Caution:
Not to be used for: children under 2 years or for patients suffering from wet or weeping skin problems or where the skin is badly broken.
Not to be used with:
Contains: coal tar, soya oil.
Other preparations:

Baltar
(Merck)

A liquid used as an antipsoriatic treatment for psoriasis, dandruff, eczema, dermatoses of the scalp.

Dose: shampoo the hair with the liquid 1-3 times a week.
Side effects:
Caution: keep out of the eyes.
Not to be used for: children under 2 years or for patients suffering from wet or weeping dermatoses or where the skin is badly broken.
Not to be used with:
Contains: coal tar.
Other preparations:

Benoxyl 5
(Stiefel)

A cream used as an antibacterial and skin softener to treat acne.

Dose: wash and dry the affected area, then apply once a day.
Side effects: irritation, peeling.
Caution: keep out of the eyes, nose, and mouth.
Not to be used for:
Not to be used with:
Contains: benzoyl peroxide.
Other preparations: Benoxyl 5 with Sulphur, Benoxyll 10, Benoxyl 10 with Sulphur.

Benzagel
(Bioglan)

A white gel used as an antibacterial and skin softener to treat acne.

Dose: wash and dry the affected area, then apply 1-2 times a day.
Side effects: irritation, peeling.
Caution: keep out of the eyes, nose, and mouth.
Not to be used for:
Not to be used with:
Contains: benzoyl peroxide.
Other preparations:

Brasivol
(Stiefel)

A paste used as an abrasive to treat acne.

Dose: wet the area, then rub in vigorously for 15-20 seconds, rinse and repeat 1-3 times a day.

Side effects:
Caution:
Not to be used for: patients suffering from visible superficial arteries or veins on the skin.
Not to be used with:
Contains: aluminium oxide.
Other preparations:

Caladryl see **Calamine lotion**

Calamine lotion

Calamine lotion is a zinc-containing pink solution which is especially useful in chicken pox to reduce itch. It can also be used in other irritating skin conditions. Other preparations of calamine include Caladryl (also contains an antihistamine and camphor) and Eczederm.

Callusolve
(Dermal)

A paint used as a skin softener to treat warts.

Dose: apply 4-5 drops of the paint to the wart, cover for 24 hours, rub away the treated part, and repeat the process.
Side effects:
Caution: apply only to warts and avoid healthy skin.
Not to be used for: treating warts on the face or anal and genital areas
Not to be used with:
Contains: benzalkonium chloride-bromine.
Other preparations:

Carbo-Dome
(Lagap)

A cream used as an antipsoriatic treatment for psoriasis.

Dose: apply to the affected area 2-3 times a day.
Side effects: irritation, sensitivity to light.
Caution:
Not to be used for: patients suffering from acute psoriasis.
Not to be used with:
Contains: coal tar.
Other preparations:

Ceanel Concentrate
(Quinoderm)

A liquid used as an antibacterial, antifungal treatment for psoriasis, seborrhoeic inflammation of the scalp.

Dose: use as a shampoo 3 times a week at first and then twice a week, or apply directly to other areas of the skin as needed.
Side effects:
Caution: keep out of the eyes.
Not to be used for:
Not to be used with:
Contains: phenylethyl alcohol.
Other preparations:

Cetavlex
(Care)

A cream used as an antiseptic to treat minor cuts and wounds, nappy rash.

Dose: apply as needed.
Side effects: irritation, peeling.

Caution:
Not to be used for:
Not to be used with:
Contains: cetrimide.
Other preparations:

Cetavlon PC
(Care)

A liquid used as a disinfectant to treat dandruff.

Dose: use as a shampoo, diluting 1 5 ml teaspoonful in 50 ml of water, once a week or more frequently if needed.
Side effects:
Caution: keep out of the eyes.
Not to be used for:
Not to be used with:
Contains: cetrimide.
Other preparations:

Cetriclens
(S & N)

A solution in a sachet used as a disinfectant for cleansing broken skin and dirty wounds.

Dose: use as needed.
Side effects:
Caution: throw away any unused solution straight away after use
Not to be used for:
Not to be used with:
Contains: chlorhexidine gluconate, cetrimide.
Other preparations: Cetriclens Forte.

Chlorasol
(Seton-Prebbles)

A solution in a sachet used as a disinfectant for cleaning and removing dead skin from ulcers.

Dose: apply to the affected areas as needed.
Side effects: irritation.
Caution: keep away from the eyes and clothes; throw away any remaining solution immediately.
Not to be used for: internal use.
Not to be used with:
Contains: sodium hypochlorite.
Other preparations:

Clearasil
(Proctor and Gamble)

Clearasil is available as a cream, gel, and soap. It contains triclosan and sulphur to clean and disinfect the skin, and is used in the treatment of acne.

Clinitar Cream
(SNP)

A cream used as an antipsoriatic treatment for psoriasis, eczema.

Dose: apply to the affected area 1-2 times a day.
Side effects: sensitivity to light.
Caution:
Not to be used for: patients suffering from pustular psoriasis
Not to be used with:
Contains: coal tar extract.
Other preparations: Clinitar Gel, Clinitar Shampoo.

Cradocap
(Napp Consumer)

A shampoo used as an antiseptic treatment for cradle cap, scurf cap.

Dose: shampoo twice a week.
Side effects: .
Caution:
Not to be used for:
Not to be used with:
Contains: cetrimide.
Other preparations:

Cuplex
(SNP)

A gel used as a skin softener to treat warts, corns, and callouses.

Dose: at night apply 1-2 drops of gel to the wart after soaking in water and drying, remove the film in the morning and repeat the process, rubbing the area with a pumice stone between treatments.
Side effects:
Caution: do not apply to healthy skin.
Not to be used for: warts on the anal or genital areas
Not to be used with:
Contains: salicylic acid, lactic acid, copper acetate.
Other preparations:

Dermacort

Dermacort contains 0.1% hydrocortisone. It can be used sparingly to treat mild itchy skin conditions such as eczema and dermatitis. Overuse of steroids on the face can cause skin thinning, and skin infections of all sorts are made worse by steroids such as hydrocortisone.

Dithrocream
(Dermal)

A cream used as an antipsoriatic treatment for psoriasis.

Dose: apply to the affected area once a day and wash off after 30-60 minutes or apply at night and wash off in the morning.
Side effects: irritation, allergy.
Caution:
Not to be used for: patients suffering from acute psoriasis.
Not to be used with:
Contains: dithranol.
Other preparations: Dithrocream Forte, Dithrocream HP, Dithrocream 2%.

Dithrolan
(Dermal)

An ointment used as an antipsoriatic and skin softener to treat psoriasis.

Dose: before going to bed, bath and then apply the ointment to the affected area.
Side effects: irritation, allergy.
Caution:
Not to be used for: patients suffering from acute psoriasis.
Not to be used with:
Contains: dithranol, salicyclic acid.
Other preparations:

Dome-Acne
(Lagap)

A cream used as a skin softener to treat acne.

Dose: apply to the affected area night and morning.
Side effects: irritation, underactive thyroid gland.
Caution: keep out of the eyes, nose, and mouth.
Not to be used for: dark-skinned patients.
Not to be used with:
Contains: sulphur, resorcinol monoacetate.
Other preparations:

Duofilm
(Stiefel)

A liquid used as a skin softener to treat warts.

Dose: apply the liquid to the wart once a day, allow to dry, and cover, rubbing down between applications.
Side effects:
Caution: do not apply to healthy skin.
Not to be used for: warts on the face or anal and genital areas.
Not to be used with:
Contains: salicylic acid, lactic acid.
Other preparations:

E45

E45 cream contains lanolin, white soft paraffin, and light liquid paraffin. It is a good cream for use in children as both a skin softener or protector, for example, in nappy rash.

Efcortelan

Efcortelan cream or ointment contains 1% hydrocortisone and is therefore ten times stronger than Dermacort. Consequently, it should be treated with even more respect. It should not be used for children.

Eskamel
(S K B)

A cream used as a skin softener to treat acne.

Dose: apply a little to the affected area once a day.
Side effects: irritation.
Caution: in patients suffering from acute local infection; keep out of the eyes, nose, and mouth.
Not to be used for:
Not to be used with:
Contains: resorcinol, sulphur.
Other preparations:

Exolan
(Dermal)

A cream used as an antipsoriatic treatment for psoriasis.

Dose: apply to the affected area 1-2 times a day.
Side effects: irritation, allergy.
Caution:
Not to be used for: patients suffering from acute psoriasis.
Not to be used with:
Contains: dithranol triacetate.
Other preparations:

Gelcosal
(Quinoderm)

A gel used as an antipsoriatic and skin softener to treat psoriasis, dermatitis, when the condition is scaling.

Dose: massage into the affected area twice a day.
Side effects:
Caution:

Not to be used for:
Not to be used with:
***Contains**:* coal tar solution, tar, salicyclic acid.
Other preparations:

Gelcotar
(Quinoderm)

A gel used as an antipsoriatic treatment for psoriasis, dermatitis.

Dose: massage into the affected area twice a day.
Side effects: irritation, sensitivity to light
Caution:
Not to be used for: patients suffering from acute psoriasis.
Not to be used with:
***Contains**:* coal tar solution, tar.
Other preparations: Gelcotar Liquid.

Genisol
(Fisons)

A liquid used as an antipsioratic and anti-dandruff treatment for psoriasis, dandruff, seborrhoeic inflammation of the scalp.

Dose: shampoo once a week or as needed.
Side effects: irritation, sensitivity to light.
Caution:
Not to be used for: patients suffering from acute psoriasis.
Not to be used with:
***Contains**:* coal tar, sodium sulphosuccinated undecylenic monoalkylomide.
Other preparations:

Glutarol
(Dermal)

A solution used as a virucidal, skin-drying agent to treat warts.

Dose: apply the solution to the wart twice a day and rub down hard skin.
Side effects: staining of the skin.
Caution: do not apply to healthy skin.
Not to be used for: warts on the face or anal and genital areas.
Not to be used with:
Contains: glutaraldehyde.
Other preparations:

Hirudoid

Hirudoid contains heparin (blood-thinning) components and is useful in dissolving skin bruises and local clots of blood. It may also reduce the tenderness in varicose veins.

Ionax
(Alcon)

A gel used as an abrasive, antibacterial preparation to clean the skin in the treatment of acne.

Dose: wet the face, then rub in once a day, and rinse.
Side effects:
Caution:
Not to be used for: children under 12 years.
Not to be used with:
Contains: polyethylene granules, benzalkonium chloride.
Other preparations:

Ionil T
(Alcon)

A shampoo used as an antipsoriatic treatment for seborrhoeic inflammation of the scalp.

Dose: shampoo once a day if needed.
Side effects: irritation, sensitivity to light.
Caution:
Not to be used for: patients suffering from acute psoriasis.
Not to be used with:
Contains: coal tar solution, salicyclic acid, benzalkonium chloride.
Other preparations:

Keralyt
(Westwood)

A gel used as a skin softener to treat thickened skin.

Dose: wet the skin for 5 minutes and then apply once a day at night.
Side effects:
Caution: keep out of the eyes, nose, and mouth.
Not to be used for:
Not to be used with:
Contains: salicyclic acid.
Other preparations:

Lenium
(Winthrop)

An anti-dandruff preparation.

Dose: twice a week for the first two weeks, once a week for two further weeks, then once every 3-6 weeks.

Side effects:
Caution: keep out of the eyes and any areas of broken skin; do not use within 48 hours of waving or colouring substances.
Not to be used for:
Not to be used with:
Contains: selenium sulphide.
Other preparations:

Meditar
(Brocades)

A waxy stick used as an antipsoriatic treatment for psoriasis, eczema.

Dose: apply to the affected area 1-2 times a day.
Side effects: irritation, sensitivity to light.
Caution:
Not to be used for: patients suffering from acute psoriasis.
Not to be used with:
Contains: coal tar.
Other preparations:

Nericur
(Schering)

A gel used as an antibacterial skin softener to treat acne.

Dose: wash and dry the affected area, then apply the gel once a day.
Side effects: irritation, peeling.
Caution: keep out of the eyes, nose, mouth.
Not to be used for: children.
Not to be used with:
Contains: benzoyl peroxide.
Other preparations:

Panoxyl
(Stiefel)

A gel used as an antibacterial skin softener to treat acne.

Dose: wash and dry the affected area, then apply once a day.
Side effects: irritation, peeling.
Caution: keep out of the eyes, nose, mouth.
Not to be used for:
Not to be used with:
Contains: benzoyl peroxide.
Other preparations: Panoxyl Aquagel, Panoxyl Wash.

Polytar Liquid
(Stiefel)

A liquid used as an antipsoriatic treatment for psoriasis of the scalp, dandruff, seborrhoea, eczema..

Dose: shampoo once or twice a week.
Side effects:
Caution:
Not to be used for:
Not to be used with:
Contains: tar, cade oil, coal tar, arachis oil, coal tar extract, oleyl alcohol.
Other preparations:

Ponoxylan
(Rorer)

A gel used as an antibacterial treatment for infection and inflammation of the skin.

Dose: apply to the affected area as needed.
Side effects:

Caution:
Not to be used for:
Not to be used with:
Contains: polynoxylin.
Other preparations:

Posalfilin
(Norgine)
An ointment used as a skin softener to treat warts.

Dose: protect healthy skin, apply the ointment to the wart, and cover; repeat 2-3 times a week.
Side effects: pain when the ointment is first applied.
Caution: do not use on healthy skin.
Not to be used for: pregnant women or on warts on the face or anal and genital areas.
Not to be used with:
Contains: salicyclic acid, podophyllum resin.
Other preparations:

Pragmatar
(Bioglan)

A cream used as an anti-itch, antiseptic, skin softener to treat scaly skin, scalp seborrhoea, and similar disorders.

Dose: apply weekly, or daily in severe cases, to wet hair.
Side effects: irritation.
Caution: dilute the cream first when using for infants.
Not to be used for:
Not to be used with:
Contains: cetyl alcohol/coal tar distillate, sulphur, salicyclic acid.
Other preparations:

Psoradrate
(Norwich Eaton)

A gel used as an antipsoriatic, drying agent to treat psoriasis.

Dose: wash and dry the area, then apply the cream twice a day.
Side effects: irritation, hypersensitivity.
Caution:
Not to be used for: pustular psoriasis.
Not to be used with:
Contains: dithranol, urea.
Other preparations:

Psoriderm
(Dermal)

An emulsion used as an antipsoriatic to treat psoriasis.

Dose: add 30 ml of the emulsion to the bath water, soak for 15 minutes, dry, then apply the cream to the affected area.
Side effects: irritation, sensitivity to light.
Caution:
Not to be used for: patients suffering from acute psoriasis.
Not to be used with:
Contains: coal tar.
Other preparations: Psoriderm Cream, Psoriderm Scalp Lotion.

Psorigel
(Alcon)

A gel used as an antipsoriatic treatment for psoriasis.

Dose: rub into the affected area and allow to dry 1-2 times a day.
Side effects: irritation, sensitivity to light.
Caution:
Not to be used for: patients suffering from acute psoriasis.

Not to be used with:
Contains: coal tar solution.
Other preparations:

Psorin
(Thames)
An ointment used as an antipsoriatic skin softener to treat psoriasis, eczema.

Dose: apply to the affected area twice a day.
Side effects:
Caution: keep out of the eyes, and avoid direct sunlight.
Not to be used for: patients suffering from unstable psoriasis.
Not to be used with:
Contains: coal tar, dithranol, salicyclic acid.
Other preparations:

Quinoderm Cream
(Quinoderm)

A cream used as an antibacterial skin softener to treat acne, acne-like eruptions, inflammation of the follicles.

Dose: massage into the affected area 1-3 times a day.
Side effects: irritation, peeling.
Caution: keep out of the eyes, nose, mouth.
Not to be used for:
Not to be used with:
Contains: potassium hydroxyquinolone sulphate, benzoyl peroxide.
Other preparations: Quinoderm Cream 5, Quinoderm Lotio-Gel, Quinoderm Lotio-Gel 5%, Quinoderm with Hydrocortisone.

Rotersept
(Roterpharma)

An aerosol used as a disinfectant for the prevention of mastitis, and to treat cracked nipples.

Dose: spray on to the breast before and after feeding.
Side effects:
Caution:
Not to be used for: children.
Not to be used with:
Contains: chlorhexidine gluconate.
Other preparations:

Salactol
(Dermal)

A paint used as a skin softener to treat warts.

Dose: apply to the wart once a day and rub down with a pumice stone.
Side effects:
Caution: do not apply to healthy skin.
Not to be used for: warts on the face or anal and genital areas.
Not to be used with:
Contains: salicyclic acid, lactic acid.
Other preparations:

Selsun
(Abbott)

A suspension used as an anti-dandruff treatment for dandruff, tinea versicolor (a scalp condition).

Dose: shampoo twice a week for 2 weeks, then once a week for 2 weeks, or apply to lesions and leave overnight.

Side effects:
Caution: keep out of the eyes or broken skin; do not use within 48 hours of using waving or colouring substances.
Not to be used for:
Not to be used with:
Contains: selenium sulphide.
Other preparations:

Synogist
(Townendale)

A shampoo used as an antifungal, antibacterial treatment for seborrhoea of the scalp.

Dose: shampoo twice a week for 4 weeks, then once a week.
Side effects:
Caution: keep out of the eyes.
Not to be used for:
Not to be used with:
Contains: sodium sulphosuccinated undecyclenic monoalkylolamide.
Other preparations:

T Gel
(Neutrogena)

A shampoo used as an antipsoriatic treatment for dandruff, seborrhoea, and psoriasis of the scalp.

Dose: shampoo 1-2 times a week.
Side effects: irritation.
Caution:
Not to be used for: patients suffering from acute psoriasis.
Not to be used with:
Contains: coal tar extract.
Other preparations:

Theraderm
(Westwood)

A gel used as an antibacterial skin softener to treat acne.

Dose: wash and dry the affected area, then apply 1-2 times a day.
Side effects: irritation, peeling.
Caution: keep out of the eyes, nose, mouth.
Not to be used for:
Not to be used with:
Contains: benzoyl peroxide.
Other preparations:

Torbetol
(Torbet Laboratories)

A lotion used as an antibacterial treatment for acne.

Dose: apply to the affected area 3 times a day.
Side effects:
Caution:
Not to be used for:
Not to be used with:
Contains: cetrimide, benzalkonium chloride, hexachlorophane.
Other preparations:

Veracur
(Typharm)

A gel used as a skin softener to treat warts.

Dose: apply to the wart twice a day and cover, rubbing down with a pumic stone between treatments.
Side effects:
Caution: do not apply to healthy skin.

Not to be used for: warts on the face or anal and genital areas.
Not to be used with:
Contains: formaldehyde.
Other preparations:

Verrugon
(Pickles)

An ointment with corn rings and plasters used as a skin softener to treat warts.

Dose: protect healthy skin, apply the ointment to the wart, and cover with a plaster, rubbing down with pumice stone between treatments.
Side effects:
Caution: do not apply to healthy skin
Not to be used for: warts on the face or anal and genital regions.
Not to be used with:
Contains: salicyclic acid.
Other preparations:

Verucasep
(Galen)

A gel used as a virucidal, anhidrotic treatment for viral warts.

Dose: apply twice a day, paring down any hard skin around the wart.
Side effects: stains the skin.
Caution: do not apply to healthy skin.
Not to be used for: warts on the face or anal and genital regions.
Not to be used with:
Contains: glutaraldehyde.
Other preparations:

Vita-E
(Bioglan)

An ointment used as an anti-oxidant to treat wounds, bed sores, burns, skin ulcers.

Dose: apply to the affected area as needed.
Side effects:
Caution:
Not to be used for: patients suffering from overactive thyroid gland.
Not to be used with: fish liver oils, digitalis, insulin.
Contains: d-alpha-tocopheryl acetate.
Other preparations:

---

witch hazel (see also **Optrex**)

witch hazel is a solution which is useful in reducing the reddening and soreness of skin inflammations.

Antiseptics

Included below is a wide variety of antiseptic creams, lotions, and solutions that are available over the counter. Many people are familiar with products, such as Savlon, TCP, and Germolene, and these skin disinfectants all do essentially the same job in the treatment of wounds, burns, nappy rash, or ulcers which may have an infective component. Your pharmacist will be able to advise which of these is appropriate in any particular situation. Severe skin infection (cellulitis) may develop into lymphangitis with red streaks appearing under the skin. These need antibiotic therapy and must be seen by a physician.

Anaflex Cream
(Geistlich)

A cream used as an antibacterial and antifungal treatment for skin infections.

Dose: apply the cream to the affected area 1-2 times a day.
Side effects:
Caution:
Not to be used for:
Not to be used with:
Contains: polynoxylin.
Other preparations: Anaflex, Anaflex Paste, Anaflex Powder, Anaflex Aerosol.

Aquasept
(Hough, Hoseason)

A solution used as a disinfectant for skin and body cleansing and disinfecting.

Dose: use as a soap.
Side effects:
Caution: keep out of the eyes.
Not to be used for:
Not to be used with:
Contains: triclosan.
Other preparations:

Bacticlens
(S & N)

A solution in a sachet used as a disinfectant to clean the skin, wounds, or broken skin.

Dose: use as needed.

Side effects: throw away any remaining solution straight away after use.
Caution:
Not to be used for:
Not to be used with:
Contains: chlorhexidine gluconate.
Other preparations:

Betadine Ointment
(Napp)

An ointment used as an antiseptic to treat ulcers.

Dose: apply to the affected area and cover once a day.
Side effects: rarely irritation.
Caution: in patients sensitive to iodine.
Not to be used for:
Not to be used with:
Contains: povidone-iodine.
Other preparations:

Betadine Scalp and Skin Cleanser
(Napp)

A solution used as an antiseptic and detergent to treat acne, seborrhoeic scalp and skin disorders.

Dose: use as a shampoo or apply directly to the skin and then cleanse properly.
Side effects: rarely irritation or sensitivity.
Caution:
Not to be used for:
Not to be used with:
Contains: povidone-iodine.
Other preparations: Betadine Skin Cleanser, Betadine Shampoo.

Betadine Spray
(Napp)

A spray used as an antiseptic to treat infected cuts, wounds, and burns.

Dose: spray on to the affected area once a day or as needed, and cover.
Side effects:
Caution: keep out of the eyes.
Not to be used for: patients suffering from non-toxic colloid goitre
Not to be used with:
Contains: povidone-iodine.
Other preparations: Betadine Dry Powder, Betadine Antiseptic Paint, Betadine Antiseptic Solution, Betadine Alcoholic Solution, Betadine Surgical Scrub.

Capitol
(Dermal)

A gel used as an antibacterial treatment for dandruff and other similar scalp disorders.

Dose: use as a shampoo.
Side effects:
Caution: in patients sensitive to iodine.
Not to be used for:
Not to be used with:
Contains: benzalkonium chloride.
Other preparations:

Chymoral Forte
(Rorer)

An orange tablet supplied at a strength of 100, 000 units and

used as an enzyme to treat acute inflammatory swelling.
Dose: 1 tablet 4 times a day before meals.
Side effects: stomach disturbance.
Caution: in patients sensitive to iodine.
Not to be used for:
Not to be used with:
Contains: trypsin, chymotrypsin.
Other preparations: Chymoral.

Conotrane
(Boehringer Ingelheim)

A cream used as an antiseptic for protecting the skin from water, nappy rash, bed sores.

Dose: apply to the affected area several times a day.
Side effects:
Caution:
Not to be used for:
Not to be used with:
Contains: benzalkonium chloride, dimethicone.
Other preparations:

CX Powder
(Bio-Medical)

A powder used as a disinfectant to clean and disinfect the skin and prevent infection.

Dose: apply to the affected area 3 times a day.
Side effects:
Caution:
Not to be used for:
Not to be used with:
Contains: chlorhexidine acetate.
Other preparations:

Debrisan
(Pharmacia)

A powder used as an absorbant to treat weeping wounds including ulcers.

Dose: wash the wound with a saline solution and, without drying first, coat with 3 mm of powder, and cover with a perforated plastic sheet; repeat before the sheet is saturated.
Side effects:
Caution:
Not to be used for:
Not to be used with:
Contains: dextranomer.
Other preparations: Debrisan Paste.

Disadine DP
(Stuart)

A powder spray used as an antiseptic for the prevention and treatment of infection in wounds such as burns, bed sores, varicose ulcers.

Dose: spray on to the affected area as needed.
Side effects:
Caution: care in treating severe burns.
Not to be used for: patients suffering from non-toxic colloid goitre.
Not to be used with:
Contains: povidone iodine.
Other preparations:

Drapolene
(Wellcome)

A cream used as an antiseptic to treat nappy rash.

Dose: apply twice a day or each time the nappy is changed.
Side effects:
Caution:
Not to be used for:
Not to be used with:
Contains: benzalkonium chloride, cetrimide.
Other preparations:

Germolene
(Smith Kline Beecham)

Germolene contains chlorhexidine, lanolin, paraffin, and salicylate and is available as a cream, ointment, or spray. It is a good general-purpose skin antiseptic useful for cleaning cuts and abrasions. Suitable for children.

Hibiscrub
(ICI)

A solution used as a disinfectant for cleansing and disinfecting skin and hands.

Dose: use as a liquid soap.
Side effects:
Caution:
Not to be used for:
Not to be used with:
Contains: chlorhexidine gluconate.
Other preparations:

Hibisol
(ICI)

A solution used as a disinfectant for cleansing and disinfecting skin and hands.

Dose: rub vigorously on to the skin until dry.
Side effects:
Caution:
Not to be used for:
Not to be used with:
Contains: chlorhexidine gluconate, isopropyl alcohol.
Other preparations:

Hibitane
(ICI)

A cream used as a disinfectant for cleansing and disinfecting hands and skin before surgery, and for prevention of infections in wounds, and after surgery.

Dose: apply freely to the affected area as needed.
Side effects:
Caution:
Not to be used for:
Not to be used with:
Contains: chlorhexidine gluconate.
Other preparations: Hibitane Obstetric Cream, Hibitane Concentrate, Hibitane 20% Gluconate.

Hioxyl
(Quinoderm)

A cream used as a disinfectant to treat minor wounds, infections, bed sores, leg ulcers.

Dose: apply freely as needed and cover with a dressing.
Side effects:
Caution:
Not to be used for:
Not to be used with:
Contains: hydrogen peroxide.

Other preparations:

Malatex
(Norton)

A solution used as an anti-inflammatory preparation to treat varicose and indolent ulcers, bed sores, burns.

Dose: cleanse the affected area with the solution and then apply the cream twice a day.
Side effects:
Caution:
Not to be used for:
Not to be used with:
Contains: propylene glycol, malic acid, benzoic acid, salicylic acid.
Other preparations: Malatex Solution

Manusept
(Hough, Hoseason)

A solution used as a disinfectant for cleansing and disinfecting skin and hands before surgery.

Dose: rub into the skin until dry.
Side effects:
Caution: keep out of the eyes.
Not to be used for:
Not to be used with:
Contains: triclosan, isopropyl alcohol.
Other preparations:

---

pHiso-Med
(Winthrop)

A solution used as a disinfectant to treat acne, and for disinfecting infants' skin, cleansing and disinfecting skin before surgery.

Dose: use as a liquid soap.
Side effects:
Caution: in newborn infants dilute 10 times.
Not to be used for:
Not to be used with:
Contains: chlorhexidine gluconate.
Other preparations:

Phytex
(Pharmax)

A paint used as an antifungal treatment for skin and nail infections.

Dose: paint on to the affected area morning and evening, and after bathing for 2-3 weeks after the symptoms have gone.
Side effects:
Caution:
Not to be used for: children under 5 years or pregnant women.
Not to be used with:
Contains: tannic acid, boric acid, salicylic acid, methyl salicylate, acetic acid.
Other preparations:

Roccal
(Winthrop)

A solution used as a disinfectant for cleansing and disinfecting the skin before surgery.

Dose: dilute the solution and use as needed.
Side effects:
Caution:

Not to be used for:
Not to be used with:
Contains: benzalkonium chloride.
Other preparations:

Savloclens
(ICI)

A solution in a sachet used as a disinfectant for cleansing and disinfecting wounds and burns.

Dose: use neat as needed.
Side effects:
Caution:
Not to be used for:
Not to be used with:
Contains: chlorhexidine gluconate, cetrimide.
Other preparations:

Savlodil
(ICI)

A solution in a sachet used as a disinfectant for cleansing and disinfecting wounds and burns.

Dose: use neat as needed.
Side effects:
Caution:
Not to be used for:
Not to be used with:
Contains: chlorhexidine gluconate, cetrimide.
Other preparations:

Savlon
(Ciba)

Savlon contains chlorhexidine and cetrimide and is available as a cream, liquid, barrier cream, nappy rash cream, sachets, and spray (containing povidine iodine). It is a useful antiseptic cream suitable for all age groups.

Savlon Hospital Concentrate
(ICI)

A solution used as a disinfectant and general antiseptic.

Dose: adequate amounts.
Side effects:
Caution:
Not to be used for:
Not to be used with:
Contains: chlorhexidine gluconate, cetrimide.
Other preparations:

Ster-Zac DC
(Hough, Hoseason)

A cream used as a disinfectant for cleansing and disinfecting the hands before surgery.

Dose: use as a liquid soap.
Side effects:
Caution: in children under 2 years.
Not to be used for:
Not to be used with:
Contains: hexachlorophane.
Other preparations:

Ster-Zac Powder
(Hough, Hoseason)

A powder used as a disinfectant for the prevention of infections in newborn infants, and to treat recurring skin infections.

Dose: adults apply to the affected area once a day; infants dust the affected area at each change of nappy.
Side effects:
Caution: in patients where the skin is broken.
Not to be used for:
Not to be used with:
Contains: hexachlorophane.
Other preparations:

TCP

TCP contains phenol and salicylate and is available as an antiseptic and lotion and ointment and throat pastilles containing blackcurrant, honey, and menthol or lemon. TCP is an efficient antiseptic which should be diluted with water to avoid too strong an astringent effect.

Tisept
(Seaton-Prebbles)

A solution in a sachet used as a disinfectant for cleansing and disinfecting wounds and burns, changing dressing, obstetrics.

Dose: use neat as needed.
Side effects:
Caution:
Not to be used for:
Not to be used with:
Contains: chlorhexidine gluconate, cetrimide.
Other preparations:

Travasept 100
(Baxter)

A solution used as an aminoglycocide antibiotic, antibacterial preparation for disinfecting wounds and burns.

Dose: use neat as needed.
Side effects:
Caution:
Not to be used for:
Not to be used with:
Contains: chlorhexidine acetate, cetrimide.
Other preparations:

Triclosept
(Hough, Hoseason)

A cream used as a disinfectant for cleansing and disinfecting the hands and skin.

Dose: rub vigorously into the affected area until the cream has been absorbed.
Side effects:
Caution:
Not to be used for:
Not to be used with:
Contains: triclosan.
Other preparations:

Unisept
(Seton-Prebbles)

A solution used as a disinfectant and general antiseptic.

Dose: use neat as needed.
Side effects:

Caution:
Not to be used for:
Not to be used with:
Contains: chlorhexidine gluconate.
Other preparations:

Videne Powder
(3M Riker)

A powder used as an antiseptic treatment for infections in wounds and burns.

Dose: dust the affected area lightly with the powder.
Side effects:
Caution:
Not to be used for:
Not to be used with:
Contains: povidone-iodine.
Other preparations: Videne Solution, Videne Tincture, Videne Surgical Scrub.

Antifungal preparations

Fortunately, there is a number of antifungal preparations available over the counter, and these are described below. Athlete's foot is caused by a fungus infection as is Dhobi itch where the sufferer has a red ring in the groin area. Circular skin complains are often due to funguses, and one particular type causes depigmentation (pale circles) in people who are suntanned. Treatment of a fungus infection with a steroid will prolong or worsen the symptoms. If in doubt, consult a doctor, but relatively little harm can be caused by trial and error.

Fungus infections can occur after a repeated course of antibiotics or in those who have low immunity, sometimes due to steroids. Internal fungus infections can be treated only by prescription medicines or by homoeopathic remedies (*see* below). Fungus infections of the nails can be persistent and may need prescribed medication.

Canesten
(Baypharm)

A solution used as an antifungal treatment for fungal inflammation and infection of the outer ear, skin, and nails.

Dose: 2-3 applications a day until 14 days after the symptoms have gone.
Side effects: local irritation.
Caution:
Not to be used for:
Not to be used with:
Contains: clotrimazole, polyethylene glycol solution.
Other preparations: Canesten Spray, Canesten Powder.

Daktarin Cream
(Janssen)

A cream used as an antifungal treatment for infections of the skin and nails.

Dose: apply 1-2 times a day until 10 days.after the wounds have healed.
Side effects:
Caution:
Not to be used for:
Not to be used with:
Contains: miconazole nitrate.
Other preparations: Daktarin Twin Pack, Daktarin Spray Powder, Daktarin Powder.

Daktarin Oral Gel
(Janssen)

A gel supplied at a strength of 25 mg and used as an antifungal treatment for fungal infections of the mouth and pharynx.

Dose: adults hold 5-10 ml of gel in the mouth 4 times a day; children under 2 years use 2.5 ml twice a day, 2-6 years 5 ml gel twice a day, over 6 years 5 ml gel 4 times a day.
Side effects: mild stomach upset.
Caution:
Not to be used for:
Not to be used with: warfarin
Contains: miconazole.
Other preparations:

Derminostat
(Cilag)

A cream used as an antifungal treatment for fungal infections of the skin and nails.

Dose: apply to the affected area twice a day until 10 days after the wounds have healed.
Side effects:
Caution:
Not to be used for:
Not to be used with:
Contains: miconazole nitrate.
Other preparations:

Ecostatin
(Squibb)

A cream used as an antifungal treatment for fungal infections of the skin.

Dose: apply to the affected area night and morning.
Side effects:
Caution:
Not to be used for:
Not to be used with:

Contains: econazole nitrate.
Other preparations: Ecostatin Lotion, Ecostatin Powder, Ecostatin Spray.

Exelderm
(ICI)

A cream used as an antifungal treatment for fungal infections of the skin.

Dose: rub into the affected area twice a day for 2-3 weeks after the wounds have healed.
Side effects:
Caution: keep out of the eyes; if the area becomes irritated, the treatment should be stopped.
Not to be used for:
Not to be used with:
Contains: sulconazole nitrate.
Other preparations:

Monphytol
(LAB)

A paint used as an antifungal treatment for athlete's foot.

Dose: paint on to the affected area twice a day at first, then once a week.
Side effects:
Caution:
Not to be used for: children or pregnant women.
Not to be used with:
Contains: chlorbutol, methyl undecoanate, salicylic acid, methyl salicylate, propyl salicylate, propyl undecoanate.
Other preparations:

Phytocil
(Fisons)

A cream used as an antifungal treatment for tinea infections.

Dose: apply to the affected area 2-3 times a day.
Side effects:
Caution:
Not to be used for:
Not to be used with:
Contains: phenoxypropanol, chlorophenoxyethanol, salicylic acid, menthol.
Other preparations: Phytocil Powder.

Quinoped
(Quinoderm)

A cream used as a steroid, antifungal, antibacterial treatment for skin disorders where there is also infection.

Dose: massage into the affected area 2-3 times a day.
Side effects: fluid retention, suppression of adrenal glands, thinning of the skin may occur.
Caution: use for short periods of time only.
Not to be used for: patients suffering from acne or any other skin infections caused by tuberculosis, ringworm, viruses, or funguses, or continuously especially in pregnant women.
Not to be used with:
Contains: potassium hydroxyquinolone sulphate, hydrocortisone.
Other preparations:

Timoped
(Reckitt & Colman)

A cream used as an antifungal treatment for athlete's foot and similar skin infections.

Dose: rub gently into the affected area and allow to dry.
Side effects:
Caution:
Not to be used for:
Not to be used with:
Contains: tolnaftate, triclosan.
Other preparations:

Tineafax
(Wellcome)

An ointment used as an antifungal treatment for athlete's foot and similar skin infections.

Dose: apply to the affected area twice a day at first, then once a day.
Side effects:
Caution:
Not to be used for:
Not to be used with:
Contains: zinc undecenoate, zinc naphthenate.
Other preparations: Tineafax Powder.

Anti-infestation preparations

Conditions such as lice and scabies are caused by infestations with insects. These can be picked up from infested bedding, often in poorly cleaned rooms. Overseas climates which are warm and moist encourage the growth of these insects. In the United Kingdom, the most commonly seen infestations are head lice in children, and pubic lice which can be transmitted venereally. Scabies is more common in down-and-out patients with poor general health and nutrition.

Ascabiol
(M & B)

An emulsion used as an insect-destroying preparation to treat scabies, pediculosis.

Dose:
Side effects: irritation.
Caution: keep out of the eyes.
Not to be used for:
Not to be used with:
Contains: benzyl benzoate.
Other preparations:

Carylderm
(Napp Consumer)

A lotion used as a pediculicide to treat lice in the head and pubic areas.

Dose: rub into the hair and allow to dry, then shampoo.
Side effects:
Caution: keep out of the eyes.
Not to be used for:
Not to be used with:
Contains: carbaryl.
Other preparations: Carylderm Liquid Shampoo.

Clinicide
(De Witt)

A liquid used as a pediculicide to treat lice in the head and pubic areas.

Dose: apply to the hair and allow to dry, then shampoo the following day.

Side effects:
Caution: keep out of the eyes.
Not to be used for:
Not to be used with:
Contains: carbaryl.
Other preparations:

Derbac-M
(International)

A liquid used as a pediculicide and scabicide to treat scabies, lice in the head and pubic areas.

Dose: apply liberally and then shampoo after 24 hours.
Side effects:
Caution: keep out of the eyes.
Not to be used for:
Not to be used with:
Contains: malathion.
Other preparations:

Derbac Shampoo
(International)

A shampoo used as a pediculicide to treat head lice.

Dose: use as a shampoo, applying twice and then leaving the second treatment for 5 minutes before rinsing and drying.
Side effects:
Caution: keep out of the eyes.
Not to be used for:
Not to be used with:
Contains: carbaryl.
Other preparations:

Eurax
(Geigy)

A lotion used as a scabicide to treat scabies.

Dose: apply to the body apart from the head and face after a hot bath.
Side effects:
Caution: keep out of the eyes.
Not to be used for: patients suffering from acute exudative dermatitis.
Not to be used with:
Contains: crotamiton.
Other preparations: Eurax Cream.

Lorexane
(Care)

A cream used as a scabicide and pediculicide to treat scabies and lice.

Dose: apply to the affected areas as directed.
Side effects:
Caution: keep out of the eyes.
Not to be used for:
Not to be used with:
Contains: lindane.
Other preparations: Lorexane Medicated Shampoo.

Prioderm
(Napp Consumer)

A lotion used as a pediculicide and scabicide to treat scabies, lice in the head and pubic areas.

Dose: rub in and shampoo after 2-12 hours; repeat after 7-9

days.
Side effects:
Caution: keep out of the eyes.
Not to be used for:
Not to be used with:
Contains: malathion.
Other preparations: Prioderm Cream Shampoo.

Quellada
(Stafford-Miller)

A lotion used as a scabicide to treat scabies.

Dose: apply as directed.
Side effects:
Caution: keep out of the eyes.
Not to be used for: infants under 1 month.
Not to be used with:
Contains: lindane.
Other preparations: Quellada Application PC.

Suleo-C
(International)

A lotion used as a pediculicide to treat head lice.

Dose: rub into the scalp as directed.
Side effects:
Caution: keep out of the eyes.
Not to be used for:
Not to be used with:
Contains: carbaryl.
Other preparations: Suleo-C Shampoo.

Suleo-M
(International)

A lotion used as a pediculicide to treat head lice.

Dose: rub into the scalp as directed.
Side effects:
Caution: keep out of the eyes.
Not to be used for:
Not to be used with:
Contains: malathion.
Other preparations:

Tetmosol
(ICI)

A solution used as a scabicide to treat scabies.

Dose: dilute and apply to the body as directed.
Side effects:
Caution: keep out of the eyes.
Not to be used for:
Not to be used with: alcohol.
Contains: monosulfiram.
Other preparations: Tetmosol Soap.

Antimalarials

Malaria is a feverish disease which can be caught in many areas of Africa, Asia, Central and South America if you are bitten by an infected mosquito. It is best to avoid being bitten by mosquitoes but, if you are planning to travel to any country within the risk areas, ask your doctor for advice. There are resistant strains of malaria in some areas, so your doctor may need to seek advice about the best prophylactic tablets for you to take.

We include here some general advice about immunization and malaria for travellers. Antimalarial preparations listed in this section can be bought over the counter. Different areas of the world have different strains of malaria, and the traveller should check which preparation is to be recommended. Medication against malaria should be started a few days before travelling and continue for four weeks after returning from overseas. Any influenza-like condition should be regarded as potential malaria in someone who has returned from an area where malaria is endemic.

Daraprim
(Wellcome)

A white, scored tablet supplied at a strength of 25 mg and used as an antimalarial drug for the prevention of malaria.

Dose: adults and children over 10 years 1 tablet a week; children 5-10 years half adult dose.
Side effects: rash, anaemia.
Caution: in pregnant women, nursing mothers, and in patients suffering from liver or kidney disease.
Not to be used for: children under 5 years.
Not to be used with: co-trimoxazole, lorazepam.
Contains: pyrimethamine.
Other preparations:

Nivaquine
(M & B)

A yellow tablet supplied at a strength of 200 mg and used as an antimalarial drug for the prevention and treatment of malaria.

Dose: adults prevention 2 tablets on the same day once a week; treatment as advised by the physician; children use Nivaquine Syrup.
Side effects: headache, stomach upset, skin eruptions, hair loss, eye disorders, blood disorders, loss of pigment.
Caution: in pregnant women, nursing mothers, and in patients suffering from porphyria (a rare blood disorder), liver or kidney disease, psoriasis. The eyes should be tested before and during prolonged treatment
Not to be used for:
Not to be used with:
Contains: chloroquine sulphate.
Other preparations: Nivaquine Syrup, Nivaquine Injection.

Paludrine
(ICI)

A white, scored tablet supplied at a strength of 100 mg and used as an antimalarial drug for the prevention of malaria.

Dose: adults and children over 12 years 1-2 tablets a day after meals; children under 1 year ¼ tablet, 1-4 years ½ tablet, 5-8 years ¾ tablet, 9-12 years 1 tablet after meals.
Side effects: stomach upset.
Caution:
Not to be used for:
Not to be used with:
Contains: proguanil hydrochloride.
Other preparations:

Gynaecological infections

Cystitis and thrush (*Candida*) are the most common gynaecological complaints, and it is reassuring to see that some preparations are available over the counter for both these conditions.

Cystitis can be treated with citrates which render the urine alkaline and thus antibacterial. In addition, Furadantin is an effective antibacterial.

Thrush responds to preparations, such as Econazole. This section also includes a number of preparations for general vaginal infections.

Vaginal bleeding or blood in the urine should be reported to a medical practitioner.

Itch can be caused by thrush and this can be provoked by antibiotic therapy or by taking the contraceptive pill. Many citrate preparations are available which can be used to treat cystitis. Allergic reactions to bath oils can occur in the genital area and can present as itch or rash. Cystitis often responds to drinking plenty of fluid and to one of the citrate preparations.

Aci-Jel
(Cilag)

A jelly with applicator used as an antiseptic to treat non-specific vaginal infection.

Dose: 1 application into the vagina twice a day.
Side effects: irritation and inflammation.
Caution:
Not to be used for: children.
Not to be used with:
Contains: acetic acid.
Other preparations:

Betadine
(Cilag)

A pessary and applicator supplied at a strength of 200 mg and used as an antiseptic to treat inflammation of the vagina.

Dose: 1 pessary to be inserted into the vagina night and morning for at least 14 days.
Side effects: irritation and sensitivity.
Caution:
Not to be used for: children.
Not to be used with:
Contains: povidone-iodine.
Other preparations: Betadine Vaginal Gel, Betadine VC Kit.

Cystemme see **Effercitrate**

Cystoleve see **Effercitrate**

Cystopurin see **Effercitrate**

Effercitrate
(Typharm)

A white effervescent tablet used as an alkalizing agent to treat cystitis.

Dose: adults and children over 6 years 2 tablets dissolved in water up to 3 times a day with meals; children 1-6 years half adult dose.
Side effects: raised potassium levels, stomach irritation, mild diuresis.
Caution: in patients suffering from kidney disease.
Not to be used for: infants under 1 year or for patients suffering from ulcerated or blocked small bowel.
Not to be used with: potassium-sparing diuretics.
Contains: citric acid, potassium bicarbonate.
Other preparations:

Furadantin
(Norwich Eaton)

A yellow, pentagonal, scored tablet supplied at strengths of 50 mg, 100 mg, and used as an antiseptic to treat infection of the urinary tract.

Dose: adults treatment 100 mg 4 times a day with food or milk, prevention 100-200 mg a day; children 3 months-2½ years one-eighth adult dose, 2½-6 years quarter adult dose, 6-11 years half adult dose, 11-14 years three-quarters adult dose.
Side effects: stomach upset, allergy, jaundice, nerve inflammation, blood changes, possible liver damage.
Caution:
Not to be used for: infants under 1 month or for patients suffering from kidney problems resulting in reduced urine output.
Not to be used with:
Contains: nitrofurantoin.

Other preparations: Furadantin Suspension.

Hiprex
(3M Riker)

A white, oblong, scored tablet supplied at a strength of 1 g and used as an antibacterial treatment for infections of the urinary tract.

Dose: adults 1 g twice a day; children 6-12 years half adult dose.
Side effects: stomach upset, rash, bladder irritation.
Caution:
Not to be used for: patients suffering from severe dehydration, severe kidney failure, or electrolyte changes.
Not to be used with: sulphonamides, alkalizing agents.
Contains: hexamine hippurate.
Other preparations:

Pevaryl
(Cilag)

A cream used as an antifungal treatment for inflammation of the penis, inflammation of the vulva, thrush-like nappy rash, other skin infections such as tinea or nail infections.

Dose: massage gently into the affected area 2-3 times a day.
Side effects: irritation.
Caution:
Not to be used for:
Not to be used with:
Contains: econazole nitrate.
Other preparations: Pevaryl Lotion, Pevaryl Spray, Pevaryl Powder.

Urisal
(Sterling Research Laboratories)

Orange-flavoured granules in sachets of 4 g used as an alkalizing agent to relieve the pain of cystitis.

Dose: the contents of 1 sachet dissolved in water 3 times a day for 3 days.
Side effects:
Caution: in patients suffereing from kidney disease.
Not to be used for: children, pregnant women, or for patients suffering from heart disease, high blood pressure, or with a history of kidney disease.
Not to be used with:
Contains: sodium citrate.
Other preparations:

Bowel disorders

Constipation, diarrhoea, and irritable bowel syndrome are the three bowel conditions for which over-the-counter preparations are available. Simple remedies for diarrhoea include kaolin formulations and Arret (Imodium). Various laxatives are available in addition to those listed below. These include Exlax, Milpar, Milk of Magnesia, Duphalac, and Dulcolax which is available as suppositories or tablets. Phenolphthalein can be bought as Brooklax. Andrews Liver Salts contain bicarbonate for indigestion, as well as citrate and magnesium sulphate which is a good, simple laxative.

Finally, there are some medications available over the counter which are used to treat haemorrhoids and anal problems. The best known of these are Preparation H (yeast cells and shark liver oil), Haemocaine cream or suppositories and Anusol cream, ointment, and suppositories.

Significant change in bowel habit, passing blood, or weight loss should be reported to the doctor.

Diarrhoea is most commonly due to gastro-enteritis; specific remedies are included here but particularly in children, replacement of minerals with Dioralyte (*see* section on Minerals below) is the most important remedy. Vague abdominal pains are often due to the irritable bowel syndrome (spastic colon) and respond to antispasm agents such as Colpermin.

Agarol
(Warner-Lambert)

An emulsion used as a lubricant and stimulant to treat constipation.

Dose: adults 5-15 ml at bedtime; children 5-12 years 5 ml at bedtime.
Side effects: allergies to phenolphthalein, blood or protein in the urine.
Caution:
Not to be used for: children under 5 years.
Not to be used with:
Contains: liquid paraffin, phenolphthalein, agar.
Other preparations:

Alophen
(Warner-Lambert)

A brown pill used as a stimulant and anticholinergic to treat constipation.

Dose: 1-3 pills at bedtime.
Side effects: allergies to phenolphthalein, skin rash, protein in the urine.
Caution:
Not to be used for: children or for patients suffering from glaucoma or inflammatory bowel disease.
Not to be used with:
Contains: aloin, phenolphthalein, ipecacuanha, belladonna extract.
Other preparations:

Arret
(Janssen)

A capsule used to treat diarrhoea.
Dose: up to 8 capsules daily.
Availability;
Side effects: rashes
Caution: in severe colitis.
Not to be used for: children.
Not to be used with:
Contains: loperamide.
Other preparations: Imodium capsules and syrup on prescription.

Colpermin
(Tillotts)

A blue capsule used as an anti-spasm treatment for irritable bowel syndrome.

Dose: 1-2 capsules 3 times a day.
 over the counter.
Side effects:
Caution:
Not to be used for: children.
Not to be used with:
Contains: peppermint oil.
Other preparations:

Dioralyte
(Rorer)

Cherry- or pineapple-flavoured powder supplied as sachets and used as a fluid and electrolyte replacement to treat acute watery diarrhoea including gastro-enteritis.

Dose: 1-2 sachets in 200-400 ml water after each occasion of diarrhoea; infants substitute equivalent volume of reconstituted powder to feeds.

Side effects:
Caution:
Not to be used for:
Not to be used with:
Contains: sodium chloride, potassium chloride, sodium bicarbonate, glucose.
Other preparations: Dioralyte Effervescent, Electrolade (Nicholas); Gluco-Lyte (Cupal); Rehidrat (Searle).

Dulcolax
(Boehringer Ingelheim)

A yellow tablet supplied at a strength of 5 mg and used as a stimulant to treat constipation and for evacuation of the bowels before surgery.

Dose: adults 2 tablets at night; children under 10 years half adult dose.
NHS (when prescribed as a generic), private prescription, over the counter.
Side effects:
Caution:
Not to be used for:
Not to be used with:
Contains: Bisacodyl.
Other preparations: Dulcolax suppositories.

Duphalac
(Duphar)

A syrup used as a laxative to treat constipation, brain disease due to liver problems.

Dose: children 0-1 year 2.5 ml twice a day; 1-4 years 5 ml twice a day; 5-10 years 10 ml twice a day; adults 15-50 ml 2-3 times a day until 2-3 soft stools are produced each day.

NHS (when prescribed as a generic), private prescription, over the counter.
Side effects:
Caution:
Not to be used for: patients suffering from galactosaemia (an inherited disorder).
Not to be used with:
Contains: lactulose.
Other preparations: lactulose solution.

Exlax
(Intercare)

Exlax contains phenolphthalein which is a powerful laxative only to be used when other simple remedies have failed.

Fybranta
(Norgine)

A mottled, pale-brown, chewable 2 g tablet used as a bulking agent in the treatment of diverticular disease, irritable colon syndrome, constipation through a diet lacking in fibre.

Dose: adults 1-3 tablets with liquid 3-4 times a day; children in proportion.
Side effects:
Caution:
Not to be used for:
Not to be used with:
Contains: bran.
Other preparations:

---

kaolin

Kaolin preparations are useful for mild diarrhoea; they are not absorbed into the body and so have limited side effects. Products containing kaolin include Kaopectate, Kaodene, Enterosan (with belladonna and morphine), and Collis Browne's (with morphine, peppermint oil, and calcium carbonate).

Milk of Magnesia

Milk of Magnesia contains magnesium hydroxide and is available in liquid and tablet form, as well as in combination with paraffin as Milpar.

Mintec
(Bridge)

A green/ivory capsule used as an anti-spasm treatment for irritable bowel syndrome, spastic colon.

Dose: adults 1-2 capsules 3 times a day before meals.
 NHS and over the counter.
Side effects:
Caution:
Not to be used for:
Not to be used with:
Contains: peppermint oil.
Other preparations:

---

senna tablets

A tablet supplied at a strength of 7.5 mg and used as a stimulant laxative to treat constipation.

Dose: adults 2-4 tablets at bedtime; children 6-12 years half adult dose.
Side effects:
Caution:

Not to be used for: pregnant women, children under 6 years.
Not to be used with:
Contains: sennosides.
Other preparations:

Senokot
(Reckitt & Colman)

A brown tablet supplied at a strength of 7.5 mg and used as a stimulant to treat constipation.

Dose: adults 2-4 tablets at bedtime; children 2-6 years 2.5-5 ml syrup (*see* below) in morning; children over 6 years half adult dose in morning.
Side effects:
Caution:
Not to be used for: infants under 2 years.
Not to be used with:
Contains: Sennoside B.
Other preparations: Senokot granules, Sennokott syrup.

Spasmonal
(Norgine)

A blue/grey capsule supplied at a strength of 60 mg and used as an anti-spasmodic treatment for irritable bowel syndrome.

Dose: 1-2 capsules 1-3 times a day.
Side effects: blurred vision, confusion, dry mouth.
Caution:
Not to be used for: children or for patients suffering from glaucoma, inflammatory bowel disease, intestinal obstruction, enlarged prostate.
Not to be used with:
Contains: alverine citrate.
Other preparations:

Anti-worm preparations

Intestinal worms are normally present with abdominal pain, weight loss, and the passage of worms through the anus. There are several medications available over the counter which can be used to treat these infections.

Alcopar
(Wellcome)

Dispersible granules in a sachet of 2.5 g used as an anti-worm treatment.

Dose: adults and children over 2 years 1 sachet dispersed in water; children under 2 years half adult dose.
Side effects: stomach upset.
Caution:
Not to be used for: patients who are continuously vomiting.
Not to be used with:
Contains: bephenium hydroxy-naphthoate.
Other preparations:

Antepar
(Wellcome)

An elixir used as an anti-worm treatment.

Dose: adults up to 30 ml as a single dose; children reduced doses.
Side effects: stomach upset, changes in the central nervous system, hypersensitivity, bruising, blood changes, liver disorder.
Caution: in nursing mothers and in patients suffering from nervous disorders.
Not to be used for: patients suffering from epilepsy, or kidney or liver disease.
Not to be used with:
Contains: piperazine hydrate, piperazine citrate.
Other preparations:

Banocide
(Wellcome)

A white, scored tablet supplied at a strength of 50 mg and used

as an anti-worm agent to treat worms in the blood and lymph channels.

Dose: as advised by the physician.
Side effects: itchy skin, eye disorders.
Caution: your doctor may advise regular eye tests.
Not to be used for: pregnant women.
Not to be used with:
Contains: diethylcarbamazine.
Other preparations:

Mintezol
(MSD)

A pink, scored, chewable tablet supplied at a strength of 500 mg and used to treat worms and other associated conditions and infections.

Dose: under 60 kg body weight 25 mg per kg twice a day with food; over 60 kg body weight 1.5 g twice a day with food.
Side effects: reduced alertness, stomach and brain disturbances, allergy, liver damage, changes to sight and hearing, low blood pressure, bed wetting.
Caution: in patients suffering from liver or kidney disease.
Not to be used for:
Not to be used with: xanthine derivatives (such as theophylline).
Contains: thiabendazole.
Other preparations:

Pripsen
(Reckitt & Colman)

A sachet used to treat worms.

Dose: adults and children over 6 years 1 sachet and then a second dose of 1 sachet after 14 days; infants 3 months-1 year

⅓ sachet then a second dose after 14 days; children 1-6 years ⅔ sachet then a second dose after 14 days.
Side effects: rarely sight disorders, vertigo.
Caution: in nursing mothers and in patients suffering from nervous disorders.
Not to be used for: patients suffering from epilepsy, liver or kidney disease.
Not to be used with:
Contains: piperazine phosphate, sennoside.
Other preparations:

Yomesan
(Bayer)

A yellow tablet supplied at a strength of 500 mg used to treat tapeworm.

Dose: as advised by the physician.
Side effects: stomach upset, lightheadedness, itch.
Caution:
Not to be used for:
Not to be used with: alcohol.
Contains: niclosamide.
Other preparations:

Stomach preparations

Most of the stomach preparations available are used to treat gastritis, ulcers, and other hyperacidity syndromes. Simple remedies, such as Rennies, contain antacid, whereas ENOs and Alka Seltzer have sodium bicarbonate. Of the preparations listed in this section, the majority are antacids which act directly to neutralize the acid in the stomach. Caved-S and De-Nol may be singled out as having more specific anti-ulcer properties.

Persistent indigestion may mean that an ulcer is present and that medical evaluation is necessary. Care should be taken not to overdose an antacid preparation.

The main complaints related to the upper gastro-intestinal system are pain, indigestion, acid reflux, distension, and wind. Loss of appetite can be treated with tonics (*see* below). Persistent vomiting may be due to acid reflux or to gastro-enteritis. If vomiting does not settle in twenty-four hours, medical advice should be sought. Upper abdominal pain can also be due to gall bladder disease.

Magnesium-containing antacids are usually laxative in nature while aluminium- and sodium-containing preparations may constipate. The simplest of antacids (alkalis) is sodium bicarbonate, but care should be taken to avoid mineral overload. For example, sodium should be avoided in those with heart conditions or high blood pressure because it can lead to heart failure. Magnesium and aluminium should be used carefully in those with kidney disorders and a combination of alkalis and milk can lead to excess calcium deposits in the kidney. Actal is an example of a sodium-containing antacid, Actonorm of a magnesium- and aluminium-containing antacid.

Actal
(Winthrop)

A white tablet supplied at a strength of 360 mg and used as an antacid to treat indigestion, dyspepsia.

Dose: 1-2 tablets when needed.
Side effects: few; sodium overload is possible.
Caution:
Not to be used for: children.
Not to be used with: tetracycline antibiotics.
Contains: alexitol sodium.
Other preparations: Actal Suspension.

Actonorm
(Wallace)

A white liquid supplied in 200 ml bottles and used as an antacid to treat indigestion, wind.

Dose: 5-20 ml after meals.
Side effects: few; occasionally constipation or diarrhoea.
Caution:
Not to be used for: children.
Not to be used with: tetracycline antibiotics.
Contains: aluminium hydroxide, magnesium hydroxide, activated dimethicone.
Other preparations:

Algicon
(Rorer)

A white tablet used as an antacid to treat heartburn, hiatus hernia indigestion.

Dose: 1-2 tablets 4 times a day after meals and at night.

Side effects: few; constipation or diarrhoea.
Caution: in patients suffering from diabetes because of sucrose content.
Not to be used for: children, or in patients suffering from kidney failure or severe debilitation.
Not to be used with: tetracycline antibiotics.
Contains: magnesium alginate, aluminium hydroxide/magnesium carbonate, magnesium carbonate, potassium bicarbonate.
Other preparations: Algicon Suspension.

Alka Seltzer
(Bayer)

Alka Seltzer contains aspirin, citric acid, and sodium bicarbonate. Although the sodium bicarbonate is an alkali, the combination with aspirin means that this preparation is not suitable for those with ulcer disease, because aspirin makes ulcers bleed. Alka Seltzer can be used for mild headache and indigestion combined, for example in those with a hangover.

Altacite Plus
(Roussel)

A white liquid supplied in 500 ml bottles and used as an antacid and anti-wind preparation to treat wind, indigestion, dyspepsia, and gastric ulcers.

Dose: adults 10 ml between meals and at bedtime; children 8-12 years half adult dose.
Side effects: few; occasional diarrhoea and constipation.
Caution:
Not to be used for: children under 8 years.
Not to be used with: tetracycline antibiotics.
Contains: hydrotalcite, activated dimethicone.
Other preparations: higher-strength suspension.and tablets.

Alu-Cap
(3M Riker)

A green/red capsule supplied at a strength of 475 mg and used as an antacid to treat hyperacidity.

Dose: 1 capsule 4 times a day and at bedtime.
Side effects: few; occasional bowel disorder such as constipation.
Caution:
Not to be used for: children.
Not to be used with: tetracycline antibiotics.
Contains: aluminium hydroxide gel.
Other preparations:

Aluhyde
(Sinclair)

A white scored tablet used as an antispasmodic and antacid to treat hyperacidity and intestinal spasm.

Dose: 2 tablets after meals.
Side effects: occasionally constipation and blurred vision.
Caution: in patients suffering from prostate enlargement.
Not to be used for: children or for patients suffering from glaucoma.
Not to be used with: tetracycline antibiotics.
Contains: aluminium hydroxide gel, magnesium trisilicate, belladonna liquid extract.
Other preparations:

Andrew's see **ENO**

Andrew's Answer see **ENO**

Andursil
(Geigy)

A white liquid supplied in 100 ml bottles and used as an antacid and anti-wind preparation to treat dyspepsia, heartburn, peptic ulcer.

Dose: 5-10 ml 3 times a day and at bedtime.
Side effects: few; possibly constipation or diarrhoea.
Caution:
Not to be used for: children.
Not to be used with: tetracycline antibiotics.
Contains: aluminium oxide, magnesium hydroxide, aluminium hydroxide/magnesium carbonate, activated dimethicone.
Other preparations: Andursil Tablets.

Asilone
(Rorer)

A white liquid used as an antacid, anti-wind preparation to treat gastritis, ulcers, dyspepsia, wind.

Dose: adults 5-10 ml before meals and at bedtime; children use infant suspension or half adult dose.
Side effects: few; occasionally constipation.
Caution:
Not to be used for: infants.
Not to be used with:
Contains: activated dimethicone, aluminium hydroxide gel, magnesium oxide.
Other preparations: Asilone Gel, Asilone Infant Suspension, Asilone Tablets; Infacol (Pharmax); Polycrol Gel and Tablets, Polycrol Forte Gel (Nicholas); Unigest (Unigreg) — private prescription and over the counter only; Siloxyl (Martindale) — private prescription and over the counter only.

Bellocarb
(Sinclair)

A beige tablet used as an antacid and anti-spasm treatment for bowel spasm, ulcers, dyspepsia.

Dose: 1-2 tablets 4 times a day.
Side effects: few; occasional constipation.
Caution: in patients suffering from enlarge prostate, heart, kidney, or liver problems.
Not to be used for: patients suffereing from glaucoma.
Not to be used with:
Contains: belladonna, magnesium trisilicate, magnesium carbonate.
Other preparations:

Carbellon
(Torbet)

A black tablet used as an anti-spasm, anti-wind, antacid preparation to treat acidity, ulcers, food poisoning.

Dose: adults 2-4 tablets 3 times a day; children 1-3 tablets a day.
Side effects: few; occasionally constipation.
Caution:
Not to be used for: patients suffering from glaucoma, pyloric stenosis, enlarged prostate.
Not to be used with:
Contains: belladonna, magnesium hydroxide, charcoal, peppermint oil.
Other preparations:

Caved-S
(Tillotts)

A brown tablet used as a cell-surface protector and antacid to treat peptic ulcer.
Dose: adults 2 tablets chewed between meals; children 10-14 years half adult dose.
Side effects: few; occasionally constipation.
Caution:
Not to be used for: infants.
Not to be used with: tetracycline antibiotics.
Contains: liquorice extract, aluminium hydroxide, magnesium carbonate, sodium bicarbonate.
Other preparations: Rabro (Sinclair).

De-Nol
(Brocades)

A white liquid used as a cell-surface protector to treat gastric and duodenal ulcer.

Dose: 10 ml diluted with 15 ml water twice a day 30 minutes before meals.
Side effects: black colour to tongue and stools.
Caution:
Not to be used for: children of for patients suffering from kidney failure.
Not to be used with:
Contains: tri-potassium dicitrato bismuthate.
Other preparations: De-Noltab

Diovol
(Pharmax)

A white suspension used as an antacid and anti-wind preparation to treat ulcers, hiatus hernias, wind, and acidity.

Dose: adults 10-20 ml as required; children over 6 years half adult dose.
Side effects: few; occasionally constipation.
Caution:
Not to be used for: infants.
Not to be used with: tetracycline antibiotics.
Contains: aluminium hydroxide, magnesium hydroxide, dimethicone.
Other preparations:

Droxalin
(Sterling Health)

A white tablet used as an antacid to treat acidity, dyspepsia, and hiatus hernia.

Dose: 1-3 tablets chewed as required, usually every 4 hours.
Side effects: few; occasionally constipation.
Caution:
Not to be used for: infants.
Not to be used with: tetracycline antibiotics.
Contains: alexitol sodium, magnesium trisilicate.
Other preparations:

ENO
(Smith Kline Beecham)

ENO contains sodium bicarbonate, tartaric acid, and citric acid and is useful as an effervescent antacid. Care should be taken to avoid sodium overload. In contrast, Andrew's (Sterling Health) contains magnesium sulphate and acts as both an antacid and laxative. Andrew's Answer is another hangover remedy which contains paracetamol, caffeine, sodium bicarbonate, and citric acid.

Gastrocote
(MCP)

A white tablet used as an antacid and reflux suppressant to treat dyspepsia, hiatus hernia, oesophagitis.
Dose: adults 1-2 tablets 4 times a day; children over 6 years as adult.
Side effects: few; occasionally constipation.
Caution:
Not to be used for: infants.
Not to be used with: tetracycline antibiotics.
Contains: alginic acid, aluminium hydroxide, magnesium trisilicate, sodium bicarbonate.
Other preparations: Gastrocote Liquid.

Gastron
(Sterling Research Laboratories)

A white tablet used as an antacid and reflux suppressant to treat reflux symptom.

Dose: 1-2 tablets 3 times a day and 2 at bedtime.
Side effects: few; occasionally constipation.
Caution: in pregnant women and in patients suffering from high blood pressure, heart or kidney failure.
Not to be used for: infants.
Not to be used with: tetracycline antibiotics.
Contains: alginic acid, aluminium hydroxide, magnesium trisilicate, sodium bicarbonate.
Other preparations:

Gaviscon
(Reckitt & Colman)

A white tablet used as an antacid and reflux suppressant to treat reflux.

Dose: adults 1-2 tablets or 10-20 ml after meals and at night; children ½ infant sachet after meals.
Side effects: few; occasionally constipation.
Caution: in pregnant women, and in patients suffering from high blood pressure, heart or kidney failure.
Not to be used for: infants.
Not to be used with: tetracycline antibiotics.
Contains: sodium alginate, sodium bicarbonate, calcium carbonate.
Other preparations: Gaviscon Liquid, Gaviscon Infant.

Gelusil
(Warner-Lambert)

A white tablet used as an antacid to treat dyspepsia, heartburn.

Dose: adults 1-2 tablets after meals; children over 6 years half adult dose.
Side effects: few; occasionally constipation.
Caution:
Not to be used for: infants.
Not to be used with: tetracycline antibiotics.
Contains: magnesium trisilicate, aluminium hydroxide.
Other preparations:

Kolanticon
(Merrell Dow)

A gel used as an antacid, anti-spasm, and anticholinergic preparation to treat bowel/stomach spasm, acidity, wind, ulcers.

Dose: 10-20 ml every 4 hours.
Side effects: occasionally constipation, blurred vision, confusion, dry mouth.
Caution:
Not to be used for: infants or for patients suffering from

glaucoma, inflammatory bowel disease, intestinal obstruction, or enlarged prostate.
Not to be used with: tetracycline antibiotics.
Contains: aluminium hydroxide, magnesium oxide, dicyclamine hydrochloride, dimethicone.
Other preparations:

Loasid
(Calmic)

A white tablet used as an antacid and anti-wind preparation to treat ulcers, oesophagitis, gastritis, hiatus hernia, heartburn.

Dose: 1-2 tablets when required.
Side effects: few; occasionally constipation.
Caution: in patients suffereing from kidney failure.
Not to be used for: infants.
Not to be used with: tetracycline antibiotics.
Contains: aluminium hydroxide, dimethicone.
Other preparations:

Maalox
(Rorer)

A white tablet used as an antacid to treat gastric and duodenal ulcer, hiatus hernias, wind, and acidity.

Dose: 1-2 tablets after meals and at bedtime.
Side effects: few; occasionally constipation.
Caution:
Not to be used for: infants.
Not to be used with: tetracycline antibiotics.
Contains: aluminium hydroxide, magnesium hydroxide.
Other preparations: Maalox Suspension, Maalox Plus Suspension and Tablets (with dimethicone), Maalox TC (higher-dose aluminium suspension and tablets); Mucogel (Pharmax).

Malinal
(Robins)

A scored, white chewable tablet supplied at a strength of 500 mg and used as an antacid to treat indigestion, ulcers, hyperacidity.

Dose: 2 tablets at mealtimes and at bedtime.
Side effects:
Caution:
Not to be used for: children.
Not to be used with: tetracycline antibiotics.
Contains: almasilate.
Other preparations:

Nulacin
(Bencard)

A beige tablet used as an antacid to treat dyspepsia, acidity, oesophagitis, hiatus hernia.

Dose: 1 or more tablets as required.
Side effects: diarrhoea.
Caution: in patients suffering from kidney impairment.
Not to be used for: children, or for patients suffering from coeliac disease.
Not to be used with: tetracycline antibiotics.
Contains: milk solids with dextrins and maltose, magnesium oxide, magnesium carbonate, magnesium trisilicate.
Other preparations:

Peptobismol

Peptobismol contains bismuth salicylate (see also De-Nol). Bismuth may colour the stools black and should be used with caution in patients suffering from kidney disease.

Roter
(Roterpharma)

A pink tablet used as an antacid and antibulking agent to treat peptic ulcer, gastritis.
Dose: 1-2 tablets 3 times a day.
Side effects: constipation, nerve damage.
Caution:
Not to be used for: infants.
Not to be used with: tetracycline antibiotics.
Contains: magnesium carbonate, bismuth subnitrate, sodium bicarbonate, frangula.
Other preparations:

Setlers

Setlers contain calcium carbonate, magnesium carbonate and hydroxide, and aluminium hydroxide. Setlers Tums contain calcium carbonate only. Various strength and flavours are available and there are liquid and tablet preparations.

Topal
(ICI)

A cream tablet used as an antacid to treat oesophagitis, heartburn, gastritis.

Dose: adults 1-3 tablets 3-4 times a day between meals and at bedtime; children half adult dose.
Side effects: occasionally constipation.
Caution:
Not to be used for: infants.
Not to be used with: tetracycline antibiotics.
Contains: aluminium hydroxide, magnesium carbonate, alginic acid.
Other preparations:

Respiratory conditions

1 Antihistamines, cough and cold remedies

Most upper respiratory conditions are caused by virus infections and allergies such as hay fever. The common cold will not respond to antibiotics unless there is an added bacterial infection. Symptomatic treatment with many of the preparations listed below will benefit many cold sufferers.Pollution and cigarette smoking will exacerbate upper respiratory symptoms.

Antihistamines are anti-allergic preparations used to treat allergies of all types. Many different over-the-counter allergy preparations are listed in this section. Allergies need not be confined to the respiratory system, and the antihistamines referred to in this section can be used for generalized skin reactions such as allergies to drugs or foods. Most antihistamines have some sedative effect; they also dry up the nasal passages so they are included in combination with other drugs in numerous cold treatments.

Triludan is a good general, non-sedating antihistamine available in tablet or syrup form. Combined antihistamine/sympathomimetic (blood-vessel constricting) preparations include Benylin, Benylin Day and Night, Contac 400, Day Nurse, and Night Nurse. Sedating antihistamines, such as promethazine, are used as over-the-counter sleeping tablets (Sominex). Travel sickness also responds to antihistamines such as hyoscine (Joy Rides) or cinnarizine (Stugeron).

Other cold treatments include the Vicks range of remedies, Karvol inhalant capsules to clear catarrh from the airways, Lem-Sip, Coldrex, and Beecham's preparations, which rely on combinations of mild analgesics, such as aspirin and paracetamol, with other drugs, such as caffeine and phenylephrine (a sympathomimetic).

Care should be taken to keep a note of the total daily dose of the preparations taken, because one may find drugs such as paracetamol building up in the body. Total daily dose of paracetamol should not exceed 4 grams for adults.

Coughing of blood should be reported to a doctor.

Actidil
(Wellcome)

A white, scored tablet supplied at a strength of 2.5 mg and used as an antihistamine to treat allergies.

Dose: adults 1-2 tablets 3 times a day; children use elixir.
Side effects: drowsiness, reduced reactions, rarely skin eruptions.
Caution: in patients suffering from liver or kidney disease.
Not to be used for:
Not to be used with: alcohol, sedatives, some antidepressants (MAOIs).
Contains: triprolidine hydrochloride.
Other preparations:

Actifed Compound
(Wellcome)

A linctus used as an antihistamine to treat cough, congestion.

Dose: adults 2 5 ml teaspoonsful 3 times a day; children 2-5 years ½ teaspoonful 3 times a day, 6-12 years 1 teaspoonful 3 times a day..
Side effects: drowsiness, reduced reactions.
Caution: in patients suffering from liver or kidney disease.
Not to be used for: children under 2 years
Not to be used with: alcohol, sedatives, some antidepressants (MAOIs).
Contains: triprolidine hydrochloride, pseudoephedrine hydrochloride, dextromethorphan hydrobromide.
Other preparations: Actifed Expectorant, Actifed Tablets, Actifed Syrup.

Avomine
(Wellcome)

A white, scored tablet supplied at a strength of 25 mg and used as an antihistamine treatment for travel sickness, nausea, vomiting, vertigo.

Dose: adults travel sickness1 tablet at bedtime before long journeys or 1-2 hours before short journeys, nausea 1 tablet 1-3 times a day; children 5-10 years half adult dose.
Side effects: drowsiness, reduced reactions, rarely skin eruptions.
Caution: in patients suffering from liver or kidney disease.
Not to be used for: children under 5 years.
Not to be used with: alcohol, sedatives, some antidepressants (MAOIs).
Contains: promethazine, theoclate.
Other preparations:

Beecham's Powders

Beecham's Powders contain aspirin and caffeine; powder capsules have paracetamol, caffeine, and phenylephrine. Beecham's Hot Lemon is paracetamol with ascorbic acid (vitamin C). The main caution is to observe total daily dose of asprin or paracetamol.

Benylin Day and Night

Benylin Day and Night contains paracetamol and is a useful tablet preparation for treating the common cold.

Side effects: drowsiness, reduced reactions.
Caution: in patients suffering from liver or kidney disease.

Benylin Expectorant
(Warner-Lambert)

A syrup used as an antihistamine, expectorant, and sputum softener to treat cough, bronchial congestion.

Dose: adults 1-2 5 ml teaspoonsful every 2-3 hours; children 1-5 years ½ teaspoonful every 3-4 hours, 6-12 years 1 teaspoonful every 3-4 hours.
Side effects:
Caution:
Not to be used for: children under 1 year.
Not to be used with:
Contains: diphenhydramine hydrochloride, ammonium chloride, sodium citrate, menthol.
Other preparations: Benylin Paediatric, Benylin Decongestant, Benylin with Codeine.

Coldrex see Lemsip

Contac 400

Contac 400 contains phenylpropanolamine as a sympathomimetic and chlorpheniramine as an antihistamine.

Side effects: drowsiness, reduced reactions.
Caution: in patients suffering from liver or kidney disease.

Copholco
(Fisons)

A linctus used as an opiate, expectorant to treat laryngitis, inflammation of the windpipe.

Dose: adults 2 5 ml teaspoonsful 4-5 times a day; children over

5 years ½-1 teaspoonful 3 times a day.
Side effects: constipation.
Caution: in patients suffering from asthma.
Not to be used for: children under 5 years, or for patients suffering from liver disease.
Not to be used with: MAOIs.
Contains: pholcodine, menthol, cineole, terpin hydrate.
Other preparations:

Copholcoids
(Fisons)

A black pastille used as an opiate, expectorant to treat dry cough.

Dose: adults 1-2 pastilles sucked 3-4 times a day; children over 5 years 1 pastille sucked 3 times a day.
Side effects: constipation.
Caution: in patients suffering from asthma.
Not to be used for: children under 5 years or for patients suffering from liver disease
Not to be used with: MAOIs.
Contains: pholcodine, menthol, cineole, terpin hydrate.
Other preparations:

Daneral SA
(Hoechst)

An orange tablet supplied at a strength of 75 mg and used as an antihistamine to treat allergies.

Dose: adults 1-2 tablets at night.
Side effects: drowsiness, reduced reactions.
Caution: in nursing mothers.
Not to be used for:
Not to be used with: sedatives, MAOIs, alcohol.

Contains: pheniramine maleate.
Other preparations:

Davenol
(Wyeth)

A linctus used as an antihistamine, sympathomimetic, and opiate preparation to treat cough.

Dose: adults 1-2 5 ml teaspoonsful 3-4 times a day; children no more than 1 teaspoonful 3-4 times a day.
Side effects: constipation, drowsiness, reduced reactions, anxiety, hands shaking, irregular or rapid heart rate, dry mouth, excitement, rarely skin eruptions.
Caution: in patients suffering from asthma, kidney disease, diabetes.
Not to be used for: children under 5 years or for patients suffering from liver disease, heart or thyroid disorders.
Not to be used with: MAOIs, alcohol, sedatives, tricyclics.
Contains: carbinoxamine maleate, ephedrine hydrochloride, pholcodine.
Other preparations:

Day Nurse

Day Nurse contains paracetamol, ascorbic acid, phenylpropanolamine, dextromethorphan, and alcohol. It is available in tablet and liquid form. Night Nurse omits the stimulant sympathomimetic. Side effects are similar to those of Actifed.

Dimotane Expectorant
(Robins)

A liquid used as an antihistamine, expectorant, and

sympathomimetic treatment for cough.

Dose: adults 1-2 5 ml teaspoonsful 3 times a day; children 2-6 years ½ teaspoonful 3 times a day, 7-12 years 1 teaspoonful 3 times a day.
Side effects: anxiety, hands shaking, rapid or abnormal heart rate, dry mouth, brain stimulation.
Caution: in patients suffering from diabetes.
Not to be used for: children under 2 years or for patients suffering from cardiovascular problems, overactive thyroid gland.
Not to be used with: MAOIs, tricyclics, alcohol, sedatives, anticholinergics.
Contains: brompheniramine maleate, guaiphenesin, pseudoephedrine hydrochloride.
Other preparations: Dimotane Co, Dimotane Co Paediatric.

Dimotane Plus
(Robins)

A liquid used as an antihistamine and sympathomimetic treatment for allergic rhinitis.

Dose: adults 2 5 ml teaspoonsful 3 times a day; children use Paediatric.
Side effects: drowsiness, reduced reactions, rarely stimulant effects.
Caution: in nursing mothers and in patients suffering from bronchial asthma.
Not to be used for: patients suffering from glaucoma, comatose states, brain damage, epilepsy, retention of urine, cardiovascular problems, overactive thyroid gland.
Not to be used with: MAOIs, tricyclics, alcohol, sedatives, anticholinergics.
Contains: brompheniramine maleate, pseudoephedrine hydrochloride.
Other preparations: Dimotane Plus Paediatric, Dimotane Plus LA, Dimotane LA, Dimotane Tablets, Dimotane Elixir.

Dimotapp LA
(Robins)

A brown tablet used as an antihistamine and sympathomimetic treatment for catarrh, allergic rhinitis, sinusitis.

Dose: adults 1-2 tablets night and morning; children use elixir.
Side effects: drowsiness, reduced reactions, rarely stimulant effects.
Caution: in nursing mothers and in patients suffering from bronchial asthma.
Not to be used for: patients suffering from glaucoma, comatose states, brain damage, epilepsy, retention of urine, cardiovascular problems, overactive thyroid gland.
Not to be used with: MAOIs, tricyclics, alcohol, sedatives, anticholinergics.
Contains: brompheniramine maleate, phenylephrine hydrochloride, phenylpropanolamine hydrochloride.
Other preparations: Dimotapp Elixir, Dimotapp Elixir Paediatric.

Dramamine
(Searle)

A white, scored tablet supplied at a strength of 50 mg and used as an antihistamine treatment for vertigo, nausea, vomiting, travel sickness.

Dose: adults 1-2 tablets 2-3 times a day; children 1-6 years ¼-½ tablet. 7-12 years ½-1 tablet 2-3 times a day.
Side effects: drowsiness, reduced reactions, rarely skin eruptions.
Caution: in patients suffering from liver or kidney disease.
Not to be used for:
Not to be used with: alcohol, sedatives, some antidepressants (MAOIs).
Contains: dimenhydrenate.
Other preparations:

Eskornade Spansule
(S K B)

A grey/clear capsule used as an antihistamine and sympathomimetic to treat congestion, running nose, and phlegm brought on by common cold, rhinitis, flu, sinusitis.

Dose: adults 1 capsule every 12 hours; children use syrup.
Side effects: drowsiness.
Caution: in patients suffering from diabetes.
Not to be used for: patients suffering from cardiovascular problems, overactive thyroid gland.
Not to be used with: MAOIs, tricyclics, alcohol.
Contains: phenylpropanolamine hydrochloride, diphenylpyraline hydrochloride.
Other preparations: Eskornade Syrup.

Expulin
(Galen)

A linctus used as an antihistamine, opiate, and sympathomimetic treatment for cough and congestion.

Dose: adults 2 5 ml teaspoonsful 4 times a day; children 2-6 years ½-1 teaspoonful 4 times a day, 7-12 years 1-2 teaspoonsful 4 times a day.
Side effects: constipation, drowsiness, reduced reactions, anxiety, hands shaking, irregular or rapid heart rate, dry mouth, excitement, rarely skin eruptions.
Caution: in patients suffering from asthma, kidney disease, diabetes.
Not to be used for: children under 5 years, or for patients suffering from liver disease, heart or thyroid disorders.
Not to be used with: MAOIs, alcohol, sedatives, tricyclics
Contains: pholcodine, pseudoephedrine hydrochloride, chlorpheniramine hydrochloride, chlorpheniramine maleate.
Other preparations: Expulin Paediatric.

Expurhin
(Galen)

A linctus used as an antihistamine and sympathomimetic treatment for congestion, phlegm, and running nose in children.

Dose: 3 months-1 year ½-1 5 ml teaspoonful twice a day, 1-5 years 1-2 teaspoonsful 3 times a day, 6-12 years 2-3 teaspoonsful 3 times a day.
Side effects: drowsiness, reduced reactions, anxiety, hands shaking, irregular or rapid heart rate, dry mouth, excitement, rarely skin eruptions.
Caution: in patients suffering from liver or kidney disease, diabetes.
Not to be used for: infants under 3 months, or for patients suffering from heart or thyroid disorders.
Not to be used with: alcohol, sedatives, some antidepressants (MAOIs), tricyclics
Contains: ephedrine hydrochloride, chlorpheniramine hydrochloride, chlorpheniramine maleate, menthol.
Other preparations:

Fenostil Retard
(Zyma)

A white tablet supplied at a strength of 2.5 mg and used as an antihistamine treatment for rhinitis, urticaria, hay fever, other allergies.

Dose: adults 1 tablet night and morning.
Side effects: drowsiness, reduced reactions.
Caution: in nursing mothers.
Not to be used for: children.
Not to be used with: alcohol, sedatives, MAOIs.
Contains: dimethindene maleate.
Other preparations:

Galcodine
(Galen)

A linctus supplied at a strength of 15 mg and used as an opiate to treat dry cough.

Dose: adults 1 5 ml teaspoonful 4 times a day; children 1-5 years ½-1 teaspoonful 3-4 times a day, 6-12 years 1 teaspoonful 3-4 times a day..
Side effects: constipation.
Caution: in patients suffering from asthma.
Not to be used for: infants under 1 year, or for patients suffering from liver disease.
Not to be used with: MAOIs.
Contains: codeine phosphate.
Other preparations: Galcodine Paediatric.

Galenphol
(Galen)

A liquid supplied at a strength of 5 mg and used as an opiate to treat dry cough.

Dose: adults 1-2 5 ml teaspoonsful 3-4 times a day; children 1-5 years ½-1 teaspoonful 3-4 times a day, 6-12 years 1 teaspoonful 3-4 times a day.
Side effects: constipation.
Caution: in patients suffering from asthma.
Not to be used for: infants under 1 year, or for patients suffering from liver disease.
Not to be used with: MAOIs.
Contains: pholcodine.
Other preparations: Galenphol Linctus Strong, Galenphol Linctus Paediatric.

Galpseud
(Galen)
A white tablet supplied at a strength of 60 mg and used as an sympathomimetic to treat congestion of the nose, sinuses, and upper respiratory tract.

Dose: adults 1 tablet 3 times a day; children use linctus.
Side effects: anxiety, hands shaking, irregular or rapid heart rate, dry mouth, excitement.
Caution: in patients suffering from diabetes.
Not to be used for: children under 2 years, or for patients suffering from heart or thyroid disorders.
Not to be used with: MAOIs, tricyclics.
Contains: pseudoephedrine hydrochloride.
Other preparations: Galpseud Linctus.

Guanor
(R P Drugs)

A liquid used as an expectorant, antihistamine, mucus softener to treat cough, bronchial congestion.

Dose: adults 1-2 5 ml teaspoonsful every 2-3 hours; children 1-5 years ½ teaspoonful every 3-4 hours, 6-12 years 1 teaspoonful every 3-4 hours.
Side effects: drowsiness, reduced reactions, rarely skin eruptions.
Caution: in patients suffering from liver or kidney disease.
Not to be used for: infants under 1 year.
Not to be used with: alcohol, sedatives, some antidepressants (MAOIs).
Contains: ammonium chloride, diphenhydramine hydrochloride, sodium citrate, menthol.
Other preparations:

Haymine
(Pharmax)

A yellow tablet used as an antihistamine and sympathomimetic treatment for allergies.

Dose: 1 tablet in the morning and 1 tablet at night if needed.
Side effects: drowsiness, reduced reactions, dizziness.
Caution:
Not to be used for: children, or for patients suffering from overactive thyroid gland, high blood pressure, coronary thrombosis.
Not to be used with: alcohol, sedatives, MAOIs.
Contains: chlorpheniramine maleate, ephedrine hydrochloride.
Other preparations:

Hayphryn
(Winthrop)

A spray used as a sympathomimetic, antihistamine treatment for blocked nose resulting from allergy.

Dose: adults 2 sprays into the nostrils every 3-4 hours; children over 7 years half adult dose.
Side effects:
Caution: in patients suffering from overactive thyroid gland, cardiovascular disease; do not use for periods longer than 7 days.
Not to be used for: children under 7 years
Not to be used with: MAOIs.
Contains: phenylephrine hydrochloride, thenyldiamine hydrochloride.
Other preparations:

Histalix
(Wallace)

A syrup used as qan antihistamine, expectorant, and sputum softener to treat bronchial and nasal congestion.

Dose: adults 1-2 5 ml teaspoonsful every 3 hours; children hald adult dose.
Side effects: drowsiness, reduced reactions, rarely skin eruptions.
Caution: in patients suffering from liver or kidney disease.
Not to be used for:
Not to be used with: alcohol, sedatives, MAOIs.
Contains: diphenhydramine hydrochloride, ammonium chloride, sodium citrate, menthol.
Other preparations:

Histryl Spansule
(S K & F)

A pink/clear capsule supplied at a strength of 5 mg and used as an antihistamine to treat rhinitis, severe allergic conditions, insect bites and stings, allergies to food or other drugs.

Dose: 1-2 capsules night and morning.
Side effects: drowsiness, reduced reactions, dry mouth, blurred vision, dizziness.
Caution: in nursing mothers.
Not to be used for: children.
Not to be used with: alcohol, sedatives, MAOIs.
Contains: diphenyl pyraline hydrochloride.
Other preparations: Histryl Paediatric.

Lemsip

Lemsip contains paracetamol, caffeine, and phenylephrine.

Mildly stimulant and pain relieving — caffeine may cause tremors. Coldrex is similar and has additional ascorbic acid.

Lergoban
(3M Riker)

An off-white tablet supplied at a strength of 5 mg and used as an antihistamine to treat allergies.

Dose: 1-2 tablets every 12 hours.
Side effects: drowsiness, reduced reactions, dizziness, headache, flushing, anorexia, dry mouth.
Caution: in nursing mothers.
Not to be used for: children.
Not to be used with: alcohol, sedatives, MAOIs.
Contains: diphenylpyraline hydrochloride.
Other preparations:

Lotussin
(Searle)

A linctus used as an antihistamine, antussive treatment for cough.

Dose: adults 2 5 ml teaspoonsful 3 times a day; children 1-5 years ½-1 teaspoonful 3 times a day, 5-12 years 1-2 teaspoonsful 3 times a day.
Side effects: drowsiness, reduced reactions, constipation, rarely skin eruptions.
Caution: in patients suffering from kidney disease, asthma.
Not to be used for: infants under 1 year, or for patients suffering from liver disease.
Not to be used with: alcohol, sedatives, some antidepressants (MAOIs).
Contains: diphenhydramine hydrochloride, dextromethorphan hydrobromide.
Other preparations:

Noradran
(Norma)

A syrup used as an antussive to treat bronchitis, bronchial asthma.
Dose: adults 2 5 ml teaspoonsful every 4 hours; children over 5 years 1 5 ml teaspoonful every 4 hours.
Side effects: sedation, dry mouth, nervousness, restlessness, hands shaking, abnormal heart rhythm, stomach upset.
Caution: in patients suffering from heart or liver disease, diabetes.
Not to be used for: children under 5 years, or for patients suffering from high blood pressure, overactive thyroid, coronary disease, cardiac asthma
Not to be used with: MAOIs, sympathomimetics, tricyclics, alcohol, cimetidine, erythomycin, interferon, ciprofloxaxin.
Contains: guaiphenesin.
Other preparations:

Optimine
(Kirby-Warrick)

A white, scored tablet supplied at a strength of 1 mg and used as an antihistamine and serotonin antagonist (hormone blocker) to treat bites and stings, itch, allergic rhinitis, urticaria.

Dose: adults 1-2 tablets twice a day; children over 1 year use syrup.
Side effects: drowsiness, reduced reactions, greater appetite, anorexia, nausea, headache, anticholinergic effects.
Caution:
Not to be used for: infants under 1 year or for patients suffering from prostate enlargement, retention of urine, glaucoma, peptic ulcer causing blockage.
Not to be used with: sedatives, MAOIs, alcohol.
Contains: azatadine maleate.
Other preparations: Optimine Syrup.

Pavacol-D
(Boehringer Ingelheim)

A mixture containing opiate and demulcents used to treat cough.

Dose: adults 1-2 5 ml teaspoonsful as needed; children 1-2 years ½ teaspoonful 3-4 times a day, 3-5 years 1 teaspoonful 3 times a day, 6-12 years 1 teaspoonful 4-5 times a day.

Side effects: constipation.

Caution: in patients suffering from asthma.

Not to be used for: infants under 1 year, or for patients suffering from liver disease.

Not to be used with: MAOIs.

Contains: pholcodine, aromatic oils.

Other preparations:

Periactin
(MSD)

A white, scored tablet supplied at a strength of 4 mg and used as an antihistamine , serotonin antagonists (hormone blocker) to improve appetite and to treat allergies, itchy skin conditions.

Dose: adults and children over 7 years 1 tablet 3-4 times a day; children 2-6 years 2 tablets a day or ½ tablet 3-4 times a day.

Side effects: anticholinergic effects, reduced reactions, drowsiness, excitement.

Caution: in pregnant women, and in patients suffering from bronchial asthma, raised eye pressure, overactive thyroid, cardiovascular disease, high blood pressure.

Not to be used for: newborn infants, nursing mothers, the elderly, or patients suffering from glaucoma, enlarged prostate, bladder obstruction, retention of urine, stomach blockage, peptic ulcer, or debilitation.

Not to be used with: alcohol, sedatives, MAOIs.

Contains: cyproheptadine hydrochloride.

Other preparations: Periactin Syrup.

Phenergan
(M & B)

A blue tablet supplied at a strength of 10 mg, 25 mg and used as an antihistamine to treat allergies.

Dose: adults 10-20 mg 2-3 times a day; children 1-5 years 5-15 mg a day, over 5 years 10-25 mg a day.
Side effects: drowsiness, reduced reactions, dizziness, disorientation, sensitivity to light, convulsions on high doses, extrapyramidal reactions (shaking and rigidity).
Caution:
Not to be used for: infants under 1 year
Not to be used with: alcohol, sedatives, MAOIs.
Contains: promethazine hydrochloride.
Other preparations: Phenergan Elixir, Phenergan Injection.

Phensedyl
(M & B)

A linctus used as an antihistamine, opiate, sympathomimetic treatment for cough.

Dose: adults 1-2 5 ml teaspoonsful 2-3 times a day; children 2-5 years ½ teaspoonful 2-3 times a day, 6-12 years ½-1 teaspoonful 2-3 times a day.
Side effects: constipation, drowsiness, reduced reactions, anxiety, hands shaking, irregular or rapid heart rate, dry mouth, excitement, rarely skin eruptions.
Caution: in patients suffering from asthma, kidney disease, diabetes.
Not to be used for: children under 2 years, or for patients suffering from liver disease, heart or thyroid disorders.
Not to be used with: MAOIs, alcohol, sedatives, tricyclics.
Contains: promethazine hydrochloride, codeine phosphate, ephedrine hydrochloride.
Other preparations: Galcodine Paediatric.

Pholcomed-D
(Galen)
A linctus used as an opiate and bronchial relaxant to treat dry, irritating cough.

Dose: adults 2-3 5 ml teaspoonsful 3-4 times a day; children under 2 years years ½ teaspoonful 3-4 times a day, 2-12 years 1 teaspoonful 3-4 times a day.
Side effects: constipation.
Caution: in patients suffering from asthma.
Not to be used for: children under 1 year, or for patients suffering from liver disease.
Not to be used with: MAOIs.
Contains: pholcodine, papaverine hydrochloride.
Other preparations: Pholcomed Capsules, Pholcomed, Pholcomed Forte, Pholcomed Forte Diabetic, Pholcomed Expectorant.

Pholtex
(3M Riker)

A liquid used as an opiate and antihistamine treatment for dry cough.

Dose: adults 1 5 ml teaspoonful 2-3 times a day; children ½-1 teaspoonful 2-3 times a day.
Side effects: constipation.
Caution: in patients suffering from asthma.
Not to be used for: children under 5 years, or for patients suffering from liver disease.
Not to be used with: MAOIs.
Contains: pholcodine, phenyltoloxamine.
Other preparations:

Piriton
(A & H)

A cream-coloured tablet supplied at a strength of 4 mg and used as an antihistamine treatment for allergies.
Dose: adults 1 tablet 3-4 times a day; children 6-12 years ½-1 tablet 3-4 times a day, under 6 years use syrup.
Side effects: drowsiness, reduced reactions, dizziness, excitation.
Caution: in nursing mothers.
Not to be used for:
Not to be used with: MAOIs, sedatives, alcohol.
Contains: chlorpheniramine maleate.
Other preparations: Piriton Syrup, Piriton Spandets, Piriton Injection.

Polleneze

Polleneze contains astemozole and is a useful antihistamine for hay fever.

Side effects: drowsiness, reduced reactions, dizziness, excitation.
Caution: in nursing mothers.

Pro-Actidil
(Wellcome)

A white tablet supplied at a strength of 10 mg and used as an antihistamine treatment for allergies.

Dose: 1 tablet a day 5-6 hours before going to bed.
Side effects: drowsiness, reduced reactions, rarely skin eruptions.
Caution: in nursing mothers, and in patients suffering from liver or kidney disease.

Not to be used for: children.
Not to be used with: MAOIs, sedatives, alcohol.
Contains: triprolidine hydrochloride.
Other preparations:

Stugeron
(Janssen)

A white, scored tablet supplied at a strength of 15 mg and used as an antihistamine treatment for vestibular disorders, travel sickness.

Dose: vestibular disorders adults 2 tablets 3 times a day; travel sickness 1 tablet 2 hours before journey, then 1 every 8 hours during the journey. Children 5-12 years half adult dose.
Side effects: drowsiness, reduced reactions, rarely skin eruptions.
Caution: in patients suffering from liver or kidney disease.
Not to be used for: children under 5 years.
Not to be used with: MAOIs, sedatives, alcohol.
Contains: cinnarizine.
Other preparations:

Sudafed
(Calmic)

A red tablet supplied at a strength of 60 mg and used as a sympathomimetic treatment to relieve congestion of the nose, sinuses, and upper respiratory tract.

Dose: adults 1 tablet 3 times a day; children use elixir.
Side effects: anxiety, tremor, rapid or abnormal heart rate, dry mouth, brain stimulation.
Caution: in patients suffering from diabetes.
Not to be used for: patients suffering from cardiovascular disorders, overactive thyroid.

Not to be used with: MAOIs, tricyclics.
Contains: pseudoephedrine.
Other preparations: Sudafed Elixir, Sudafed SA, Sudafed-Co, Sudafed Expectorant.

Sudafed Plus
(Calmic)

A white, scored tablet used as an antihistamine, sympathomimetic treatment for allergic rhinitis.

Dose: adults 1 tablet 3 times a day; children over 2 years use Syrup.
Side effects: drowsiness, rash, disturbed sleep, rarely hallucinations.
Caution: in patients suffering from raised eye pressure, enlarged prostate.
Not to be used for: infants under 2 years, or for patients suffering from severe high blood pressure, coronary artery disease, overactive thyroid.
Not to be used with: MAOIs, sympathomimetics, furazolidone alcohol.
Contains: triprolidine hydrochloride, pseudoephedrine hydrochloride.
Other preparations: Sudafed Plus Syrup.

Tavegil
(Sandoz)

A white, scored tablet supplied at a strength of 1 mg and used as an antihistamine treatment for allergic rhinitis, dermatoses, urticaria, allergy to other drugs.

Dose: adults 1 tablet night and morning; children ½-1 tablet night and morning.
Side effects: drowsiness, reduced reactions, rarely dizziness,

dry mouth, palpitations, gastro-intestinal disturbances.
Caution:
Not to be used for:
Not to be used with: MAOIs, sedatives, alcohol.
Contains: clemastine.
Other preparations: Tavegil Elixir.

Tercoda
(Sinclair)

A syrup used as an opiate, expectorant, antussive, sputum softener to treat bronchitis.

Dose: 1-2 5 ml teaspoonsful 3 times a day.
Side effects: constipation.
Caution: in patients suffering from asthma.
Not to be used for: children, or for patients suffering from liver disease.
Not to be used with: MAOIs.
Contains: codeine phosphate, terpin hydrate, cineole, menthol, peppermint oil, pumilio pine oil.
Other preparations:

Terpoin
(Hough, Hoseason)

An elixir used as an opiate treatment for dry cough.

Dose: 1 5 ml teaspoonful every 3 hours.
Side effects: constipation.
Caution: in patients suffering from asthma.
Not to be used for: children under 5 years, or for patients suffering from liver disease.
Not to be used with: MAOIs.
Contains: codeine phosphate, cineole, menthol.
Other preparations:

Thephorin
(Sinclair)

A white tablet supplied at a strength of 25 mg and used as an antihistamine to treat allergies.

Dose: 1-2 tablets 3 times a day before 4.00 in the afternoon.
Side effects: dry mouth, stomach upset, rarely drowsiness.
Caution:
Not to be used for: children.
Not to be used with: MAOIs, sedatives, alcohol, anticholinergics.
Contains: phenindamine tartrate.
Other preparations:

Triludan
(Merrell Dow)

A white, scored tablet supplied at a strength of 60 mg and used as an antihistamine treatment for allergies including hay fever and rhinitis.

Dose: adults 1 tablet twice a day or 2 tablets once a day; children 6-12 years ½ tablet twice a day.
Side effects: rash, sweating, headache, mild stomach disturbances.
Caution:
Not to be used for: children under 6 years.
Not to be used with:
Contains: terfenadine.
Other preparations: Triludan Forte, Triludan Suspension.

Uniflu & Gregovite C
(Unigreg)

A red, oblong tablet and a yellow tablet used as an analgesic, opiate, antussive, xanthine, antihistamine treatment for cold and flu symptoms.

Dose: 1 each of the tablets every 4 hours up to a maximum of 6 of each tablets in 24 hours.

Side effects: constipation, drowsiness, reduced reactions, anxiety, hands shaking, irregular or rapid heart rate, dry mouth, excitement, rarely skin eruptions.

Caution: in patients suffering from asthma, kidney disease, diabetes.

Not to be used for: children, or for patients suffering from liver disease, heart or thyroid disorders.

Not to be used with: MAOIs, sedatives, alcohol, tricyclics.

Contains: paracetamol, codeine phosphate, caffeine, diphenhydramine hydrochloride, phenylphrine hydrochloride, ascorbic acid.

Other preparations:

Vick

Vicks preparations contain basic ingredients similar to Day Nurse. In addition, there is an expectorant which contains guaiphenesin and citrate, and a Medinite preparation which has ephedrine, doxylamine, and alcohol. Vicks Sinex spray contains oxymetalozine, menthol, camphor and eucalyptol. Vicks throat spray and vapour rub are also available. The side effects of these preparations depend upon the main ingredients but they should be treated similarly to Actifed.

Respiratory conditions

2 Nose drops and sprays

Runny nose is usually due to allergy such as hay fever or the common cold — *see* section above. Sinusitis may present as persistent runny nose. Persistent nasal drip responds to sympathomimetic drugs which narrow the blood vessels and restrict leaking of fluid into the nose. These drugs should not be used in excess or for prolonged periods continuously.

Afrazine
(Kirby-Warrick)

A spray or nasal drops used as a sympathomimetic treatment for blocked nose.

Dose: adults and children over 5 years 2-3 sprays or drops in each nostril 2-3 times a day; children under 5 years use Paediatric drops.
Side effects: itching nose, headache, sleeplessness, rapid heart rate.
Caution: in patients suffering from overactive thyroid gland, diabetes, coronary disease. Do not use for extended periods.
Not to be used for:
Not to be used with: MAOIs.
Contains: oxymetazoline hydrochloride.
Other preparations: Afrazine Paediatric.

Neophryn
(Winthrop)

A spray or nasal drops used as a sympathomimetic treatment for blocked nose.

Dose: adults 2-3 drops or 2 sprays in each nostril every 3-4 hours; children over 7 years 1-2 drops into each nostril every 3-4 hours.
Side effects:
Caution: in patients suffering from cardiovascular disease or overactive thyroid. Do not use for longer than 7 days.
Not to be used for: children under 7 years
Not to be used with: MAOIs.
Contains: phenylephrine hydrochloride.
Other preparations:

Otrivine-Antistin
(Ciba)

A spray or drops used as a sympathomimetic, antihistamine treatment for hay fever, allergic rhinitis.

Dose: 2-3 drops or 1 spray into each nostril 2-3 times a day.
Side effects: itching nose, headache, sleeplessness, rapid heart rate.
Caution: Do not use for extended periods.
Not to be used for: children.
Not to be used with: MAOIs.
Contains: xylometazoline hydrochloride, antazoline sulphate.
Other preparations:

Respiratory conditions

3 Bronchodilators

Bronchodilators containing theophylline or aminophylline open up respiratory muscles controlling the size of the bronchi in the chest. They may thus improve breathing in asthma and related conditions. There is a number of these preparations available over the counter and they are listed below.

In addition, Rynacrom Spray is used where there is an allergic component and Visclair helps to clear mucus from the system.

Overdose of aminophylline-type drugs causes palpitations and tremor, and their use should be monitored.

Biophylline
(Delandale)

A syrup used as a bronchodilator to treat bronchial spasm.

Dose: adults 1-2 5 ml teaspoonsful every 6-8 hours; children 2-6 years ½ 5 ml teaspoonsful every 6-8 hours, 6-12 years ½-1 5 ml teaspoonful every 6-8 hours.
Side effects: rapid heart rate, stomach upset, headache, sleeplessness, nausea, abnormal rhythms.
Caution: in the elderly, pregnant women, nursing mothers, and in patients suffering from heart or liver disease or peptic ulcer.
Not to be used for:
Not to be used with: cimetidine, erythromycin, ciprofloxacin, interferon.
Contains: theophylline hydrate.
Other preparations:

Brovon
(Torbet)

A solution used as a bronchodilator to treat bronchial spasm brought on by chronic bronchitis, bronchial asthma, emphysema.

Dose: inhale 1-2 times a day and once at night.
Side effects: nervousness, tremor, dry mouth, abnormal heart rhythms.
Caution: in patients suffering from diabetes.
Not to be used for: children or for patients suffering from heart disease, high blood pressure, overactive thyroid gland.
Not to be used with: sympathomimetics.
Contains: adrenaline, atropine methonitrate, papaverine hydrochloride.
Other preparations:

Cam
(Rybar)

A syrup used as a bronchodilator to treat bronchial spasm.

Dose: adults 4 5 ml teaspoonsful 3-4 times a day; children under 2 years ½ 5 ml teaspoonsful 3-4 times a day, 2-4 years 1 5 ml teaspoonful 3-4 times a day, over 4 years 2 5 ml teaspoonsful 3-4 times a day.
Side effects: nervousness, sleeplessness, restlessness, dry mouth, cold hands and feet, abnormal heart rhythms.
Caution: in patients suffering from diabetes.
Not to be used for: patients suffering from heart disease, high blood pressure, overactive thyroid gland.
Not to be used with: MAOIs.
Contains: ephedrine hydrochloride, butethamate citrate.
Other preparations:

Choledyl
(Parke-Davis)

A pink tablet or a yellow tablet according to strengths of 100 mg, 200 mg and used as a bronchodilator to treat bronchial spasm brought on by chronic bronchitis or asthma.

Dose: adults 100-400 mg 4 times a day; children 3-6 years use syrup, 6-12 years 100 mg 3-4 times a day.
Side effects: rapid heart rate, stomach upset, sleeplessness, nausea, change in heart rhythms.
Caution: in pregnant women, nursing mothers, and in patients suffering from heart or liver disease or peptic ulcer. Diabetics should avoid syrup.
Not to be used for: children under 3 years.
Not to be used with: cimetidine, erythromycin, ciprofloxacin, interferon.
Contains: choline theophyllinate.
Other preparations: Choledyl Syrup.

Rynacrom Spray
(Fisons)

A spray used as an anti-allergy treatment for allergic rhinitis.

Dose: 1 spray into each nostril 4-6 times a day.
Side effects: temporary itching nose, rarely bronchial spasm.
Caution:
Not to be used for:
Not to be used with:
Contains: sodium cromoglycate.
Other preparations: Rynacrom Nasal Drops, Rynacrom Cartridges, Rynacrom Compound.

Theodrox
(3M Riker)

A white tablet used as a bronchodilator to treat bronchial spasm brought on by asthma, chronic bronchitis.

Dose: 1 tablet 4 times a day including 1 tablet at night.
Side effects: rapid heart rate, stomach upset, headache, sleeplessness, abnormal heart rhythms.
Caution: in the elderly, pregnant women, nursing mothers, and in patients suffering from heart or liver disease or peptic ulcer.
Not to be used for: children.
Not to be used with: cimetidine, erythromycin, ciprofloxacin, interferon.
Contains: aminophylline, aluminium hydroxide gel.
Other preparations:

Visclair
(Sinclair)

A yellow tablet supplied at a strength of 100 mg and used as a mucus softener to treat bronchitis, phlegm.

Dose: adults 2 tablets 3-4 times a day for 6 weeks then 2 tablets twice a day; children over 5 years 1 tablet 3 times a day.
Side effects: stomach upset.
Caution:
Not to be used for: children under 5 years.
Not to be used with:
Contains: methylcysteine hydrochloride.
Other preparations:

Rheumatic conditions

Sprains, strains, sports injuries, and other rheumatic conditions, such as frozen shoulder, fibrositis, and lumbago, respond to simple pain killers or analgesics (*see* **Simple pain killers** below) or the application of a local preparation. Algipan and Algispray, Radicin B and Transvasin are similar to those listed below. The effect of these preparations is to relax muscle spasm and to have a local anaesthetic effect. Nurofen (*see* below) is a good general anti-inflammatory which is also available as a cream (Proflex). Crampex contains calcium gluconate, nicotinic acid, and ergocalciferol, and is used for persistent leg cramps.

Hot, swollen joints may indicate arthritis which should be investigated full by a medical practitioner.

Algesal
(Duphar)

A cream used as an analgesic rub to treat rheumatic conditions.

Dose: massage into the affected area 3 times a day.
Side effects:
Caution:
Not to be used for: children under 6 years.
Not to be used with:
Contains: diethylamine salicylate.
Other preparations:

Aradolene
(Fisons)

A cream used as an analgesic rub to treat rheumatic conditions.

Dose: massage into the affected area 2-3 times a day.
Side effects: may be irritant
Caution:
Not to be used for: areas such as near the eyes, on broken or inflamed skin, or on membranes (such as the mouth).
Not to be used with:
Contains: diethylamine salicylate, capsicum oleoresin, camphor oil, menthol.
Other preparations:

Aspellin
(Fisons)

A liniment or a spray used as a topical analgesic to treat muscular rheumatism, sciatica, lumbago, fibrositis, chilblains.

Dose: massage gently into the affected area every 3-4 hours.
Side effects: may be irritant.

Caution:
Not to be used for: areas near the eyes, or where the skin is broken or inflamed, or on membranes (such as the mouth).
Not to be used with:
Contains: aspirin, menthol, camphor, methyl salicylate.
Other preparations:

Balmosa
(Pharmax)

A cream used as an analgesic rub to treat muscular rheumatism, fibrositis, lumbago, sciatica, unbroken chilblains.

Dose: massage into the affected area as needed.
Side effects: may be irritant
Caution:
Not to be used for: areas near the eyes, on broken or inflamed skin, or on membranes (such as the mouth).
Not to be used with:
Contains: menthol, camphor, methyl salicylate, capsicum oleoresin.
Other preparations:

Bayolin
(Bayer)

A cream used as an analgesic rub to treat rheumatism, fibrositis, lumbago, sciatica.

Dose: massage gently into the affected area 2-3 times a day.
Side effects: may be irritant.
Caution:
Not to be used for: areas near the eyes, broken or inflamed skin, or on membranes (such as the mouth).
Not to be used with:
Contains: heparinoid, glycol salicylate, benzyl nicotinate.
Other preparations:

Cremalgin
(Rorer)

A balm used as an analgesic rub to treat rheumatism, fibrositis, lumbago, sciatica.

Dose: massage into the affected area 2-3 times a day.
Side effects: may be irritant.
Caution:
Not to be used for: areas near the eyes, broken or inflamed skin, or on membranes (such as the mouth).
Not to be used with:
Contains: methyl nicotinate, glycol salicylate, capsicum oleoresin.
Other preparations:

Difflam
(3M Riker)

A cream used as an anti-inflammatory and analgesic rub to relieve muscular and skeletal pain.

Dose: massage gently into the affected area 3-6 times a day.
Side effects: may be irritant.
Caution:
Not to be used for: areas near the eyes, broken or inflamed skin, or on membranes (such as the mouth).
Not to be used with:
Contains: benzydamine hydrochloride.
Other preparations:

Dubam
(Norma)

An aerosol used as a topical analgesic to relieve muscular pain.

Dose: spray on to the affected area for 2 seconds up to 4 times a day.
Side effects: may be irritant.
Caution:
Not to be used for: areas near the eyes, broken or inflamed skin, or on membranes (such as the mouth).
Not to be used with:
Contains: glycol salicylate, methyl salicylate, ethyl salicylate, methyl nicotinate.
Other preparations:

Finalgon
(Boehringer Ingelheim)

An ointment supplied with an applicator and used as an analgesic rub to relieve muscular and skeletal pain.

Dose: massage gently into the affected area as needed.
Side effects: may be irritant.
Caution:
Not to be used for: areas near the eyes, broken or inflamed skin, or on membranes (such as the mouth).
Not to be used with:
Contains: nonivamide, butoxyethyl nicotinate.
Other preparations:

Intralgin
(3M Riker)

A gel used as an analgesic rub to treat muscle strains, sprains.

Dose: massage gently into the affected area as needed.
Side effects: may be irritant.
Caution:
Not to be used for: areas near the eyes, broken or inflamed skin, or on membranes (such as the mouth).

Contains: salicylamide, benzocaine.
Other preparations:

Salonair
(Salonpas)

An aerosol used as an analgesic rub to relieve muscular and rheumatic pain.

Dose: spray on to the affected area 1-2 times a day.
Side effects: may be irritant.
Caution:
Not to be used for: areas near the eyes, broken or inflamed skin, or on membranes (such as the mouth).
Not to be used with:
Contains: glycol salicylate, menthol, camphor, squalane, benzyl nicotinate.
Other preparations:

Transvasin
(Lloyds)

A cream used as an analgesic rub for the relief of rheumatic and muscular pain.

Dose: massage into the affected area at least twice a day.
Side effects:
Caution:
Not to be used for:
Not to be used with:
Contains: thurfyl salicylate, ethyl nicotinate, n-hexyl nicotinate, benzocaine.
Other preparations:

Simple pain killers

Drugs, such as aspirin, paracetamol, or codeine, form the basis of this section of over-the-counter preparations. Other items listed include Nurofen (ibuprofen) and migraine treatments. Many analgesics are combined with caffeine.

Analgesics should be taken only for short treatment courses for conditions such as headache, backache, period pain, and simple rheumatic conditions. They are also useful for the treatment of fevers. Total daily dose should be monitored carefully, and manufacturers' recommendations should be followed. Aspirin should be avoided in children and by those suffering from stomach conditions; paracetamol should not be used by anyone with liver problems.

aspirin

A white tablet supplied at a strength of 300 mg and used as an analgesic to relieve pain and reduce fever.

Dose: 1-3 tablets every 4-6 hours as needed to a maximum of 12 tablets a day.
Side effects: stomach upsets, allergy, asthma.
Caution: in pregnant women, the elderly, or in patients with a history of allergy to aspirin, asthma, impaired kidney or liver function, indigestion.
Not to be used for: children, nursing mothers, or for patients suffering from haemophilia or ulcers.
Not to be used with: anticoagulants (blood-thinning drugs), some antidiabetic drugs, anti-inflammatory agents, methotrexate, spironolactone, steroids, some antacids, some uric-acid lowering drugs.
Contains:
Other preparations: dispersible aspirin.

Cafadol
(Typharm)

A yellow, scored tablet used as an analgesic to relieve pain including period pain.

Dose: adults 2 tablets every 3-4 hours; children 5-12 years half adult dose.
Side effects:
Caution: in patients with liver or kidney disease.
Not to be used for: children under 5 years.
Not to be used with:
Contains: paracetamol, caffeine.
Other preparations:

Caprin
(Sinclair)

A pink tablet supplied at a strength of 324 mg and used as an analgesic to treat rheumatic and associated conditions.

Dose: 3 tablets 3-4 times a day.
Side effects: stomach upsets, allergy, asthma.
Caution: in pregnant women, the elderly, and in patients with a history of allergy to aspirin, asthma, impaired kidney or liver function, indigestion.
Not to be used for: children, nursing mothers, or for patients suffering from haemophilia or ulcers.
Not to be used with: anticoagulants (blood-thinning drugs), some antidiabetic drugs, anti-inflammatory agents, methotrexate, spironolactone, steroids, some antacids, some uric-acid lowering drugs.
Contains: aspirin.
Other preparations:

Co-Codamol

A tablet used as an analgesic to relieve pain.

Dose: adults 1-2 tablets every 4-6 hours to a maximum of 8 tablets a day; children 7-12 years ½-1 tablet every 4-6 hours to a maximum of 4 tablets a day.
Side effects:
Caution: in patients suffering from kidney or liver disease.
Not to be used for: children under 7 years.
Not to be used with:
Contains: codeine phosphate, paracetamol.
Other preparations:

Co-Codaprin Dispersible

A dispersible tablet used as an analgesic to relieve pain.

Dose: 1-2 tablets in water every 4-6 hours as needed.
Side effects: stomach upsets, allergy, asthma.
Caution: in pregnant women, the elderly, and in patients with a history of allergy to aspirin, asthma, impaired kidney or liver function, indigestion.
Not to be used for: children, nursing mothers, or for patients suffering from haemophilia or ulcers.
Not to be used with: anticoagulants (blood-thinning drugs), some antidiabetic drugs, anti-inflammatory agents, methotrexate, spironolactone, steroids, some antacids, some uric-acid lowering drugs.
Contains: aspirin, codeine phosphate.
Other preparations: Co-Codaprin.

Disprol Paed
(Reckitt & Colman)

A suspensions supplied at a strength of 120 mg/5 ml teaspoonful and used as an analgesic to relieve pain and fever in children.

Dose: 3 months-1 year ½ 5 ml teaspoonful 4 times a day if needed, 1-6 years 1-2 teaspoonsful 4 times a day if needed, 6-12 years 2-4 teaspoonsful 4 times a day if needed.
Side effects:
Caution: in children suffering from liver or kidney disease.
Not to be used for:
Not to be used with:
Contains: paracetamol.
Other preparations:

Femerital
(MCP)

A white, scored tablet used as an antispasmodic and analgesic for the relief of period pain.

Dose: 1-2 tablets 2-3 times a day beginning 2 days before the start of the period.
Side effects:
Caution: in patients suffering from liver or kidney disease.
Not to be used for: children.
Not to be used with:
Contains: ambucetamide, paracetamol.
Other preparations:

Midrid
(Sinclair)

A red capsule used as an analgesic to treat migraine.

Dose: 2 capsules at the beginning of the migraine attack, then 1 capsule every hour to a maximum of 5 capsules in 12 hours.
Side effects: dizziness.
Caution: in pregnant women and nursing mothers.
Not to be used for: children, or for patients suffering from severe kidney, liver, or heart disease, gastritis, severe high blood pressure, or glaucoma.
Not to be used with: MAOIs.
Contains: isometheptene mucate, paracetamol.
Other preparations:

Migraleve
(International)

A pink tablet and a yellow tablet according to strength and contents and used as an analgesic, antihistamine treatment for migraine.

Dose: adults and children over 10 years 2 pink tablets at the beginning of the attack and then 2 yellow tablets every 4 hours if needed to a maximum of 2 pink tablets and 6 yellow tablets in 24 hours.

Side effects: drowsiness.
Caution: in patients suffering from liver or kidney disease.
Not to be used for: children under 10 years.
Not to be used with: .
Contains: pink: buclizine hydrochloride, paracetamol, codeine phosphate; yellow: paracetamol, codeine phosphate.
Other preparations:

Nurofen
(Boots)

A magenta-coloured, oval tablet supplied at strengths of 200 mg, 400 mg, 600 mg, and used as a non-steroid anti-inflammatory drug to treat pain, rheumatoid arthritis, ankylosing spondylitis, osteoarthritis, seronegative arthritis, peri-articular disorders, soft tissue injuries.

Dose: adults 1200-1800 mg a day in divided doses, to a maximum of 2400 mg a day; children 20 mg per kg body weight a day.
Side effects: dyspepsia, stomach bleeding, rash, rarely low blood platelet levels.
Caution: in pregnant women, and in patients suffering from asthma or allergy to aspirin or anti-inflammatory drugs.
Not to be used for: patients suffering from peptic ulcer.
Not to be used with:
Contains: ibuprofen.
Other preparations: Apsifen (APS), Brufen (Boots), Ebufac (DDSA), Lidifen (Berk), Motrin (Upjohn), Paxofen (Steinhard).

Palaprin Forte
(Nicholas)

An orange, oval, scored tablet supplied at a strength of 600 mg and used as a non-steroid anti-inflammatory drug to treat rheumatoid arthritis, osteoarthritis, spondylitis.

Dose: 1 tablet per 6.5 kg body weight a day in divided doses dispersed in water, sucked, chewed, or swallowed.
Side effects: stomach upsets, allergy, asthma.
Caution: in pregnant women, the elderly, and in patients with a history of allergy to aspirin, asthma, impaired kidney or liver function, indigestion.
Not to be used for: children, nursing mothers, or for patients suffering from haemophilia or ulcers.
Not to be used with: anticoagulants (blood-thinning drugs), some antidiabetic drugs, anti-inflammatory agents, methotrexate, spironolactone, steroids, some antacids, some uric-acid lowering drugs.
Contains: aloxiprin.
Other preparations:

---

paracetamol tablets

A tablet supplied at a strength of 500 mg and used as an analgesic to relieve pain and reduce fever.

Dose: adults 1-2 tablets 4 times a day; children 6-12 years ½-1 tablet 4 times a day.
Side effects:
Caution: in patients suffering from kidney or liver disease.
Not to be used for: children under 6 years.
Not to be used with:
Contains:
Other preparations: paracetamol soluble, paracetamol elixir, Panadol (Winthrop), Panasorb (Winthrop).

Paracodol
(Fisons)

A white, effervescent tablet used as an analgesic to relieve pain.

Dose: adults 1-2 tablets in water every 4-6 hours to a maximum of 8 tablets in 24 hours; children 6-12 years ½-1 tablet to a maximum of 4 doses in 24 hours.
Side effects:
Caution: in patients suffering from kidney or liver disease, or who are on a limited consumption of salt.
Not to be used for: children under 6 years.
Not to be used with:
Contains: paracetamol, codeine phosphate.
Other preparations:

Parahypon
(Calmic)

A pink, scored tablet used as an analgesic to relieve pain.

Dose: adults 1-2 tablets 4 times a day; children 6-12 years half adult dose.
Side effects:
Caution: in patients suffering from kidney or liver disease.
Not to be used for: children under 6 years.
Not to be used with:
Contains: paracetamol, caffeine, codeine phosphate.
Other preparations:

Parake
(Galen)

A white tablet used as an analgesic to relieve pain and reduce fever.

Dose: 2 tablets every 4 hours to a maximum of 8 tablets in 24 hours.
Side effects:
Caution: in patients suffering from kidney or liver disease.
Not to be used for: children.

Not to be used with:
Contains: paracetamol, codeine phosphate.
Other preparations:

Pardale
(Martindale)

A white, scored tablet used as an analgesic to relieve headache, rheumatism, period pain.

Dose: 1-2 tablets 3-4 times a day.
Side effects:
Caution: in patients suffering from kidney or liver disease.
Not to be used for: children.
Not to be used with:
Contains: paracetamol, caffeine hydrate, codeine phosphate.
Other preparations:

Paynocil
(S K B)

A white, scored tablet used as an analgesic to relieve pain, reduce fever, and to treat rheumatoid arthritis and other rheumatic conditions.

Dose: 1 tablet dissolved on the tongue every 4-6 hours. For rheumatic conditions 2-3 tablets 3 times a day for 2-3 weeks reducing to 1-2 tablets 3 times a day.
Side effects: stomach upsets, allergy, asthma.
Caution: in pregnant women, the elderly, or in patients with a history of allergy to aspirin, asthma, impaired kidney or liver function, indigestion.
Not to be used for: children, nursing mothers, or for patients suffering from haemophilia or ulcers.
Not to be used with: anticoagulants (blood-thinning drugs), some antidiabetic drugs, anti-inflammatory agents,

methotrexate, spironolactone, steroids, some antacids, some uric-acid lowering drugs.
Contains: aspirin, glycine.
Other preparations:

Propain
(Panpharma)

A yellow, scored tablet used as an analgesic, antihistamine treatment for headache, migraine, muscle pain, period pain.

Dose: 1-2 tablets every 4 hours to a maximum of 10 tablets in 24 hours.
Side effects: drowsiness.
Caution: in patients suffering from liver or kidney disease.
Not to be used for: children.
Not to be used with: alcohol, sedatives.
Contains: codeine phosphate, diphenhydramine hydrochloride, paracetamol, caffeine.
Other preparations:

Salzone
(Wallace)

A syrup supplied at a strength of 120 mg/5 ml teaspoonful and used as an analgesic to relieve pain and reduce fever.

Dose: children ½-2 5 ml teaspoonsful every 4 hours according to age.
Side effects:
Caution: in children suffering from liver or kidney disease.
Not to be used for:
Not to be used with:
Contains: paracetamol.
Other preparations:

Solpadeine
(Sterling Research Laboratories)

A white, effervescent tablet used as an analgesic to relieve rheumatic, muscle, bone pain, headache, sinusitis, influenza.

Dose: adults 2 tablets in water 3-4 times a day; children 7-12 ½-1 tablet 3-4 times a day.
Side effects: constipation.
Caution: in patients suffering from liver or kidney disease, or who have a restricted salt consumption.
Not to be used for: children under 7 years.
Not to be used with:
Contains: paracetamol, codeine phosphate, caffeine.
Other preparations:

Solprin
(Reckitt & Colman)

A white, soluble tablet supplied at a strength of 300 mg used as an analgesic to relieve pain and to treat rheumatic conditions.

Dose: 1-3 tablets in water every 4 hours to a maximum of 12 tablets in 24 hours; higher doses for rheumatoid arthritis.
Side effects:
Caution:
Not to be used for: children.
Not to be used with:
Contains: aspirin.
Other preparations: Solprin 75 mg.

Syndol
(Merrell Dow)

A yellow, scored tablet used as an analgesic, antihistamine treatment for tension headache after dental or other surgery.

Dose: 1-2 tablets every 4-6 hours up to a maximum of 8 tablets in 24 hours.

Side effects: drowsiness, constipation.

Caution: in patients suffering from liver or kidney disease.

Not to be used for: children.

Not to be used with: alcohol, sedatives.

Contains: paracetamol, codeine phosphate, doxylamine succinate, caffeine.

Other preparations:

Tonics

(*See also* sections on Vitamins and Minerals as well as the section on Homoeopathic Medicines.)

Tonics are generally given to improve appetite. Those listed here contain a variety of minerals and other preparations which are claimed to improve the desire to eat and produce a feeling of well-being.

Eating disorders, such as anorexia nervosa or bulimia, require professional care.

Effico
(Pharmax)

Effico is a good general tonic which contains nicotinamide, thiamine, caffeine, and gentian. Caffeine excess can lead to palpitations — the preparation Proplus is concentrated caffeine which is a stimulant but may also cause insomnia and palpitations.

---

gentian mixture, acid

A tonic used to improve appetite.

Dose: 2-4 5 ml teaspoonsful ½ hour before a meal.
Side effects:
Caution:
Not to be used for: children.
Not to be used with:
Contains:
Other preparations: gentian mixture, alkaline.

Glykola
(Sinclair)

A liquid used as a tonic.

Dose: 1-2 5 ml teaspoonsful 3 times a day.
Side effects:
Caution: in patients with a history of peptic ulcer.
Not to be used for: children.
Not to be used with:
Contains: caffeine, calcium glycerophosphate, kola liquid extract, chloroform suspension, alcohol, ferrous perchloride liquid.
Other preparations:

Labiton
(LAB)

A liquid used as a tonic.

Dose: 2-4 5 ml teaspoonsful twice a day.
Side effects:
Caution:
Not to be used for: children, or for patients suffering from hepatitis or who are taking sedatives.
Not to be used with:
Contains: thiamine hydrochloride, p-aminobenzoic acid, kola nut dried extract, alcohol, caffeine.
Other preparations:

Metatone
(Warner-Lambert)

A liquid used as a source of vitamin B1 and minerals and used as a tonic.

Dose: adults 1-2 5 ml teaspoonsful twice a day.
Side effects:
Caution:
Not to be used for: children under 6 years.
Not to be used with:
Contains: thiamine hydrochloride, calcium glycerophosphate, manganese, potassium, sodium.
Other preparations:

Vitamin preparations

Many vitamin preparations are available over the counter. Some are combined with minerals (*see* next section), and many appear as homoeopathic remedies (*see* **Homoeopathic remedies**). True deficiency states of vitamins are rare but are seen occasionally nowadays, particularly B_{12} deficiency in vegetarians and those with pernicious anaemia, scurvy in elderly people who also do not eat enough fruit, and variations of rickets (vitamin D deficiency) are still seen. B_6 deficiency is said to occur in the premenstrual syndrome.

It is uncertain whether healthy people benefit from vitamin supplements. Controversially, some claim that children do better academically when taking vitamin supplements. Pregnant women routinely take folic acid and iron. Overdoses of vitamins can occur (*see* table).

THE MAIN TOXIC EFFECTS OF AN OVERDOSEAGE OF VITAMINS

Deficiency States	Vitamin	Administration	Toxic Dose (mass/units per day)	Signs and Symptoms of Toxicity
Night Blindness	A	acute	over 30 mg over 100 000 units	anorexia, vomiting, hyperirritability, raised intercranial pressure, peeling skin
		chronic	over 6 mg over 20 000 units	erythema, eczema, pruritus, bleeding lips, alopecia, tiredness, anorexia, nausea, muscle soreness, bone pain, raised intercranial pressure, liver damage, effects leading to foetal abnormalities
		injection	over 30 mg over 100 000 units	local pain, erythema, itching, skin discoloration
Rickets	D		over 0.125 mg over 50 000 units	muscle weakness, nausea, vomiting, constipation, polyuria, pruritus, hypercalcaemia, kidney and bladder stones
Bleeding	K	oral		itching, haemolytic anaemia, liver disease
		injection		neonatal jaundice and and kernicterus in new born; tender plaques in adults
	E	oral		fatigue, muscle weakness and myopathy, thrombophlebitis, thromboembolism, raised blood pressure
		injection		death (in infants)
	B_3, nicotinic acid		over 300 mg	anorexia, pruritus, glucose intolerance, hyperuricaemia, tachycardia, abnormal heart rhythms, liver failure
	B_6, pyridoxine		over 100 mg	clumsiness, ataxia, numbness around the mouth, sensory neuropathy (permanent)
Scurvy	C (ascorbic acid)		over 1 g	kidney stones, dependency, and withdrawal scurvy
Beri-Beri Anaemia	B_1, B_2, B_{12} folic acid			toxicity very low when taken by mouth; isolated (anecdotal) cases only

Abidec
(Warner-Lambert)

Drops used as a multivitamin preparation to treat vitamin deficiencies.

Dose: adults and children over 1 year 0.6 ml a day; infants under 1 year half adult dose.
Side effects:
Caution:
Not to be used for:
Not to be used with: levodopa.
Contains: calciferol, thiamine hydrochloride, riboflavine, pyridoxine hydrochloride, nicotinamide, ascorbic acid.
Other preparations: Abidec Capsules (not available on NHS).

Allbee with C
(Robins)

A green/yellow capsule used as a multivitamin treatment for vitamin B and vitamin C deficiencies.

Dose: adults 1-3 capsules a day; children 1 capsule a day.
Side effects:
Caution:
Not to be used for:
Not to be used with: levodopa.
Contains: thiamine mononitrate, riboflavine, pyridoxine hydrochloride, nicotinamide, calcium pantothenate, ascorbic acid.
Other preparations:

AT 10
(Sterling Research Laboratories)

A solution used as a source of vitamin D to treat vitamin D deficiency.

Dose: 1-7 ml taken by mouth each week.
Side effects: loss of appetite, listlessness, vertigo, stupor, nausea, urgent need to urinate.
Caution: in nursing mothers. Your doctor may advise that your calcium levels should be checked regularly.
Not to be used for: children.
Not to be used with:
Contains: dihydrotachysterol.
Other preparations:

BC 500
(Wyeth)

An orange, oblong tablet used as a multivitamin preparation to treat vitamin B and vitamin C deficiencies, and to aid recovery from illness, long-term alcoholism, long-term antibiotic treatment.

Dose: 1 tablet a day.
Side effects:
Caution:
Not to be used for: children.
Not to be used with: levodopa.
Contains: thiamine mononitrate, riboflavine, pyridoxine hydrochloride, nicotinamide, calcium pantothenate, ascorbic acid, cyanocoblamin.
Other preparations:

BC 500 with Iron
(Wyeth)

A red tablet used as a vitamin and iron supplement to treat iron deficiency anaemia.

Dose: 1 tablet a day.
Side effects: nausea, constipation.
Caution:

Not to be used for: children.
Not to be used with: tetracyclines, levodopa.
Contains: ferrous fumarate, thiamine mononitrate, riboflavine, pyridoxine hydrochloride, nicotinamide, calcium pantothenate, ascorbic acid.
Other preparations:

Becosym
(Roche)

A brown tablet used as a source of B vitamins to treat vitamin B deficiencies.

Dose: adults 1-3 tablets a day; children use syrup.
Side effects:
Caution:
Not to be used for:
Not to be used with: levodopa.
Contains: thiamine, riboflavine, pyridoxine, nicotinamide.
Other preparations: Becosym Syrup (not available on NHS), Becosym Forte Tablets (not available on NHS).

Benerva
(Roche)

A white tablet supplied in strengths of 25 mg, 50 mg, 100 mg and used as a source of vitamin B_1 to treat beri-beri, neuritis.

Dose: 25-50 mg a day.
Side effects:
Caution:
Not to be used for:
Not to be used with: levodopa.
Contains: thiamine hydrochloride.
Other preparations: Benerva Compound.

Ce-Cobalin
(Paines & Byrne)

A syrup used as a multivitamin preparation to treat anorexia, recovery from long-term illness.

Dose: adults 1-2 5 ml teaspoonsful 3 times a day; children 1 teaspoonful 3 times a day.
Side effects:
Caution:
Not to be used for:
Not to be used with:
Contains: cyanocoblamin.
Other preparations:

Comploment Continus
(Napp)

A yellow tablet supplied at a strength of 100 mg and used as a source of vitamin B_6 to treat vitamin B_6 deficiency including that developed by the contraceptive pill.

Dose: 1 tablet a day.
Side effects:
Caution:
Not to be used for: children.
Not to be used with: levodopa.
Contains: pyridoxine hydrochloride.
Other preparations:

Concavit
(Wallace)

A capsule used as a multivitamin treatment for vitamin deficiencies.

Dose: 1 capsule a day.
Side effects:
Caution:
Not to be used for:
Not to be used with: levodopa.
Contains: vitamin A, thiamine, riboflavine, pyridoxine, calciferol, vitamin E, nicotinamide, calcium pantothenate, ascorbic acid, cyanocoblamin.
Other preparations: Concavit Drops, Concavit Syrup.

Cytacon
(Duncan, Flockhart)

A white tablet supplied at a strength of 50 micrograms and used as a source of vitamin B_{12} to treat undernourishment, vitamin deficiencies, some types of anaemia, vitamin B_{12} deficiency after stomach surgery.

Dose: adults 1-3 tablet a day up to a maximum of 6 tablets a day for pernicious anaemia; children use liquid.
Side effects: rarely allergy
Caution:
Not to be used for:
Not to be used with: para-aminosalicylic acid, methyldopa, colchicine, cholestyramine, neomycin, biguanides, potassium chloride, cimetidine.
Contains: cyanocoblamin.
Other preparations: Cytacon Liquid.

Dalivit Drops
(Paines & Byrne)

Drops used as a multivitamin preparation in the prevention and treatment of vitamin deficiency in children.

Dose: 0-1 year 7 drops a day, over 1 year 14 drops a day.

Side effects:
Caution:
Not to be used for:
Not to be used with: levodopa.
Contains: vitamin A, ergocalciferol, thiamine, riboflavine, pyridoxine, nicotinamide, ascorbic acid
Other preparations:

Ephynal
(Roche)

A white tablet or a white, scored tablet according to strengths of 10 mg, 50 mg, 200 mg, and used as a source of vitamin E to treat vitamin E deficiency, tropical vitamin E deficiency.

Dose: adults 10-15 mg a day; children 1-10 mg per kg body weight a day.
Side effects:
Caution:
Not to be used for:
Not to be used with:
Contains: tocopheryl acetate.
Other preparations:

Forceval
(Unigreg)

A brown/red capsule used as a source of multivitamins and minerals to treat vitamin and mineral deficiencies.

Dose: adults 1 capsule a day; children over 5 years use Forceval Junior.
Side effects:
Caution:
Not to be used for: children under 5 years.
Not to be used with: levodopa.

Contains: multivitamins and minerals.
Other preparations: Forceval Junior.

Gevral
(Lederle)

A brown capsule used as a source of multivitamins and minerals to treat vitamin and mineral deficiencies.

Dose: 1 capsule a day.
Side effects:
Caution:
Not to be used for:
Not to be used with: levodopa.
Contains: multivitamins and minerals.
Other preparations:

Givitol
(Galen)

A maroon/red capsule used as an iron, folic acid, and vitamin supplement to treat iron and folic acid deficiences in pregnancy where vitamin supplements are also needed.

Dose: 1 capsule a day before food.
Side effects: nausea, constipation.
Caution:
Not to be used for: children.
Not to be used with: tatracyclines, levodopa.
Contains: ferrous fumarate, ascorbic acid, riboflavine, pyridoxine hydrochloride, nicotinamide, folic acid.
Other preparations:

Halycitrol
(LAB)

An emulsion used as a multivitamin preparation to treat vitamin A and vitamin D deficiencies.

Dose: adults and children over 6 months 1 5 ml teaspoonful a day; infants under 6 months ½ teaspoonful a day.
Side effects: vitamin poisoning
Caution: in patients suffering from kidney disease, sarcoidosis (a chest disease that affects calcium levels).
Not to be used for:
Not to be used with:
Contains: vitamin A, vitamin D.
Other preparations:

Lipoflavonoid
(Lipomed)

A black/pink capsule used as a multivitamin treatment for vitamin B deficiency.

Dose: 3 capsules 3 times a day for 2-3 months reducing to 2 capsules 3 times a day.
Side effects:
Caution:
Not to be used for: children.
Not to be used with:
Contains: choline bitartrate, inositol, methionine, ascorbic acid, lemon bioflavonoid complex, thiamine, riboflavine, nicotinamide, pyridoxine, panthenol, hydroxocobalamin.
Other preparations:

Lipotriad
(Lipomed)

A clear/pink capsule used as a multivitamin treatment for vitamin B deficiency.

Dose: 3 capsules 3 times a day for 2-3 months reducing to 2 capsules 3 times a day.
Side effects:
Caution:
Not to be used for: children.
Not to be used with: levodopa.
Contains: choline bitartrate, inositol, di-methionine, thiamine, riboflavine, nicotinamide, pyridoxine, panthenol, hydroxocobalamin.
Other preparations: Lipotriad Liquid.

Multivite
(Duncan, Flockhart)

A brown pellet used as a multivitamin treatment for vitamin deficiencies.

Dose: adults 2 pellets a day; children 1 pellet a day.
Side effects:
Caution:
Not to be used for:
Not to be used with:
Contains: vitamin A, thiamine, calciferol, ascorbic acid.
Other preparations:

Octovit
(S K B)

A maroon, oblong tablet used as a multivitamin treatment for vitamin and mineral deficiencies.

Dose: 1 tablet a day.
Side effects:

Caution:
Not to be used for: children
Not to be used with: tetracyclines, levodopa.
Contains: vitamin A, thiamine, riboflavine, nicotinamide, pyridoxine, cyanocoblamin, ascorbic acid, cholecalciferol, tocopheryl acetate, calcium hydrogen phosphate, ferrous sulphate, magnesium hydroxide, zinc.
Other preparations:

Orovite
(Bencard)

A maroon tablet used as a source of multivitamins to aid recovery from feverish illness, infection or surgery, and to treat confusion in the elderly, mild alcoholic disorders, or for treatment after intravenous vitamin therapy.

Dose: adults 1 tablet 3 times a day; children use syrup.
Side effects:
Caution:
Not to be used for:
Not to be used with: levodopa.
Contains: thiamine, riboflavine, pyridoxine, nicotinamide, ascorbic acid.
Other preparations: Orovite Syrup.

Orovite 7
(Bencard)

Granules in a sachet used as a multivitamin treatment for vitamin deficiencies.

Dose: 1 sachet in water once a day.
Side effects:
Caution:
Not to be used for: children under 5 years.

Not to be used with: levodopa.
Contains: vitamin A palmitate, calciferol, thiamine, riboflavine, pyridoxine, nicotinamide, ascorbic acid.
Other preparations:

Polyvite
(Medo)

A red, oval capsule used as a multivitamin treatment for vitamin deficiencies.

Dose: 1-2 capsules a day.
Side effects:
Caution:
Not to be used for:
Not to be used with: levodopa.
Contains: vitamin A, calciferol, thiamine, riboflavine, pyridoxine, ascorbic acid, calcium pantothenate, nicotinamide.
Other preparations:

Redoxon
(Roche)

A white tablet supplied at strengths of 25 mg, 50 mg, 200 mg, and used as a vitamin C treatment for scurvy, and as an additional treatment for wounds and infections.

Dose: adults 500 mg-1 g 2-3 times a day; children under 4 years quarter adult dose, 4-12 years half adult dose, 12-14 years three-quarters adult dose.
Side effects: diarrhoea.
Caution:
Not to be used for:
Not to be used with:
Contains: ascorbic acid.
Other preparations: Redoxon Effervescent.

Surbex T
(Abbott)

An orange, oval tablet used as a multivitamin treatment for vitamin B and vitamin C deficiencies.

Dose: adults 1 or more tablets a day; children 6-12 years 1 tablet a day.
Side effects:
Caution:
Not to be used for: children under 6 years.
Not to be used with: levodopa.
Contains: thiamine, riboflavine, nicotinamide, pyridoxine, ascorbic acid.
Other preparations:

Tachyrol
(Duphar)

A white, scored tablet supplied at a strength of 0.2 mg and used as a source of vitamin D to treat rickets, osteomalacia, underactive parathyroid gland, kidney osteodystrophy (bone problems due to kidney disease).

Dose: adults 1 tablet a day at first, adjusted as needed; children as advised by a physician.
Side effects: raised blood or urine clacium levels.
Caution: in patients suffering from kidney disease. Blood calcium should be checked regularly.
Not to be used for:
Not to be used with: barbiturates, anticonvulsant drugs.
Contains: dihydrotachysterol.
Other preparations:

Tonivitan
(Medo)

A brown capsule used as a multivitamin treatment for vitamin deficiencies.

Dose: 1-3 capsules 3 times a day.
Side effects:
Caution:
Not to be used for:
Not to be used with:
Contains: vitamin A, thiamine, nicotinic acid, ascorbic acid, calciferol, dried yeast.
Other preparations:

Tonivitan A & D
(Medo)

A syrup used as a source of vitamins A and D and minerals, and used as a tonic.

Dose: adults and children over 10 years 2 5 ml teaspoonsful 3 times a day; infants under 1 year ½ teaspoonful 3 times a day, 1-10 years 1 teaspoonful 3 times a day.
Side effects:
Caution:
Not to be used for:
Not to be used with:
Contains: vitamin A, thiamine, calciferol, ferric ammonium citrate, calcium glycerophosphate, manganese glycerophosphate, copper sulphate.
Other preparations:

Tonivitan B
(Medo)

A syrup used as a source of vitamin B and minerals, and used as a tonic.

Dose: adults 1-2 5 ml teaspoonsful 3 times a day; children as advised by a physician.

Side effects:

Caution:

Not to be used for:

Not to be used with: levodopa.

Contains: thiamine hydrochloride, riboflavine, pyridoxine hydrochloride, nicotinamide, calcium glycerophosphate, manganese glycerophosphate.

Other preparations:

Verdiviton
(Squibb)

A liquid used as a source of vitamin B complex for maintaining vitamin B complex levels.

Dose: 3 5 ml teaspoonsful 3 times a day before food.

Side effects:

Caution:

Not to be used for: children, or for patients suffering from hepatitis, alcoholism

Not to be used with: levodopa

Contains: glycerophosphates of calcium, sodium, potassium, manganese, cyanocobalamin, d-panthenol, nicotinamide, pyridoxine, riboflavine, thiamine, alcohol.

Other preparations:

Minerals

Minerals supplements are often combined with vitamins (*see* above) and also appear in the section on homoeopathic remedies (*see* below). Iron deficiency occurs in pregnant and nursing women, the elderly, and in vegetarians. Other minerals included in this section are potassium (which may be depleted with overuse of diuretic tablets), sodium depleted in hot weather), and calcium (depleted in the elderly and in some bone conditions). There are also preparations included here to treat elevated levels of potassium and calcium. There is some interest in zinc deficiency, and some zinc preparations are available over the counter.

Overdose can occur with these minerals and their use should be monitored.

Calcichew
(Shire)

A white, chewable tablet supplied at a strength of 500 mg and used as a calcium supplement to treat calcium deficiency.

Dose: 1 tablet chewed 3 times a day.
Side effects: constipation, wind.
Caution:
Not to be used for: children, or for patients suffering from overactive parathyroid glands, severe kidney disease, decalcifying tumours.
Not to be used with: tetracyclines.
Contains: calcium carbonate.
Other preparations:

Calcimax
(Wallace)

A brown syrup used as a calcium and vitamin supplement to treat calcium deficiency where vitamins are also needed.

Dose: adults 4 5 ml teaspoonsful 2-3 times a day; children 1-2 5 ml teaspoonsful 3 times a day.
Side effects:
Caution:
Not to be used for: children, or for patients suffering from overactive parathyroid glands, severe kidney disease, decalcifying tumours.
Not to be used with:
Contains: calcium glycine hydrochloride, calciferol, thiamine, riboflavine, pyridoxine, cyanocobalamin, calcium panthothenate.
Other preparations:

Calcisorb
(3M Riker)

A powder in a sachet of 4.7 g and used as an ion-exchange compound to treat raised calcium levels in the urine, recurring kidney stones, osteoporosis.

Dose: adults 1 sachet dispersed in water with meals or sprinkled on to food 3 times a day; children 2 sachets a day in 3 divided doses with food.
Side effects: diarrhoea.
Caution: treatment of children should be monitored, and the treatments should be accompanied by a low-calcium diet with foods rich in oxalates.
Not to be used for: pregnant women, nursing mothers, or for patients suffering from kidney disease, congestive heart disease, or any other conditions in which a low-sodium diet is needed.
Not to be used with:
Contains: sodium cellulose phosphate.
Other preparations:

Calcium Resonium
(Winthrop)

A powder used as an ion-exchange resin to treat raised potassium levels.

Dose: adults 15 g 3-4 times a day; children 1 g per kg body weight a day in divided doses.
Side effects: hyper calcaemia (raised calcium levels).
Caution: potassium and calcium levels should be checked.
Not to be used for: patients suffering from overactive parathyroid glands, multiple myeloma (a bone marrow tumour), sarcoidosis (a disease causing raised calcium levels), certain forms of cancer with kidney failure and hypercalcaemia.
Not to be used with:
Contains: calcium polystyrene sulphonate.
Other preparations:

Chocovite
(Shire)

A buff-coloured tablet used as a calcium and vitamin D$_2$ supplement to treat calcium deficiency.

Dose: 1-3 tablets sucked 3 times a day.
Side effects:
Caution:
Not to be used for:
Not to be used with:
Contains: calcium gluconate, calciferol.
Other preparations:

Citrical
(Shire)

Orange-flavoured granules supplied in sachets of 500 mg and used as a calcium supplement to treat calcium deficiency.

Dose: 1 sachet dissolved in water 3 times a day.
Side effects: constipation, wind.
Caution:
Not to be used for: children, or for patients suffering from overactive parathyroid glands, severe kidney disease, decalcifying tumours.
Not to be used with: tetracyclines.
Contains: calcium carbonate.
Other preparations:

Dioralyte
(Rorer)

Cherry- or pineapple-flavoured powder supplied as sachets and used as a fluid and electrolyte replacement to treat acute watery diarrhoea including gastro-enteritis.

Dose: 1-2 sachets in 200-400 ml water after each occasion of diarrhoea; infants substitute equivalent volume of reconstituted powder to feeds.
Side effects:
Caution:
Not to be used for:
Not to be used with:
Contains: sodium chloride, potassium chloride, sodium bicarbonate, glucose.
Other preparations: Dioralyte Effervescent, Electrolade (Nicholas); Gluco-Lyte (Cupal); Rehidrat (Searle).

Fefol Spansule
(S K & F)

A clear/green capsule used for the prevention of iron and folic acid deficiency in pregnancy.

Dose: 1 capsule a day.
Side effects: mild stomach upset.
Caution:
Not to be used for: children.
Not to be used with: tetracyclines.
Contains: ferrous sulphate, folic acid.
Other preparations:

Fefol Z Spansule
(S K & F)

A clear/blue capsule used for the prevention of iron and folic acid deficiency in pregnancy where zinc supplement is also needed.

Dose: 1 capsule a day.
Side effects: mild stomach upset.
Caution: in patients suffering from kidney disease

Not to be used for: children.
Not to be used with: tetracyclines.
Contains: ferrous sulphate, folic acid, zinc sulphate monohydrate.
Other preparations:

Fefol-Vit Spansule
(S K & F)

A clear/white capsule used for the prevention of iron, folic acid, and vitamin deficiency in pregnancy.

Dose: 1 capsule a day.
Side effects: mild stomach upset.
Caution:
Not to be used for: children.
Not to be used with: tetracyclines.
Contains: ferrous sulphate, folic acid, thiamine mononitrate, riboflavine, pyridoxine hydrochloride, nicotinamide, ascorbic acid.
Other preparations:

Feospan Spansule
(S K B)

A clear/red capsule supplied at a strength of 150 mg and used as an iron supplement to treat iron deficiency, anaemia.

Dose: adults 1-2 capsules a day; children 1-12 years 1 capsule a day.
Side effects: mild stomach upset.
Caution:
Not to be used for: infants under 1 year.
Not to be used with: tetracyclines.
Contains: ferrous sulphate.
Other preparations:

Fergon
(Winthrop)

A red tablet supplied at a strength of 300 mg and used as an iron supplement to treat iron deficiency, anaemia.

Dose: adults treatment 4-8 tablets a day in divided doses 1 hour before food, prevention 2 tablets a day; children 6-12 years 1-3 tablets a day.
Side effects: nausea, constipation.
Caution:
Not to be used for: children under 6 years.
Not to be used with: tetracyclines.
Contains: ferrous gluconate.
Other preparations:

Ferrocontin Continus
(Degussa)

A red tablet supplied at a strength of 100 mg and used as an iron supplement to treat iron deficiency, anaemia.

Dose: 1 tablet a day.
Side effects:
Caution:
Not to be used for: children.
Not to be used with: tetracyclines.
Contains: ferrous glycine sulphate.
Other preparations: Ferrocontin Folic Continus.

Ferrograd
(Abbott)

A red tablet supplied at a strength of 325 mg and used as an iron supplement to treat iron deficiency, anaemia.

Dose: 1 tablet a day before food.
Side effects:
Caution: in patients suffering from slow bowel actions.
Not to be used for: children, or for patients suffering from diverticular disease, blocked intestine.
Not to be used with: tetracyclines.
Contains: ferrous sulphate.
Other preparations:

Ferrograd C
(Abbott)

A red, oblong tablet used as an iron supplement to treat iron deficiency, anaemia where absorption is difficult.

Dose: 1 tablet a day before food.
Side effects:
Caution: in patients suffering from slow bowel action.
Not to be used for: children, or for patients suffering from diverticular disease, blocked intestine.
Not to be used with: tetracyclines, Clinistix urine test.
Contains: ferrous sulphate, ascorbic acid.
Other preparations:

Ferrograd Folic
(Abbott)

A red yellow/tablet used as an iron supplement to treat anaemia in pregnancy.

Dose: 1 tablet a day before food.
Side effects:
Caution: in patients suffering from slow bowel movments.
Not to be used for: children, or for patients suffering from diverticular disease, intestinal blockage, vitamin B_{12} deficiency.
Not to be used with: tetracyclines.

Contains: ferrous sulphate, folic acid.
Other preparations:

Ferromyn
(Calmic)

An elixir used as an iron supplement to treat iron deficiency anaemia.

Dose: adults and children over 10 years 1 5 ml teaspoonful 3 times a day; children up to 2 years 1 ml twice a day, 2-5 years ½ teaspoonful 3 times a day, 5-10 years 1 teaspoonful twice a day.
Side effects: stomach upset.
Caution:
Not to be used for:
Not to be used with: tetracyclines, antacids.
Contains: ferrous succinate.
Other preparations:

Fersaday
(Duncan, Flockhart)

A brown tablet supplied at a strength of 100 mg and used as an iron supplement to treat iron deficiency.

Dose: 1 tablet 1-2 times a day.
Side effects: stomach upset.
Caution: in patients with a history of peptic ulcer
Not to be used for: children.
Not to be used with: tetracyclines, antacids.
Contains: ferrous fumarate.
Other preparations:

Fersamal
(Duncan, Flockhart)

A brown tablet supplied at a strength of 65 mg and used as an iron supplement to treat iron deficiency, anaemia.

Dose: adults 1 tablet 3 times a day; children use Fersamal Syrup.
Side effects: stomach upset.
Caution: in patients with a history of peptic ulcer.
Not to be used for:
Not to be used with: tetracyclines, antacids.
Contains: ferrous fumarate.
Other preparations: Fersamal Syrup, Ferrocap (Consolidated).

Fesovit Spansule
(S K B)

A yellow/clear capsule used as an iron and vitamin supplement to treat iron deficiency anaemia needing vitamins B and C.

Dose: adults 1 capsule 1-2 times a day; children 1-12 years 1 capsule a day.
Side effects: mild stomach upset.
Caution:
Not to be used for: infants under 1 year.
Not to be used with: tetracyclines.
Contains: ferrous sulphate, ascorbic acid, thiamine mononitrate, riboflavine, pyridoxine hydrochloride, nicotinamide.
Other preparations:

Fesovit Z Spansule
(S K B)

An orange/clear capsule used as an iron, zinc, and vitamin supplement to treat iron deficiency anaemia where vitamins B and C and zinc are needed.

Dose: adults 1-2 capsules a day; children 1-12 years 1 capsule a day.
Side effects: mild stomach upset.
Caution: in patients suffering from kidney disease.
Not to be used for: infants under 1 year.
Not to be used with: tetracyclines.
Contains: ferrous sulphate, zinc sulphate monohydrate, ascorbic acid, thiamine mononitrate, riboflavine, pyridoxine hydrochloride, nicotinamide.
Other preparations:

Folex-350
(Rybar)

A pink tablet used as an iron supplement for the prevention of iron and folic acid deficiency in pregnancy.

Dose: 1 tablet a day.
Side effects: nausea, constipation.
Caution:
Not to be used for: children, or for patients suffering from megaloblastic anaemia.
Not to be used with: tetracyclines.
Contains: ferrous fumarate, folic acid.
Other preparations:

Fosfor
(Chancellor)

A syrup used as a food supplement.

Dose: adults 4 5 ml teaspoonsful 3 times a day; children half adult dose.
Side effects:

Caution:
Not to be used for:
Not to be used with:
Contains: phosphorylcolamine.
Other preparations:

Galfer
(Galen)

A green/red capsule supplied at a strength of 290 mg and used as an iron supplement to treat iron deficiency anaemia.

Dose: adults 1 capsule a day before food; children as advised by a physician.
Side effects: nausea, constipation.
Caution:
Not to be used for:
Not to be used with: tetracyclines.
Contains: ferrous fumarate.
Other preparations:

Galfervit
(Galen)

An orange/maroon capsule used as an iron and vitamin supplement to treat iron deficiency anaemia where a vitamin supplement is also needed.

Dose: adults 1 capsule 1-2 times a day; children as advised by a physician.
Side effects: nausea, constipation.
Caution:
Not to be used for:
Not to be used with: tetracyclines, levodopa.
Contains: ferrous fumarate, ascorbic acid, thiamine mononitrate, riboflavine, pyridoxine hydrochloride, nicotinamide.

Other preparations:

Irofol C
(Abbott)

A red, oblong tablet used as an iron, folic acid, and vitamin supplement for the prevention and treatment of iron and folic acid deficiency in pregnancy where vitamin supplement is also needed.

Dose: 1 tablet a day before food.
Side effects:
Caution: in patients suffering from slow bowel action.
Not to be used for: children or for patients suffering from megaloblastic anaemia, diverticular disease, intestinal blockage.
Not to be used with: tetracyclines, Clinistix urine test.
Contains: ferrous sulphate, folic acid, ascorbic acid.
Other preparations:

Kloref
(Cox)

A white effervescent tablet used as a potassium supplement to treat potassium deficiency.

Dose: adults 1-2 tablets in water 3 times a day; children as advised by a physician.
Side effects:
Caution: in patients suffering from kidney disease.
Not to be used for: patients suffering from increased chloride levels or other rare metabolic disorders.
Not to be used with:
Contains: betaine hydrochloride, potassium bezoate, potassium bicarbonate, potassium chloride.
Other preparations: Kloref-S.

Leo K
(Leo)

A white, oval tablet used as a potassium supplement to treat potassium deficiency.

Dose: adults 3-5 tablets a day in divided doses; children as advised by a physician.
Side effects: ulcers or blockage in the small bowel.
Caution: in patients suffering from kidney disease.
Not to be used for:
Not to be used with:
Contains: potassium chloride.
Other preparations:

Minamino
(Chancellor)

A syrup used as a source of amino acids, B vitamins, and minerals to treat vitamin and mineral deficiences.

Dose: adults 4 5 ml teaspoonsful 3 times a day; children half adult dose.
Side effects:
Caution:
Not to be used for:
Not to be used with: levodopa.
Contains: multivitamins and minerals.
Other preparations:

Niferex
(Tillotts)

An elixir used as an iron supplement to treat iron deficiency anaemia.

Dose: adults treatment s 5 ml teaspoonful 1-2 times a day, prevention ½ teaspoonful a day; children 0-2 years 1 drop per 0.45 kg body weight a day, 2-6 years ½ 5 ml teaspoonful a day, 6-12 years 1 teaspoonful a day.
Side effects:
Caution: in patients with a history of peptic ulcer.
Not to be used for:
Not to be used with: tetracyclines.
Contains: polysaccharide-iron complex.
Other preparations: Niferex Tablets, Niferex-150.

Nu-K
(Consolidated)

A blue capsule supplied at a strength of 600 mg and used as a potassium supplement to treat potassium deficiency.

Dose: 1-6 capsules a day in divided doses after food..
Side effects: ulcers or blockage in the small bowel.
Caution:
Not to be used for: children or for patients suffering from advanced kidney disease.
Not to be used with:
Contains: potassium chloride.
Other preparations:

Ossopan 800
(Sanofi)

A buff-coloured tablet supplied at a strength of 830 mg and used as a calcium-phosphorus supplement to treat osteoporosis, rickets, osteomalacia (bone disorders).

Dose: adults 4-8 tablets a day in divided doses before food; children as advised by a physician.
Side effects:

Caution: in patients suffering from kidney disease, severe loss of movement, or a history of kidney stones.
Not to be used for: patients suffering from raised blood or urine calcium.
Not to be used with:
Contains: hydroxyapatite compound.
Other preparations: Ossopan Powder.

Paedialyte RS
(Abbott)

A solution used to supply electrolytes in the treatment of dehydration.

Dose: adults dose as required; children equivalent amount to estimated fluid loss in divided doses given over 6-8 hours.
Side effects:
Caution: in patients suffering from dehydration.
Not to be used for: patients suffering from kidney disease with kidney failure, blocked intestine, bowel paralysis, severe vomiting, severe dehydration where intravenous fluid treatment is needed.
Not to be used with:
Contains: glucose, sodium chloride, sodium citrate, potassium citrate.
Other preparations:

Phosphate
(Sandoz)

A white, effervescent tablet used as a phosphate supplement to treat elevated calcium levels.

Dose: adults and children over 5 years up to 6 tablets a day; children under 5 years half adult dose.
Side effects: diarrhoea.

Caution: in patients suffering from kidney disease, congestive heart disease, high blood pressure.
Not to be used for: patients on a low sodium diet.
Not to be used with: antacids.
Contains: sodium acid phosphate, sodium bicarbonate, potassium bicarbonate.
Other preparations:

Plesmet
(Napp)

A syrup used as an iron supplement to treat iron-deficiency anaemia.

Dose: adults 1-2 5 ml teaspoonsful 3 times a day; children ½-1 teaspoonful 2-3 times a day.
Side effects:
Caution:
Not to be used for:
Not to be used with: tetracyclines.
Contains: ferrous glycine sulphate.
Other preparations:

Pregaday
(Duncan, Flockhart)

A brownish-red tablet used as an iron and folic acid supplement in the prevention of iron and folic acid deficiency in pregnancy.

Dose: 1 tablet a day.
Side effects: stomach upset, allergy.
Caution: in patients with a history of peptic ulcer or who are in the first three months of pregnancy..
Not to be used for: patients suffering from vitamin B_{12} deficiency.
Not to be used with: tetracyclines, antacids, anticonvulsant

drugs, co-trimoxazole.
Contains: ferrous fumarate, folic acid.
Other preparations:

Pregnavite Forte F
(Bencard)

A lilac-coloured tablet used as an iron, folic acid, and vitamin supplement to treat iron and vitamin deficiencies.

Dose: 1 tablet 3 times a day after meals starting at least 1 month before conception and continuing at least until the second missed period date.
Side effects: stomach upset.
Caution:
Not to be used for: children or for patients suffering from megaloblastic anaemia.
Not to be used with: tetracyclines, levodopa.
Contains: ferrous sulphate, folic acid, calciferol, thiamine hydrochloride, riboflavine, pyridoxine hydrochloride, nicotinamide, ascorbic acid, calcium phosphate.
Other preparations:

Rehidrat
(Searle)

A lemon and lime, and orange-flavoured powder used to provide electrolytes in fluid and electrolyte loss.

Dose: adults and children until thirst is quenched: infants substitute for feeds or after breast feeding.
Side effects:
Caution:
Not to be used for: patients suffering from kidney disease, blocked intestine, bowel paralysis.
Not to be used with:

Contains: sodium chloride, potassium chloride, sodium bicarbonate, citric acid, glucose, sucrose, laevulose.
Other preparations:

Resonium-A
(Winthrop)

A powder used for ion-exchange to lower potassium levels.

Dose: 15 g 3-4 times a day.
Side effects:
Caution: potassium and sodium levels should be checked regularly.
Not to be used for:
Not to be used with:
Contains: sodium polystyrene sulphonate.
Other preparations:

Sando-K
(Sandoz)

A white effervescent tablet used as a potassium supplement to treat potassium deficiency.

Dose: 2-4 tablets a day dissolved in water.
Side effects: stomach upset
Caution: in patients suffering from kidney disease.
Not to be used for: children.
Not to be used with:
Contains: potassium bicarbonate, potassium chloride.
Other preparations: Kloref-S.

Sandocal
(Sandoz)

An orange effervescent tablet used as a calcium supplement in additional treatment for osteoporosis, osteomalacia, rickets, pregnancy, lactation, undernourishment, and after gastric surgery when absorption is poor.

Dose: adults 3-4 tablets a day dissolved in water; children 1-2 tablets a day dissolved in water.
Side effects: diarrhoea, nausea, flushes.
Caution: in patients suffering from kidney disease, unbalanced electrolyte levels, congestive heart failure. Your doctor may advise that calcium levels should be checked regularly.
Not to be used for: patients suffering from raised calcium levels in the blood or urine, severe kidney failure, kidney stones, galactosaemia.
Not to be used with: thiazides, tetracyclines.
Contains: calcium lactate gluconate, sodium bicarbonate, potassium bicarbonate.
Other preparations: Calcium Sandoz Syrup, Calcium Sandoz Injection.

Selora
(Winthrop)

Fine white grabules used as a common salt substitute for patients on low-sodium diets.

Dose: normal salt use.
Side effects:
Caution:
Not to be used for: patients suffering from kidney disease.
Not to be used with:
Contains: potassium chloride.
Other preparations:

Slow Sodium
(Ciba)

A white tablet supplied at a strength of 600 mg and used as a salt supplement to treat salt deficiency.

Dose: adults 4-20 tablets times a day; children in proportion to dose for 70 kg adult.
Side effects:
Caution:
Not to be used for: patients suffering from fluid retention, heart disease, heart failure.
Not to be used with: diuretics, lithium.
Contains: sodium chloride.
Other preparations:

Slow-Fe
(Ciba)

An off-white tablet supplied at a strength of 160 mg and used as an iron supplement to treat iron-deficiency anaemia.

Dose: adults 1-2 tablets a day; children 6-12 years 1 tablet a day.
Side effects: nausea, constipation.
Caution:
Not to be used for: children under 6 years.
Not to be used with: tetracyclines.
Contains: ferrous sulphate.
Other preparations:

Slow-K
(Ciba)

An orange tablet supplied at a strength of 600 mg and used as a potassium supplement to treat potassium deficiency.

Dose: adults 2-6 tablets a day or every other day after food; children as advised by a physician.
Side effects: blocked or ulcerated small bowel.
Caution: in patients suffering from kidney disease or peptic ulcer.
Not to be used for: patients suffering from advanced kidney disease.
Not to be used with:
Contains: potassium chloride.
Other preparations:

Solvazinc
(Thames)

An off-white effervescent tablet supplied at a strength of 200 mg and used as a zinc supplement to treat zinc deficiency.

Dose: adults and children over 30 kg body weight 1 tablet dissolved in water 1-3 times a day after food; children under 10 kg body weight ½ tablet in water once a day after food, 10-30 kg half adult dose.
Side effects: stomach upset.
Caution: in patients suffering from kidney failure.
Not to be used for:
Not to be used with: tetracyclines.
Contains: zinc sulphate.
Other preparations:

Sytron
(Parke-Davis)

An elixir used as an iron supplement to treat iron-deficiency anaemia.

Dose: adults 1 5 ml teaspoonful 3 times a day at first increasing gradually to 2 teaspoonsful 3 times a day; children 0-1 year ½

teaspoonful twice a day, 1-5 years ½ teaspoonful 3 times a day, 6-12 years 1 teaspoonful 3 times a day.
Side effects: nausea, diarrhoea.
Caution:
Not to be used for:
Not to be used with: tetracyclines.
Contains: sodium iron edetate.
Other preparations:

Titralac
(3M Riker)

A white tablet used as a calcium supplement.

Dose: to be adjusted for individuals.
Side effects:
Caution:
Not to be used for:
Not to be used with:
Contains: calcium carbonate, glycine.
Other preparations: Kloref-S.

Z Span Spansule
(S K & F)

A blue/clear capsule used as a zinc supplement for the prevention and treatment of zinc deficiency.

Dose: adults and children over 1 year 1 capsule 1-3 times a day.
Side effects: stomach upset.
Caution: in patients suffering from kidney failure.
Not to be used for: infants under 1 year.
Not to be used with: tetracyclines.
Contains: zinc sulphate monohydrate.
Other preparations:

Food products

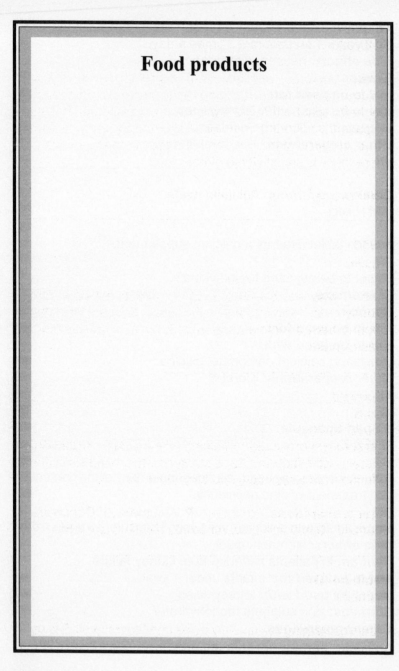

Aglutella
(Nutricia)

Gluten-, sucrose-, and lactose-free protein which is low in sodium and potassium. It is supplied as macaroni, pasta spirals, spaghetti, spaghetti rings, tagliatelle, and semolina. It is used for patients suffering from phenylketonuria, chronic kidney failure, cirrhosis of the liver, and diseases of the digestive tract where there is sensitivity to gluten.

Other preparations: Aglutella Azeta

Al 110
(Nestle)

Gluten-, and sucrose-free powder containing fat, protein, carbohydrate, vitamins, and minerals. It is used for patients suffering from an intolerance to lactose, and galactosaemia, galactokinase.

Albumaid
(S.H.S.)

Beef serum hydrolysate containing amino acids, carbohydrate, minerals, vitamins, and trace elements. It is used for patients suffering from tyrosinosis and tyrosinaemia.

Other preparations: Albumaid XP, Albumaid XP Concentrate, Albumaid Methionine Low, Albumaid RVHB Complete.

Alembicol D
(Alembic)

A liquid containing mainly fatty acids from coconut oil. It is used in diluted form for patients suffering from impaired ability to absorb fats.

Alfare
(Nestle)

A powder containing fat, protein, carbohydrate, vitamins, and minerals. It is used for patients suffering from an intolerance to protein.

Aminex
(Cow & Gate)

Sucrose- and lactose-free biscuit which is low in protein, sodium, phenylalanine, and potassium. It is used for patients suffering from phenylketonuria, chronic kidney failure, cirrhosis of the liver, and lactose with sucrose intolerance.

Aminogran
(UCB)

Phenylalanine-free powder supplying essential and non-essential amino acids. It is used for patients suffering from phenylketonuria.

Other preparations: Aminogran Mineral Mixture.

Analog
(S.H.S.)

Phenylalanine-free powder supplying proteins, fats, vitamins, minerals, and trace elements. It is used for infants suffering from phenylketonuria.

Other preparations: Analog MSUD; Analog RVHB; Analog

Aproten
(Ultrapharm)

Low-protein, gluten-free preparation supplied as anellini, ditalini, rigatoni, tagliatelle, biscuits, crispbread, flour, bread mix, and cake mix. It is used for patients suffering from phenylketonuria, kidney and liver failure, cirrhosis of the liver, and gastro-enteritic diseases where sensitivity to gluten is present.

Bi-Aglut
(Ultrapharm)

Gluten-free preparation supplied as a biscuit. It is used for patients suffering from gastro-enteritic diseases where sensitivity to gluten is present.

Other preparations: Bi-Aglut Cracker Toast.

Calogen
(S.H.S.)

A low-electrolyte emulsion of arachis oil in water. It is used for patients suffering from kidney failure and other conditions where a diet high in energy but low in fluid and electrolytes is needed.

Caloreen
(Roussel)

A low-electrolyte, protein-, gluten-, lactose-, sucrose-, galactose-, and fructose-free glucose polymer powder. It is used for patients suffering from chronic kidney failure, amino acid disorders, hypoglycaemia, and other conditions where a high-energy, low-fluid, and low-electrolyte diet is needed.

Carbel Instant
(Cow & Gate)

An instant carob bean gum preparation used for patients suffering from persistent vomiting and regurgitation of food.

Casilan
(Farley)

A powder used as a low-electrolyte, gluten-free protein for patients suffering from hypoproteinaemia.

Clinifeed Favour
(UCB)

A gluten- and lactose-free liquid feed used to supply protein, carbohydrate, vitamins, and minerals. It is used for patients suffering from short bowel syndrome, intractable malabsorption, inflammatory bowel disease, dysphagia, bowel fistulas, anorexia nervosa, cachexia, and for preparing undernourished patients prior to surgery or following complete gastrectomy.

Caution: unsuitable as the only source of nutrition for children under 5 years.
Not to be used for: infants under 1 year.
Other preparations: Clinifeed 400; Clinifeed Protein Rich; Clinifeed Iso.

Dialamine
(S.H.S.)

Low-electrolyte, gluten-, galactose-, and lactose-free, orange-flavoured powder used as a source of essential amino acids, carbohydrate, ascorbic acid, certain minerals and trace elements for patients suffering from kidney failure, hypoproteinaemia, wound fistula leakage where there is loss of protein, and those patients who are on a diet where the nitrogen intake must be controlled.

Duocal Super Soluble
(S.H.S.)

Low-electrolyte, gluten-, protein-, and lactose-free powder used as a source of carbohydrate and fat for patients suffering from kidney failure, cirrhosis of the liver, intolerance to disaccharides, amino acid metabolic disorders, intolerance to whole protein, poor absorption states, and other conditions where a high-energy, low-fluid diet is needed.

Elemental 028
(S.H.S.)

An orange or flavour-free powder used as a source of amino acids, carbohydrate, fat, electrolytes, vitamins, and minerals for patients suffering from short bowel syndrome, intractable poor absorption, inflammatory bowel disease, bowel fistulas.

Caution: unsuitable as the only source of nutrition for children under 5 years.
Not to be used for: infants under 1 year.

Ener-G
(General Designs)

Gluten-free preparation supplied as brown rice bread or tapioca bread used for patients suffering from disorders of the digestive system in which there is sensitivity to gluten, including herpetiformis, steatorrhoea, coeliac disease, dermatitis.

Enrich
(Abbott)

Gluten- and lactose-free, vanilla-flavoured liquid feed used as a source of protein, carbohydrate, dietary fibre, fat, vitamins, and minerals for patients suffering from short bowel syndrome, intractable poor absorption, dysphagia, bowel fistulas, cachexia, anorexia nervosa, or for undernourished patients before surgery or after complete gastrectomy.

Caution: unsuitable as the only source of nutrition for children under 5 years.
Not to be used for: infants under 1 year.

Ensure
(Abbott)

Low-electrolyte, gluten- and lactose-free, vanilla-flavoured liquid feed used as a source of protein, carbohydrate, fat, vitamins, and minerals for patients suffering from short bowel syndrome, intractable poor absorption, dysphagia, bowel fistulas, cachexia, anorexia nervosa, or for undernourished patients before surgery or after complete gastrectomy.

Caution: unsuitable as the only source of nutrition for children under 5 years.
Not to be used for: infants under 1 year.
Other preparations: Ensure Savoury; Ensure Plus.

Flexical
(Mead Johnson)

Gluten- and lactose-free powder used as a source of protein, carbohydrate, fat, vitamins, and minerals for patients suffering from short bowel syndrome, intractable poor absorption, bowel fistulas, cachexia, anorexia nervosa, or for undernourished patients before surgery or after complete gastrectomy.

Caution: unsuitable as the only source of nutrition for children under 5 years.
Not to be used for: infants under 1 year.

Forceval Protein
(Unigreg)

Low-sodium, low-fat, galactose-, gluten- and lactose-free, natural-, vanilla-, orange-, or strawberry-flavoured powder used as a source of protein, carbohydrate, fat, vitamins, and minerals for patients suffering from short bowel syndrome, intractable poor absorption, dysphagia, inflammatory bowel disease, bowel fistulas, or for undernourished patients before surgery or after complete gastrectomy, where a low salt intake is needed.

Caution: unsuitable as the only source of nutrition for children under 5 years.
Not to be used for: infants under 1 year.

Formula MCT (1)
(Cow & Gate)

Lactose-low powder used as a source of fatty acids, protein, carbohydrate, minerals, and electrolytes for patients suffering from liver failure, steatorrhoea with cystic fibrosis of the pancreas, intestinal lymphangiectasis, or in intestinal surgery.

Formula S
(Cow & Gate)

Gluten-, fructose-, sucrose- and lactose-free powder used as a source of protein, carbohydrate, fat, vitamins, and minerals for patients suffering from milk intolerance, lactose intolerance, galactosaemia, and low galactokinase.

Fortical
(Cow & Gate)

Low-electrolyte, gluten-, galactose-, sucrose-, lactose-, and protein-free liquid used as a source of high-energy carbohydrate for patients suffering from kidney failure, cirrhosis of the liver, or any conditions where a low-fluid, low-electrolyte, high-energy diet is needed.

Fortisip
(Cow & Gate)

Gluten-free and lactose-low, neutral-, banana-, orange-, tropical fruits-, mushroom-, or vanilla-flavoured liquid feed used as a source of protein, carbohydrate, vitamins, and minerals for patients suffering from short bowel syndrome, intractable poor absorption, dysphagia, bowel fistulas, cachexia, anorexia nervosa, inflammatory bowel disease, or for undernourished patients before surgery or after complete gastrectomy.

Caution: unsuitable as the only source of nutrition for children under 5 years.
Not to be used for: infants under 1 year.

Fortison
(Cow & Gate)

Lactose-low and gluten-free liquid feed used as a source of protein, carbohydrate, fat, vitamins, and minerals for patients suffering from short bowel syndrome, intractable poor absorption, dysphagia, bowel fistulas, cachexia, anorexia nervosa, inflammatory bowel disease, cystic fibrosis, or for undernourished patients before surgery or after complete gastrectomy.

Caution: unsuitable as the only source of nutrition for children under 5 years (except Fortison Paediatric).
Not to be used for: infants under 1 year.
Other preparations: Fortison Energy Plus; Fortison Fibre; Fortison Paediatric; Fortison Soya.

Fresubin
(Fresenius)

Low-electrolyte, low-lactose, gluten-free, vanilla-, peach-, nut-, mocha-, and chocolate-flavoured liquid feed used as a source of protein, carbohydrate, fat, vitamins, and minerals for patients suffering from short bowel syndrome, intractable poor absorption, dysphagia, bowel fistulas, cachexia, anorexia nervosa, or for undernourished patients before surgery or after complete gastrectomy.

Caution: unsuitable as the only source of nutrition for children under 5 years.
Not to be used for: infants under 1 year.
Other preparations: Fresubin Plus F.

Galactomin 17
(Cow & Gate)

Lactose-low, gluten-free powder used as a source of glucose, caseinates, vegetable oils, vitamins, minerals, and trace elements for patients suffering from galactosaemia and low galactokinase where there is also lactose intolerance.

Other preparations: Galactomin 19.

Generaid
(S.H.S.)

A powder used as source of protein, carbohydrate, and minerals for patients suffering from chronic liver disease, porto-hepatic encephalopathy.

Glutafin
(Nutricia)

Gluten-free preparation supplied as biscuits, macaroni, spaghetti, pasta spirals for patients with digestive conditions that are sensitive to gluten.

Glutenex
(Cow & Gate)

Gluten- and milk-free biscuit used as a source of protein and sucrose for patients with digestive conditions sensitive to gluten.

Hepatic Aid II
(Kendall)

Chocolate-, chocolate mint-, custard-, or egg nog-flavoured powder used as a source of amino acids, fat, oil, and lecithin for patients suffering from chronic liver disease where the diet must be controlled.

Caution: blood ammonia, BUN levels, serum electrolytes, glucose, and liver should be monitored regularly.

Not to be used for: children or for patients suffering from severe encephalopathy, coma caused by liver failure, phenylketonuria, or other malfunctions of amino acid metabolism.

Hycal
(Beecham Products)

Low-electrolyte, lactose-, sucrose-, fructose-, and protein-free, flavoured liquid feed used as a source of carbohydrate for patients suffering from kidney failure, cirrhosis of the liver, or any conditions where a high-energy, low-electrolyte, low-fluid diet is needed.

Isocal
(Mead Johnson)

Lactose- and gluten-free liquid feed used as a source of protein, carbohydrate, fat, vitamins, and minerals for patients suffering from short bowel syndrome, intractable poor absorption, dysphagia, bowel fistulas, cachexia, anorexia nervosa, or for undernourished patients before surgery or after complete gastrectomy.

Caution: unsuitable as the only source of nutrition for children under 5 years.
Not to be used for: infants under 1 year.

Isomil
(Abbott)

Milk protein-, gluten- and lactose-free powder used as a source of protein, carbohydrate, fat, vitamins, and minerals for patients suffering from galactosaemia, intolerance to lactose and milk, low galactokinase.

Juvela
(Nutricia)
Gluten-free preparation supplied as loaf, fibre loaf, and mixes for patients with digestive conditions sensitive to gluten.

Other preparations: Juvela Low Protein.

Liga
(Cow & Gate)

Gluten-free rusks used for patients with digestive conditions sensitive to gluten.

Liquigen
(S.H.S.)

Low-electrolyte emulsion used as milk substitute to supply triglycerides for patients suffering from steatorrhoea with cystic fibrosis of the pancreas, intestinal lymphangiectasis, chronic liver disease, cirrhosis of the liver, poor absorption, and in intestinal surgery or where a ketogenic diet is needed for control of epilepsy and Type 1 hyperlipoproteinaemia.

Liquisorb
(Merck)

Gluten-free and lactose-low, plain, chocolate-, strawberry-, banana-, or vanilla-flavoured liquid feed used as a source of protein, carbohydrate, fat, vitamins, minerals, and trace elements for patients suffering from short bowel syndrome, intractable poor absorption, dysphagia, bowel fistulas, inflammatory bowel disease, cachexia, anorexia nervosa, or for undernourished patients before surgery or after complete gastrectomy.

Caution: unsuitable as the only source of nutrition for children

under 5 years.
Not to be used for: infants under 1 year.

Liquisorb MCT
(Merck)

Gluten- and fructose-free, low-lactose, plain, chocolate-, strawberry-, or vanilla-flavoured liquid feed used as a source of protein, carbohydrate, fat, vitamins, minerals, and trace elements for patients suffering from short bowel syndrome, intractable poor absorption, dysphagia, bowel fistulas, inflammatory bowel disease, cachexia, anorexia nervosa, or for undernourished patients before surgery or after complete gastrectomy.

Caution: unsuitable as the only source of nutrition for children under 5 years.
Not to be used for: infants under 1 year.

Locasol
(Cow & Gate)

Low-calcium food product used for patients needing calcium-controlled diets.

Lofenlac
(Mead Johnson)

A low-phenylalanine, gluten-, and lactose-free powder used as a source of protein, carbohydrate, fat, vitamins, and minerals for patients suffering from phenylketonuria.

M.S.U.D. Aid
(S.H.S.)

A leucine-, isoleucine-, and valine-free powder used as a source of amino acids, vitamins, minerals, and trace elements for patients suffering from maple syrup urine disease.

Maxamaid
(S.H.S.)

Leucine, isoleucine, and valine-free powder used as a source of amino acids, carbohydrate, vitamins, minerals, and trace elements for patients suffering from maple syrup urine disease.

Not to be used for: children under 2 years.
Other preparations: Maxamaid RVHB; Maxamaid XLYS TRY; Maxamaid XMET, THRE, VAL, ISOLEU; Maxamaid XPHEN, TYR: Maxamaid XP; Maxamaid XP BAR.

Maxamum XP
(S.H.S.)

Phenylalanine-free, orange- or unflavoured powder used as a source of amino acids, carbohydrate, minerals, vitamins, and trace elements for patients suffering from phenylketonuria.

Not to be used for: children under 8 years.

Maxijul Super Sol
(S.H.S.)

Gluten-, sucrose-, galactose-, fructose-, and lactose-free powder used as a source of polyglucose polymer, sodium, and potassium for patients suffering from kidney failure, cirrhosis of the liver, intolerance of disaccharide, amino acid metabolic disorders, poor absorption, and hypoglycaemia where a high-energy, low-fluid diet is needed.

Other preparations: Maxijul Liquid; Maxijul LE.

Maxipro HBV Super Soluble
(S.H.S.)
A protein powder used for patients suffering from hypoproteinaemia, short bowel syndrome, intractable poor absorption, inflammatory bowel disease, bowel fistulas, dysphagia, and for undernourished patients before surgery or in complete gastrectomy where salt intake must be reduced.

Caution: unsuitable as the only source of nutrition for children under 5 years.
Not to be used for: infants under 1 year.

MCT Pepdite
(S.H.S.)

Gluten-, sucrose-, and lactose-free powder used as a source of protein, carbohydrate, fat, vitamins, minerals, and trace elements for patients suffering from intolerance to whole protein, short bowel syndrome, intractable poor absorption, bowel fistulas, inflammatory bowel disease, where fat is difficult to absorb.

Caution: use correct formulation depending upon the patient's age.
Other preparations: MCT Pepdite 2+.

Milupa lpd
(Milupa)

Low-protein, demineralized powder used as a source of vegetable oil, starch, sucrose, monoglycerides, potassium citrate, and calcium phosphate for children suffering from amino acid disorders.

Not to be used for: infants under 1 year.

Minafen
(Cow & Gate)

Low-phenylalanine powder used as a source of protein, carbohydrate, fat, vitamins, and minerals for infants and young children suffering from phenylketonuria.

Modjul Flavour
(S.H.S.)

A blackcurrant-, pineapple-, orange-, or tomato-flavoured carbohydrate, saccharin, citric and malic acid powder used to flavour unflavoured preparations for patients where metabolic disorders need dietary control.

Neocate
(S.H.S.)

Gluten-, sucrose-, and lactose-free preparation used as a source of protein, carbohydrate, fat, vitamins, minerals, and trace elements for patients suffering from intolerance to whole protein, inflammatory bowel disease, bowel fistulas.

Nestargel
(Nestle)

A carob seed flour, calcium lactate preparation used for patients suffering from vomiting and regurgitation.

Nutramigen
(Mead Johnson)

Gluten-, fructose-, and lactose-free powder used as a source of protein, carbohydrate, fat, vitamins, and minerals for patients suffering from sensitivity to milk, intolerance to lactose, galactosaemia, or low galactokinase.

Osmolite
(Abbott)

Gluten- and lactose-free liquid feed used as a source of protein, carbohydrate, fat, vitamins, and minerals for patients suffering from short bowel syndrome, intractable poor absorption, dysphagia, bowel fistulas, inflammatory bowel disease, cachexia, anorexia nervosa, or for undernourished patients before surgery or after complete gastrectomy.

Caution: unsuitable as the only source of nutrition for children under 5 years.
Not to be used for: infants under 1 year.

Ostersoy
(Farley)

Milk protein-, gluten-, sucrose-, and lactose-free powder used as a source of protein, carbohydrate, fat, vitamins, and minerals for patients suffering from intolerance of cow's milk, lactose, or sucrose, or galactosaemia, or low galactokinase.

Paediasure
(Abbott)

A preparation used as a source of protein, carbohydrate, fat, vitamins, minerals, and trace elements for patients suffering from short bowel syndrome, intractable poor absorption, dysphagia, bowel fistulas, inflammatory bowel disease, cachexia, or for undernourished patients before surgery.

Not to be used for: adults or for infants under 1 year.

Pepdite
(S.H.S.)

Gluten-, sucrose-, and lactose-free powder used as a source of protein, carbohydrate, fat, vitamins, minerals, and trace elements for patients suffering from intolerance to whole protein or lactose, short bowel syndrome, intractable poor absorption, bowel fistulas, inflammatory bowel disease.

Caution: use the formulation suitable for the age of the patient.
Other preparations: Pepdite 2+.

Peptamen
(Clintec)

A preparation used as a source of protein, carbohydrate, fat, vitamins, minerals, and trace elements for patients suffering from short bowel syndrome, intractable poor absorption, dysphagia, bowel fistulas, inflammatory bowel disease, cachexia, anorexia nervosa, or for undernourished patients before surgery or after complete gastrectomy.

Caution: unsuitable as the only source of nutrition for children under 5 years.
Not to be used for: infants under 1 year.

Pepti-2000 LF
(Cow & Gate)

Powder used as a source of protein, carbohydrate, fat, vitamins, and minerals for patients suffering from intractable poor absorption, bowel fistulas, cachexia, and after complete gastrectomy.

Caution: unsuitable as the only source of nutrition for children under 5 years.
Not to be used for: infants under 1 year.
Other preparations: Pepti-2000 LF Liquid.

Pepti-Junior
(Cow & Gate)

Low-lactose powder used as a source of protein, carbohydrate, fat, vitamins, and minerals for patients suffering from intolerance to lactose and sucrose with protein intolerance in steatorrhoea associated with cystic fibrosis and other poor absorption conditions.

Peptisorb
(Merck)

Gluten- and fructose-free, low-lactose liquid used as a source of protein, carbohydrate, fat, vitamins, minerals, and trace elements for patients suffering from intractable poor absorption, bowel fistulas, cachexia, or after complete gastrectomy.

Not to be used for: children.

Peptisorbon
(Merck)

Low-lactose, gluten-, sucrose, fructose, and galactose-free powder used as a source of protein, carbohydrate, fat, vitamins, minerals, and trace elements for patients suffering from intractable poor absorption, bowel fistulas, cachexia, or after complete gastrectomy.

Caution: unsuitable as the only source of nutrition for children under 5 years.
Not to be used for: infants under 1 year.

PK Aid III
(S.H.S.)

Phenylalanine-free preparation used as a source of amino acids for patients suffering from phenylketonuria.

PKU 2
(Milupa)

Phenylalanine-free, vanilla-flavoured granules used as a source of amino acids, carbohydrate, vitamins, minerals, and trace elements for patients suffering from phenylketonuria.

Not to be used for: infants under 1 year.
Other preparations: PKU 3.

PKU Drink
(Nutricia)

Phenylalanine-low milk substitute used for patients suffering from phenylketonuria.

Polial
(Ultrapharm)

Gluten-, wheat starch-, milk protein-, egg-, and lactose-free, biscuit used for patients suffering from gluten-sensitive digestive disorders.

Polycal
(Cow & Gate)

A carbohydrate powder used for patients suffering from kidney failure, cirrhosis of the liver, intolerance of disaccharide and protein, hypoglycaemia, amino acid metabolic disorders, and poor absorption conditions where a high-energy, low-fluid diet is needed.

Caution: do not give to infants without diluting.

Portagen
(Mead Johnson)

Gluten-, fructose-, and lactose-free powder used as a source of protein, carbohydrate, fat, vitamins, and minerals for patients suffering from poor fat absorption with intolerance of lactose, cachexia..

Pregestimil
(Mead Johnson)

Gluten-, sucrose-, fructose-, and lactose-free powder used as a source of protein, carbohydrate, fat, vitamins, and minerals for patients suffering from galactosaemia, low galactokinase, intolerance of sucrose and lactose, poor fat absorption, intolerance of protein, cachexia.

Prejomin
(Milupa)

Gluten-, sucrose-, galactose-, fructose-, lactose-, and casein residue-free powder used as a source of protein, carbohydrate, fat, vitamins, minerals, and trace elements for patients suffering from galactosaemia, low galactokinase, intolerance of sucrose, fructose, lactose, or protein.

Promod
(Abbott)

Powder used as a source of protein and carbohydrate for patients suffering from hypoproteinaemia.

Prosobee Liquid
(Mead Johnson)

Gluten-, sucrose-, fructose-, and lactose-free, liquid used as a source of protein, carbohydrate, fat, vitamins, minerals, and trace elements for young children suffering from intolerance to lactose, sucrose, and cow's milk, and galactosaemia, and low galactokinase.

Caution: dilute the liquid.
Other preparations: Prosobee Powder.

Protifar
(Cow & Gate)

Protein powder used for patients suffering from hypoproteinaemia.

Reabilan
(Roussel)

Gluten- and lactose-free liquid feed used as a source of oligopeptides, carbohydrate, fat, vitamins, minerals and trace elements used as a complete nutrition for patients suffering from short bowel syndrome, intractable poor absorption, dysphagia, bowel fistulas, Inflammatory bowel syndrome, cachexia, or for undernourished patients before surgery or after complete gastrectomy.

Caution: unsuitable as the only source of nutrition for children under 5 years.
Not to be used for: infants under 1 year.

Rite-Diet gluten-free
(Nutricia)

Gluten-free preparation supplied as high-fibre crackers, biscuits, pasta, flour mix, baking mix, white bread mix, brown bread mix, white loaf, high-fibre loaf, brown bread, canned white loaf and used for patients suffering coeliac disease or other digestive disorders where sensitivity to gluten occurs.

Caution: unsuitable for low-protein diets, phenylketonuria, galactosaemia (except pasta, low-protein flour mix, and canned white bread.

Rite-Diet low protein
(Nutricia)

Low-phenylalanine, low-electrolyte, gluten- and lactose-free preparation supplied as flour mix, baking mix, canned bread, white bread, flavoured wafers, biscuits, and pasta for patients suffering from phenylketonuria and other conditions where there is intolerance to amino acids, kidney and liver failure, cirrhosis of the liver, and digestive disorders where there is sensitivity to gluten.

Caution: biscuits and wafers are not suitable for gluten-sensitive digestive disorders.

Rite-Diet low-sodium bread
(Nutricia)

Bread containing carbohydrate, minerals, vitamins, and trace elements and used for patients needing low-sodium diets.

Seravit Paediatric
(S.H.S.)

Low-sodium and potassium powder used as a source of carbohydrate, minerals, vitamins, and trace elements for infants and children where supplements are needed in special diets.

Triosorbon
(Merck)

Gluten-, sucrose-, fructose-, and galactose-free, low-lactose powder used as a source of protein, carbohydrate, fat, vitamins, and minerals for patients suffering from short bowel syndrome, intractable poor absorption, dysphagia, inflammatory bowel disease, cachexia, anorexia nervosa, or for undernourished patients before surgery or after complete gastrectomy.

Caution: unsuitable as the only source of nutrition for children under 5 years.
Not to be used for: infants under 1 year.

Tritamyl
(Procea)

Gluten- and lactose-free, starch-based self-raising flour used for patients suffering from coeliac disease, dermatitis herpetiformes, and digestive disorders sensitive to gluten.

Other preparations: Tritamyl PK

Trufree
(Cantassium)

Various gluten-free flours used for patients suffering from digestive disorders sensitive to gluten.

Wysoy
(Wyeth)

Gluten-, milk protein-, and lactose-free powder used as a source of protein, carbohydrate, fat, vitamins, minerals, and trace elements for patients suffering from galactosaemia, low galactokinase, intolerance to milk or lactose.

Miscellaneous

There is an interesting collection of medications available over the counter for a variety of conditions. Some of those listed below are bulking agents to treat obesity — they work by filling the stomach with an inactive substance.

Many contraceptive products, including condoms, contraceptive foams, diaphragms, spermicidal gels, C-Film contraceptives, and a contraceptive sponge, are available over the counter. Pregnancy testing kits and ovulation predicters are also available.

Circulatory disorders may be treated with Paroven, Cyclospasmol, and Hexopal, all of which are prescribed by doctors but are also available from pharmacies without a prescription. Similarly, many anti-anginal preparations are also available — Transiderm-Nitro, Suscard Buccal, Isordil, Sorbitrate, glyceryl trinitrate, Cedocard, Elantan.

Diuretics, such as Aquaban and Cascade, can also be purchased to remove excess fluid, particularly in premenstrual women.

Nicobrevin, used to stop addiction to smoking, contains quinine and methyl valerianate, and is available over the counter although its counterpart, Nicorette (nicotine chewing gum) is available on private prescription and over the counter.

Curiously, insulin used by diabetic patients to control blood sugar, can be purchased at pharmacies without a prescription. Similarly, blood glucose and urine sugar testing equipment can be bought over the counter.

Homoeopathic remedies (*see* below) to treat a wide variety of conditions are also available over the counter.

Carbomix
(Penn)

Granules used as an adsorbent to treat acute poisoning, overdose of drugs.

Dose: adults dissolve the contents of the bottle in water and take by mouth as soon as possible after poisoning; children usually take half adult dose.
Side effects:
Caution: your doctor may advise additional treatment for certain overdoses.
Not to be used for:
Not to be used with: antidotes or emetics taken by mouth.
Contains: activated charcoal.
Other preparations:

Cedocard
(Tillotts)

A blue, scored tablet or a green, scored tablet according to strengths of 20 mg, 40 mg and used as a nitrate treatment for severe congestive heart failure.

Dose: 10-40 mg 3-4 times a day.
Side effects: headache, flushes, dizziness.
Caution:
Not to be used for: children, or for patients suffering from severe low blood pressure, heart shock, severe anaemia, brain haemorrhage.
Not to be used with:
Contains: isosorbide dinitrate.
Other preparations: Cedocard I.V.

Cyclospasmol
(SNP)

Drops used as an anticholinergic agent in ophthalmic procedures.

Dose: 1 or more drops into the eye as needed.
Side effects:
Caution:
Not to be used for: patients suffering from narrow angle glaucoma.
Not to be used with:
Contains: cyclopentolate hydrochloride.
Other preparations:

Elantan
(Schwarz)

A white, scored tablet supplied at strengths of 10 mg, 20 mg, 40 mg and used as a nitrate treatment for the prevention of angina, and in addition to other treatments for congestive heart failure.

Dose: 10 mg twice a day at first increasing to 40-80 mg a day in 2 or 3 divided doses after meals to a maximum of 120 mg a day.
Side effects: headache, flushes, dizziness.
Caution:
Not to be used for: children.
Not to be used with:
Contains: isosorbide mononitrate.
Other preparations: Elantan LA, Imdur (Astra).

Glucotard
(MCP)

Mini-tablets in 5 g sachets used as a bulking agent to treat diabetes.

Dose: 1 sachet taken with water 1-3 times a day before main meals.
Side effects: wind swollen abdomen.
Caution: glucose levels should be checked initially.
Not to be used for: children or for patients suffering from blocked intestine, oesophageal disease.
Not to be used with:
Contains: guar gum.
Other preparations:

Guarem
(Rybar)

Dispersible granules in a 5 g sachet used as a bulking agent to treat diabetes.

Dose: 1 sachet taken with water 1-3 times a day before main meals.
Side effects: wind swollen abdomen.
Caution: glucose levels should be checked.
Not to be used for: children or for patients suffering from blocked intestine, oesophageal disease.
Not to be used with:
Contains: guar gum.
Other preparations: Guarina (Norgine).

Hexopal
(Winthrop)

A white, scored tablet supplied at a strength of 500 mg and used as a vasodilator to treat Raynaud's phenomenon (a condition caused by spasm of the blood vessels), intermittent claudication (difficulty walking caused by circulation disorders).

Dose: 2 tablets 3-4 times a day.
Side effects:

Caution: in pregnant women.
Not to be used for: children.
Not to be used with:
Contains: inositol nicotinate.
Other preparations: Hexopal Forte, Hexopal Suspension.

Isordil
(Wyeth)

A white, scored tablet supplied at strengths of 10 mg, 30 mg and used as a nitrate for the prevention of angina, acute congestive heart failure.

Dose: 5-15 mg under the tongue every 2-3 hours at first, then 10-60 mg swallowed 4 times a day. 40-120 mg for the prevention of angina.
Side effects: headache, flushes, dizziness, may make chest pain worse.
Caution: heart function should be checked in the case of heart failure.
Not to be used for: children.
Not to be used with:
Contains: isosorbide dinitrate.
Other preparations: Isordil Sublingual, Isordil Tembids.

Medicoal
(Lundbeck)

Effervescent granules used as an adsorbent to treat acute poisoning, overdose of drugs.

Dose: 5-10 g in 100 ml of water, repeat up to a maximum of 50 g.
Side effects:
Caution:
Not to be used for: poisoning where there is a known antidote or for poisoning by acids, alkalis, iron salts, cyanides, malathion,

DDT, sulphonylureas.
Not to be used with: drugs taken by mouth.
Contains: activated charcoal.
Other preparations:

Nicorette
(Lundbeck)

Chewing gum supplied at strengths of 2 mg and 4 mg, and used as an alkaloid to end smoking addiction.

Dose: 1 when required.
Side effects: addiction, hiccoughs, indigestion, irritated throat.
Caution: in patients suffering from coronary disease, angina, gastritis, peptic ulcer.
Not to be used for: children or pregnant women.
Not to be used with:
Contains: nicotine.
Other preparations:

Nilstim
(De Witt)

A green tablet used as a bulking agent to treat obesity.

Dose: 2 tablets to be broken into pieces and taken with liquid 15 minutes before meals.
Side effects:
Caution:
Not to be used for: children or for patients suffering from blocked intestine.
Not to be used with:
Contains: cellulose, methyl cellulose.
Other preparations:

Paroven
(Zyma)

A yellow capsule supplied at a strength of 250 mg and used as a vein constrictor to treat ankle swelling, varicose veins.

Dose: 3-4 capsules a day with food at first, then reduce.
Side effects: stomach disturbances, flushes, headache.
Caution:
Not to be used for: children.
Not to be used with:
Contains: oxerutins.
Other preparations:

Prefil
(Norgine)

Brown granules used as a bulking agent to treat obesity.

Dose: 2 5 ml teaspoonsful swallowed with water ½-1 hour before eating.
Side effects:
Caution:
Not to be used for: patients suffering from blocked intestine.
Not to be used with:
Contains: sterculia.
Other preparations:

Rowatinex
(Tillotts)

Volatile oils used to treat urinary stones, kidney disorders, prevention of urinary stones.

Dose: 3-5 drops 4-5 times a day before food.
Side effects:

Caution:
Not to be used for: children.
Not to be used with:
Contains: pinene, camphene, anethol, fenchone, cineole, olive oil.
Other preparations:

Sorbitrate
(Stuart)

A yellow, oval, scored tablet or a blue, oval, scored tablet according to strengths of 10 mg, 20 mg and used as a nitrate for the prevention of angina.

Dose: 10-40 mg 3-4 times a day.
Side effects: headache, flushes, dizziness.
Caution:
Not to be used for: children.
Not to be used with:
Contains: isosorbide dinitrate.
Other preparations:

Suscard Buccal
(Pharmax)

A white tablet supplied at strengths of 1 mg, 2 mg, 3 mg, 5 mg and used as a nitrate to treat angina, acute heart failure, congestive heart failure.

Dose: 5 mg 3 times a day at first or repeated until symptoms are relieved, allowing tablet to dissolve between upper lip and gum. For angina 1 mg as required or 1 mg 3 times a day increasing strength and frequency as needed.
Side effects: headache, flushes.
Caution:
Not to be used for: children.

Not to be used with:
Contains: glyceryl trinitrate.
Other preparations:

Transiderm-Nitro
(Ciba)

Patches supplied at strengths of 5 mg, 10 mg and used as a nitrate for the prevention of angina..

Dose: apply a patch to a hairless part of the chest every 24 hours on a different place each time.
Side effects: headache, rash, dizziness.
Caution: the treatment should be reduced gradually and replaced with decreasing doses of oral nitrate.
Not to be used for: children.
Not to be used with:
Contains: glyceryl trinitrate.
Other preparations:

PART 2

ALTERNATIVE THERAPIES

As orthodox medical practitioners, we rarely recommend or prescribe alternative or natural remedies. Having said this, we often use multivitamin preparations in recovery from viral infections such as ME (myalgic encephalomyelitis). Until recently, we used tryptophan in high doses to treat depression, but this has now fallen into disrepute since one particular source of this amino acid caused a side effect known as EMS (eosinophilic myalgic syndrome). This is a reminder to us that alternative remedies, which use small quantities of proteins, minerals, vitamins, and herbs, may still cause allergic reactions, and some suppliers have better quality control than others.

Many of the vitamins and minerals are included in their appropriate section earlier in this book; thus, vitamins and minerals span the divide between orthodox and alternative medicine.

Because an increasing number of people are turning to alternative therapies, we have included this list of alternative preparations. We are not in a position to recommend any particular treatment, and readers are advised to consult an alternative medicine practitioner or to discuss their treatment with their health food shop. We can, however, give a few points of guidance.

Many of the herbal preparations have names which give a clue to their use. Thus Feverfew is an anti-fever treatment, and Waterfall a diuretic. There is a sedative called Forte-Winx which indicates its hypnotic potential. Arnica is an anti-inflammatory herb and comfrey is often used in the treatment of rheumatic disorders. There are herbal remedies for weight loss and weight gain. Herbal extracts, such as kelp (seaweed), may often be rich in minerals.

Although most alternative remedies have not undergone formal clinical trials, there are some areas where herbal remedies have achieved generally accepted success.

Ipecacuanha is a good emetic and it is used to treat poisoning by causing emptying of the stomach. Garlic is felt to be responsible for the low incidence of heart disease in French people. Peppermint oil is used to treat irritable bowel (see Colpermin) and bran to treat bowel disorders. Yoghurt extracts may treat candida (thrush). In France, doctors routinely prescribe acidophiles, bacterial extracts with antibiotics, to prevent thrush but, in the United Kingdom, the only such preparation is available as an alternative therapy. Many rheumatologists see patients who claim to have benefited from either mussel extracts or cod liver oil. Similarly, many women take evening primrose oil or vitamin B6 for premenstrual symptoms.

Mineral preparations, such as selenium, germanium, magnesium, or zinc have been included in alternative remedies to treat apparent deficiencies. Recently, the use of germanium has come under some attack because it may cause toxicity. It is worth remembering that side effects can occur with all treatments, whether orthodox or alternative. Specific vitamin or mineral deficiencies do occur, Scurvy due to lack of vitamin C, anaemia due to iron deficiency, and rickets due to vitamin D and calcium deficiency are still seen, particularly in the elderly and in those on special diet. Vegetarians, in particular, may become anaemic because of deficiencies in iron or vitamin B_{12}. Pregnant women may be deficient in iron or folic acid.

Many of the alternative remedies are amino acid or protein extracts. Amino acids are the building blocks of proteins, and they cannot be stored in the body. True deficiency is rare but many people believe that one can build up muscle and lose fat by taking high-protein supplements. These proteins may have an antidepressant effect.

Herbal remedies and medicines

Herbs have a longer history of use than any other form of medicine, and more than 25 per cent of existing medicinal drugs are extracted from or have originated from plant materials.

The preparations included here are all licensed under the Medicines Act of 1968. This means that they are entitled to be called medicines and that there are specific controls over what the product contains, where it may be sold, in what form, and with what recommendations for use. Manufacture is subject to Department of Health inspection and the licence is a guarantee of quality control. The PL number that you will see on the product packet indicates that the medicine holds either a Full Product Licence or a Product Licence of Right (as is the case with most homoeopathic remedies).

There are many other herbal preparations to be found in health food shops and pharmacies. If they do not hold a licence, however, they may only describe themselves as food supplements and not as medicines. The licensing procedure is costly and so many smaller companies may choose not to apply for licensing for financial reasons. Many of these supplements may be excellent and may be closely comparable to their licensed counterparts as, for example, with the various brands of Evening Primrose Oil available.

It is important not to treat herbs lightly simply because they are 'natural'. Many of them may be toxic in high doses and the manufacturer's directions must be followed accurately. Remember that there is always the possibility of allergic reaction. If you are already taking medication, you should consult your doctor or medical herbalist regarding the advisability of taking a herbal medicine. Advice should always be sought before taking herbs during pregnancy or breastfeeding, or giving them to young children.

Please note that the letters B.P. after a medicine means that it has been prepared according to British Pharmacopoeia specifications; B.P.C. that it has been prepared according to British Pharmaceutical Codex specifications. And throughout the following texts 'excipients' refers to the non-active ingredients used to convey the medicine.

Acidosis
(Potters)

Dose: 2 tablets 3 times a day after meals.
Product licence: No. 0250/5190R.
Constituents: meadowsweet (*Filipendula ulmaria*), vegetable charcoal, rhubarb (*Rheum officinale*), aniseed oil (*Pimpinella anisum*), caraway oil (*Carum carvi*), cardamom (*Elattaria cardamom*), cinnamon (*Cinnamomum verum*), excipients.
Uses: indigestion, hyperacidity, heartburn.
Special notes:
Caution: not recommended for children.

Aluminium-free Indigestion Tablets
(Larkhall)
'Cantassium'

Dose: 1-4 tablets to be taken as required after meals.
Product licence: No. PL0912/5238R.
Constituents: calcium carbonate 75 mg, cinnamon (*Cinnamomum verum*) 30 mg, nutmeg (*Myristica*) 24 mg, clove (*Caryophyllin*) 12 mg, cardamom (*Elattaria cardamom*) seed 9 mg, mannitol 20 mg, calcium sulphate dihydrate 0.4 g, potato starch 40 mg, stearic acid (palm oil) 3 mg, gum acacia.
Uses: indigestion relief without risk from aluminium.
Special notes: vegan, hypoallergenic.
Caution: not recommended during pregnancy or breastfeeding without practitioner supervision. May antidote any homoeopathic remedies which you are taking.

Anased Pain Relief Tablets
(Potters)

Dose: 1-2 tablets 3 times daily and 2 at bedtime.
Product licence: No. 0250/5223R.
Constituents: hops (*Humulus lupulus*), Jamaica dogwood

(*Piscidia erythrina*), wild lettuce (*Lactuca virosa*), passionflower (*Passiflora*), wind anemone (*Pulsatilla*), excipients.
Uses: sedative, analgesic, relief of minor aches, tension headaches, insomnia, irritability.
Special notes:
Caution: not recommended during pregnancy or breastfeeding, nor for children.

Antibron Tablets
(Potters)

Dose: 2 tablets 3 times a day; children over 7 years 1 tablet 3 times a day.
Product licence: No. 0250/5177R.
Constituents: lobelia (*Lobelia inflata*), wild lettuce (*Lactuca virosa*) extracts, coltsfoot (*Tussilago farfara*), *Euphorbia hirta*, pleurisy root (*Asclepias tuberosa*), snake root (*Polygala senega*), liquorice (*Glycyrrhiza glabra*), capsicum, excipients.
Uses: expectorant, antispasmodic, anti-asthmatic, sedative, to relieve coughs.
Special notes:
Caution: do not exceed the stated dose — *Lobelia* may cause nausea and vomiting in high doses.

Antifect
(Potters)

Dose: 2 tablets 3 times a day; children over 8 years half the adult dose.
Product licence: No. 0250/5222R.
Constituents: garlic (*Allium sativum*), garlic oil, coneflower (*Echinacea angustifolia*) extract, vegetable charcoal, excipients.
Uses: expectorant, antibiotic, antibacterial, antiviral, for catarrh, rhinitis, nasal congestion, sinusitis, hayfever.
Special notes:
Caution:

Antiglan Tablets
(Potters)

Dose: elderly males 2 tablets 3 times a day, in severe cases 3 tablets 3 times a day.
Product licence: No. 0250/5076R.
Constituents: kava (*Piper methysticum*), saw palmetto (*Serenoa repens*), horsetail (*Equisetum*), *Hydrangea arboresens*, excipients.
Uses: short-term relief of mild bladder discomfort; may help with enlarged prostate glands — holding the condition and, in some cases, edging it back — helpful for those waiting for a prostate operation.
Special notes:
Caution:

Anti-smoking
(Larkhall)
'Cantassium'

Dose: 1 tablet to be swallowed with water when craving a smoke. Do not take more than 9 tablets in 24 hours.
Product licence: No. PL/0912/5977R.
Constituents: kolanuts (*Cola acuminata*) 20 mg, lobelia (*Lobelia inflata*) 65 mg, dicalcium phosphate 0.55 g, icing sugar 95 mg, magnesium trisilicate 30 mg, quassia (*Picrasma excelsa*) powder 25 mg, sago flour 20.3 mg, talc 3 mg, industrial methylated spirits 0.05 ml, stearic acid (palm oil) 2 mg.
Uses: a smoking deterrent preparation.
Special notes: vegan, hypoallergenic.
Caution: not to be taken during pregnancy or breastfeeding. Do not exceed the stated dose — higher doses may produce nausea and vomiting.

Antismoking Tablets
(Potters)

Dose: 1 tablet to be taken every hour all day; each tablet should be sucked for half-a-minute, then swallowed whole.
Product licence: No. PL/0250/5178.
Constituents: lobelia (*Lobelia inflata*), excipients.
Uses: to reduce addiction to tobacco smoking.
Special notes:
Caution: do not exceed the stated dose; higher doses may produce nausea and vomiting. Not to be taken during pregnancy or breastfeeding.

Antitis Tablets
(Potters)

Dose: 2 tablets 3 times a day.
Product licence: No. 0250/5224R.
Constituents: buchu (*Agathosma betulina*), clivers (*Galium aparine*), couchgrass (*Agropyron repens*), horsetail (*Equisetum*), shepherd's purse (*Capsella bursa-pastoris*), uva ursi (*Arctostaphylos uva-ursi*), excipients.
Uses: diuretic, antiseptic, to relieve cystitis.
Special notes: Potter's recommend increasing fluid intake, and that drinks containing bicarbonate of soda are especially useful.
Caution: not recommended for children.

Appetiser Mixture (formerly Tonic and Nervine Essence)
(Potters)

Dose: 1 5 ml teaspoonful 3 times a day in a little water before meals.
Product licence: No. P/L0250/5106R.
Constituents: camomile (*Chamaemelium nobile*), calumba (*Jateorhiza palmata*) root, gentian (*Gentiana lutea*), excipients.
Uses: tonic, to promote appetite and relieve symptoms of flatulence.
Special notes:

Caution: not recommended during pregnancy or breastfeeding, nor for children.

Artichoke Formula
(Bio-Strath: imported by Cedar Health Ltd)

Dose: 20 drops (0.6 ml) in a little water 3 times a day before meals.
Product licence: No. PL4210/0004.
Constituents: artichoke (*Cynara scolymus*) leaf extract 22.5 %, thistle seed (*Carduus marianus*) extract 22.5 %, peppermint (*Mentha piperita*) leaf extract 5 %, *Torula utilis* yeast plasmolysate 50 %, (ethanol content 38 % v/v approx.).
Uses: to relieve the symptoms of indigestion after eating fatty foods
Special notes:
Caution: may antidote any homoeopathic remedies which you are taking.

Athera
(Modern Health)

Dose: 2-3 tablets to be taken 3 times a day after meals.
Product licence: No. 2452/5001R.
Constituents: parsley (*Petroselinum crispum*) 60 mg, vervain (*Verbena officinalus*) 10 mg, vervain extract 90 mg, clivers (*Galium aparine*) extract 60 mg, senna leaf 4 mg, senna extract 10 mg, excipients.
Uses: for menopausal symptoms, to ease fluid retention, soothe the stomach, relax, increase vitality, tone the system, maintain healthy bowel action.
Special notes: not tested on animals.
Caution: may occasionally cause diarrhoea, not recommended for children or during pregnancy or breastfeeding. Senna is not to be used in colitis or spastic colon. Senna may harmlessly colour the urine or stools.

Avena Sativa Comp.
(Weleda)

Dose: 10-20 drops to be taken in water half an hour before going to bed. If necessary this dose may be repeated; children: half the adult dose.
Product licence: No. PL0298/5473.
Constituents: per 100 ml: oats (*Avena sativa*) tincture 25 ml, hops (*Humulus lupulus*) 1x 4 ml, passionflower (*Passiflora incarnata*) tincture 7.5 ml, valerian (*Valeriana officinalis*) tincture 30 ml, *Coffea tosta* 60x 15 ml, nominal ethanol content 45 % v/v.
Uses: to aid relaxation at the end of the day.
Special notes:
Caution: may cause sleepiness. Not recommended during pregnancy or breastfeeding.

Backache Tablets
(Potters)

Dose: 2 tablets 3 times a day.
Product licence: No. 0250/5182R
Constituents: gravel root (*Eupatorium purpureum*), hydrangea (*Hydrangea arborescens*) root, buchu (*Agathosma betulina*), uva ursi (*Arctostaphylos uva-ursi*), excipients.
Uses: relief of backache; this formula arises from the herbalist's view that the urinary system must also be toned effectively to deal with backache.
Special notes:
Caution: not recommended during pregnancy nor for children.

Balm of Gilead
(Potters)

Dose: adults: 2 5 ml teaspoonsful 3-4 times a day; children over 5 years 1 5 ml teaspoonful, which may be diluted with water if necessary, 3-4 times a day.

Product licence: No. P/L0250/5085R.
Constituents: acetum scillae (squill vinegar), lobelia (*Lobelia inflata*)tincture, balm of Gilead (*Populus candicans*), lungwort, (*Pulmonaria officinalis*), excipients.
Uses: expectorant, to relieve symptoms of coughs and colds.
Special notes: sugar-free base — concentrated apple juice is used as sweetener.
Caution: shake bottle before use. Not recommended during pregnancy or breastfeeding nor for children under 5 years. Do not exceed the stated dose — high doses of *Lobelia* may cause nausea and vomiting.

Balm of Gilead Cough Mixture
(Booker)
'Heath & Heather'

Dose: 2 5 ml teaspoonsful 3 times a day.
Product licence: No. PL1713/5083R.
Constituents: per 10 ml balm of Gilead (*Populus candicans*) liquid extract 0.8 ml, squill tincture 0.25 ml, lobelia (*Lobelia inflata*) tincture 0.2 ml, sugar syrup, xanthum gum, nipastat sodium.
Uses: to relieve symptoms of coughs and catarrh.
Special notes: vegan, yeast free.
Caution: shake before use. Not recommended during pregnancy or breastfeeding nor for children. Do not exceed the stated dose — high doses of *Lobelia* may cause nausea and vomiting.

Balm of Gilead Cough Pastilles
(Booker)
'Heath & Heather'

Dose: allow a pastille to dissolve in the mouth when needed. Not more than 12 to be taken in 24 hours.
Product licence: No. P/L1713/5084R.
Constituents: balm of Gilead (*Populus candicans*) buds 8 %,

squill (*Drimia maritima*) tincture 2.5 %, lobelia (*Lobelia inflata*) tincture 2 %, sugar, liquid glucose, gelatin, liquorice (*Glycyrrhiza glabra*), beetroot red as colouring, anise oil as flavouring, peppermint oil, caramel, vegetable fat.
Uses: to relieve the symptoms of coughs and catarrh.
Special notes: yeast free.
Caution: not recommended for children or during pregnancy or breastfeeding. Do not exceed the stated dose — high doses of *Lobelia* may cause nausea and vomiting. May antidote any homoeopathic remedies you are taking.

Becalm
(Heath & Heather)

Dose: 1 tablet 3 times a day with water.
Product licence: P/L1713/500R.
Constituents: valerian (*Valeriana officinalis*) extract equivalent to 160 mg, hops (*Humulus lupulus*) extract equivalent to 200 mg, passionflower (*Passiflora*) extract equivalent to 130 mg, dicalcium phosphate, microcrystalline cellulose, stearic acid, magnesium stearate; coating titanium dioxide, iron oxide, polyethylene glycol.
Uses: sedative, to aid relaxation and calm.
Special notes: vegan, yeast free.
Caution: not recommended for children or during pregnancy or breastfeeding. May cause drowsiness, if affected do not drive or operate machinery and avoid alcohol.

Biobalm Powder
(Modern Health)

Dose: 1-2 level teaspoons to be taken up to 4 times a day; children 5-12 years half the above dosage.
Product licence: No. 1146/5004R.
Constituents: per 100 g slippery elm bark (*Ulmus rubra*) 13 g, marshmallow root (*Althaea officinalis*) 8 g, Irish moss (*Chondrus*

crispus) 6 g, barley flour, excipients.
Uses: indigestion, flatulence, soothes gastro-intestinal lining.
Special notes: vegetarian.
Caution:

Biophyllin
(Gerard House)

Dose: 2 tablets after meals 3 times a day.
Product licence: No. 1661/5000R.
Constituents: valerian (*Valeriana officinalis*) 150 mg, scullcap (*Scutellaria lateriflora*)108 mg, Jamaican dogwood (*Piscidia erythrina*) 9 mg, black cohosh (*Cimicifuga racemosa*) 30 mg, cayenne (*Capsicum frutescens*) 3 mg, malto-dextrin 140 mg, calcium phosphate 50 mg, sugar 40 mg, sodium starch glycollate 20 mg, magnesium stearate 2 mg, talc 8 mg.
Uses: nervousness, tension, restlessness, irritability.
Special notes: vegan, yeast free.
Caution: not to be used during pregnancy or breastfeeding, not recommended for children under 12 years.

Blue Flag Root Compound
(Gerard House)

Dose: 1 tablet after meals 3 times a day.
Product licence: No. 1661/5002R.
Constituents: blue flag (flag lily) (*Iris versicolor*)90 mg, burdock (*Arctium lappa*) extract 46 mg, sarsaparilla (*Smilax ornata*) extract 35 mg, sugar 100 mg, lactose 40 mg, sodium starch glycollate 10 mg, talc 3.8 mg, magnesium stearate 0.9 mg, starch 1500 2.8 mg.
Uses: minor acne, eczema, dermatitis.
Special notes: vegetarian, yeast free.
Caution: not recommended for children under 12 years, not to be used in pregnancy.

Boldo Herbal Aid for Slimmers
(Larkhall)
'Cantassium'

Dose: 1-2 tablets 3 times a day after meals.
Product licence: No. PLO912/7342R.
Constituents: boldo (*Peumus boldus*) extract 64.8 mg, clivers (*Galium aparine*) extract 24.4 mg, dandelion (*Taraxacum officinale*) root 24.4 mg, uva ursi (*Arctostaphylos uva-ursi*) extract 32.4 mg, bladderwrack (*Fucus vesiculosus*) 45.8 mg, dicalcium phosphate 0.2358 g, magnesium stearate 1.6 mg, stearic acid (palm oil) 1.6 mg, potato starch 15 mg, talc 5 mg.
Uses: for women who experience water retention.
Special notes: vegan, yeast free, hypoallergenic.
Caution: not to be used in pregnancy or breastfeeding without practitioner supervision. Not recommended for children. Do not exceed the stated dose, large doses of boldo cause vomiting.

Boldo Herbal Aid to Slimming
(Potters)

Dose: 1-2 tablets 3 times a day; elderly: 1 tablet 3-4 times a day.
Product licence: No. 0250/5200R.
Constituents: dandelion root (*Taraxacum officinale*), butternut bark (*Juglans cinerea*), boldo (*Peumus boldus*), bladderwrack (*Fucus*), excipients.
Uses: increases the activity of the digestive organs, diuretic, use as an aid to slimming in conjunction with a calorie controlled diet.
Special notes:
Caution: do not exceed the stated dose. Large doses of boldo cause vomiting. Not recommended for children.

Buchu Compound
(Gerard House)

Dose: 2 tablets with water 3 times a day.
Product licence: No. 1661/5015R.
Constituents: dandelion root (*Taraxacum officinale*) 60 mg, buchu extract (*Agathosma betulina*) 20 mg, uva ursi (*Arctostaphylos uva-ursi*) extract 20 mg, clivers (*Galium aparine*) extract 4 mg, cayenne (*Capsicum frutescens*) 15 mg, sugar 45 mg, sodium starch glycollate 9 mg, magnesium stearate 1 mg, lactose 52 mg, talc 4 mg, iron oxide as a coating.
Uses: diuretic; buchu acts as an antiseptic to the urinary tract — helpful for recurring cystitis and fluid retention.
Special notes: vegetarian, yeast free.
Caution: not recommended for children. Not to be used in pregnancy or breastfeeding without practitioner supervision.

Calm Night (previously known as Restful Night)
(Seven Seas)

Dose: 1 tablet to be taken 3 times daily after food, plus 3 tablets before going to bed, or 3 tablets with the evening meal and 3 tablets before going to bed.
Product licence: No. PL1907/5015.
Constituents: wild lettuce (*Lactuca virosa*) 10 mg, passionflower (*Passiflora incarnata*) 90 mg, Jamaica dogwood (*Piscidia erythrina*) bark 45 mg, hops (*Humulus lupulus*) 30 mg, aqueous extractives from wild lettuce 90 mg, dicalcium phosphate, maize starch, hydroxypropylmethylcellulose, talc, silica, ethylcellulose, titanium dioxide, iron oxide, glycerol.
Uses: insomnia.
Special notes:
Caution: may cause drowsiness, if affected do not drive or operate machinery. Avoid alcoholic drinks. Should not be taken with other sedatives without consulting medical advice. Those patients with a known hypersensitivity to the Compositae family of plants should exercise caution taking these tablets. Not to be

used for children or during pregnancy or lactation.

Calming Tablets (previously known as Nerve Tablets)
(Seven Seas)

Dose: 2 tablets to be taken 3 times a day with meals.
Product licence: No. PL2210/5066.
Constituents: asafoetida BPC (*Ferula foetida*) oleoresin 24 mg, valerian (*Valerian officinalis*) root 3.02 mg, *Teucrium canadense* 2.16 mg, gentian (*Gentian lutea*) root 1.51 mg, plus aqueous extractives from: scullcap 28 mg, gentian 19 mg, valerian 31.4 mg. Excipients dicalcium phosphate, maize starch, hydroxypropylmethylcellulose, magnesium stearate, talc, silica, ethylcellulose, titanium dioxide, iron oxides, glycerol.
Uses: to reduce anxiety, worry, and nervous tension.
Special notes:
Caution: may cause drowsiness, if affected do not drive or operate machinery. Avoid alcoholic drinks. Should not be taken with other sedatives. If you are already receiving medical treatment, tell your doctor you are taking this product. Not to be used for children or during pregnancy or breastfeeding.

Cascade
(Modern Health)

Dose: 2 tablets to be taken 3 times a day before meals.
Product licence: No. 1146/5005R.
Constituents: burdock root (*Arctium lappa*) 50 mg, uva ursi (*Arctostaphylos uva-ursi*) 75 mg, clivers (*Galium aparine*) 75mg.
Uses: diuretic, antiseptic, soothes, strengthens, and tones urinary tract, for premenstrual water retention, cystitis.
Special notes: not tested on animals.
Caution: prolonged use of uva ursi may cause constipation. Not recommended for children under 12 years or during pregnancy or breastfeeding unless prescribed.

Catarrh Mixture
(Potters)

Dose: adults 1 5 ml teaspoonful 3 times a day;
children over 7 years 1 5 ml teaspoonful morning and evening.
Product licence: No. P/L0250/5051R.
Constituents: boneset (*Eupatorium perfoliatum*), blue flag (*Iris versicolor*), burdock root (*Arctium lappa*), hyssop (*Hyssopus officinalis*), capsicum, excipients.
Uses: to relieve the symptoms of nasal catarrh and catarrh of the throat.
Special notes: sugar free.
Caution:

Catarrh Naturtabs
(Larkhall)
'Cantassium'

Dose: 1-2 tablets 3 times a day with water, preferably after a meal.
Product licence: No. PL0912/7178R.
Constituents: Yarrow (*Achillea millefolium*) extract 6 mg, vervain (*Verbena officinalis*) extract 5 mg, white horehound extract (*Marrubium vulgare*) 6 mg, sage (*Salvia officinalis*) extract 4 mg, calcium phosphate tribasic, calcium sulphate dihydrate, potato starch, vegetable fatty acid.
Uses: upper respiratory tract discomfort and catarrh, especially in winter.
Special notes: vegan, yeast free, hypoallergenic.
Caution: not to be taken by pregnant women, or by anyone being treated for high blood pressure.

Catarrh Pastilles
(Booker)
'Heath & Heather'

Dose: allow a pastille to dissolve in the mouth when needed. Not more than 12 to be taken in 24 hours.

Product licence: P/L1713/5088R.

Constituents: squill vinegar 9.4 %, pumilio pine (*Pinus mugo*) oil 0.6 %, eucalyptus (*Eucalyptus globulus*) oil 0.5 %, sugar, liquid glucose, crystal gum, menthol, beetroot red as colouring, caramel, vegetable fat.

Uses: expectorant, decongestant, to relieve the symptoms of coughs, colds, sore throats, and catarrh.

Special notes: vegan, yeast free.

Caution: not recommended for children. May antidote any homoeopathic remedies you are taking.

Catarrh Tablets
(Booker)
'Heath & Heather'

Dose: 1 tablet 3 times a day.

Product licence: No. P/L1713/509R.

Constituents: white horehound extract (*Marrubium vulgare*) 500 mg, squill (*Drimia maritima*) 30 mg, dicalcium phosphate, microcrystalline cellulose, stearic acid, magnesium stearate; coating: hypromellose, polyethylene glycol, copper chlorophyllin, titanium dioxide.

Uses: to relieve the symptoms of coughs and catarrh.

Special notes: vegan, yeast free.

Caution: not to be taken during pregnancy without practitioner supervision.

Catarrh Tablets
(Seven Seas)

Dose: 2 tablets 3 times a day with meals.

Product licence: No. PL2210/5020.

Constituents: lobelia (*Lobelia inflata*) 31.7 mg, yarrow (*Achillea millefolium*) 3.17 mg, red sage (*Salvia officinalis*) 3.17 mg, boneset (*Eupatorium perfoliatum*) 3.17 mg, white horehound (*Marrubium vulgare*) 3.17 mg, capsicum minimum oleoresin BPC 0.5 mg; plus aqueous extractives from: yarrow 33 mg, vervain (*Verbena officinalis*) 33 mg, red sage 33 mg, boneset 33 mg, white horehound 28.5 mg; excipients dicalcium phosphate, maize starch, hydroxypropylmethylcellulose, talc, silica, ethyl cellulose, titanium dioxide, iron oxides, glycerol.

Uses: the relief of sinus obstruction and catarrh, particulary associated with hayfever.

Special notes:

Caution: do not exceed the stated dose. Should not be used in the presence of any cardiac disease or gastric hyperacidity. Individuals with a known hypersensitivity to yarrow or other members of the Compositae family should exercise caution when taking the tablets, although no instances of a reaction have been reported. Should not be used during pregnancy or breastfeeding. Not recommended for children.

Celery Seed Tablets
(Booker)
'Heath & Heather'

Dose: 1 tablet 3 times a day.
Product licence: No. P/L1713/5026R.
Constituents: celery seed (*Apium graveolens*) extract 600 mg, microcrystalline cellulose, dicalcium phosphate, stearic acid, magnesium stearate; coating hypromellose, glycerin, copper chlorophyllin, curcumin, iron oxide, titanium dioxide.
Uses: relief of rheumatic pain, lumbago, and fibrositis.
Special notes: vegan, yeast free.
Caution: not to be taken in pregnancy without practitioner supervision.

Chamomile Formula
(Bio-Strath: imported by Cedar Health Ltd)

Dose: 10-20 drops (0.3 to 0.6 ml) in a little water every 2 hours.
Product licence: No. PL04210/0001.
Constituents: German camomile flower (*Matricaria chamomilla*) extract 25 %, sage leaf (*Salvia officinalis*) extract 25 %, *Torula utilis* yeast plasmolysate 50 %, (ethanol content 37.6 % v/v approx.).
Uses: to relieve minor acute painful conditions of the mouth and throat — ulcers, gum disorders, irritating dryness of mouth and tongue.
Special notes:
Caution: not recommended during pregnancy without practitioner supervision.

Charcoal
(Potters)

Dose: 1-4 tablets after meals; children over 5 years 1-2 tablets.
Product licence: 0250/5194R.
Constituents: medicinal vegetable charcoal (herbal source).
Uses: acts as an absorbent which is particularly useful for stomach gases; helps flatulence, indigestion, heartburn, dyspepsia.
Special notes:
Caution: may affect absorbtion of other drugs you are taking.

Chest Mixture
(Potters)

Dose: 1 5 ml teaspoonful every 3 hours.
Product licence: No. P/L0250/5000R.
Constituents: horehound (*Marrubium vulgare*), pleurisy root (*Asclepias tuberosa*), senega (*Polygala senega*), lobelia (*Lobelia inflata*), squill (*Drimia maritima*) vinegar.
Uses: expectorant, soothing, to relieve the symptoms of coughs and catarrh of the upper respiratory tract.
Special notes:

Caution: not recommended for children or during pregnancy or breastfeeding. Do not exceed the stated dose, *Lobelia* may cause nausea and vomiting in high doses.

Chlorophyll Tablets
(Potters)

Dose: 1-2 tablets 3 times a day.
Product licence: No. 0250/5126R.
Constituents: kola nut (*Cola acuminata*), chlorophyll, excipients.
Uses: kola nut is used in the manufacture of cola-type drinks. It contains caffeine to give extra energy and relief from temporary tiredness. Chlorophyll was once considered to be a tonic and attracted interest because it bears a chemical similarity to haemoglobin. It is no longer thought to play any active role.
Special notes:
Caution: if tiredness persists, seek medical advice. Stimulants such as caffeine exhaust the body in prolonged use.

Cleansing Herb
(Potters)

Dose: half a level teaspoonful night and morning when required. Vary the dose as required. Place the herb in a mug. Add boiling water. Allow to stand, covered, for 15 minutes. Then drink all of it.
Product licence: No. PL0250/5143R.
Constituents: buckthorn bark (*Rhamnus catharticus*), psyllium (*Plantago ovata*) seeds light, senna leaves tinnevelly (*Cassia angustifolia*).
Uses: the relief of occasional constipation.
Special notes:
Caution: should not be used for prolonged periods without medical advice. Not recommended for children or during pregnancy or breastfeeding. Senna is not to be used in colitis or spastic colon. Senna may colour urine or stools.

Cough Drops
(Weleda)

Dose: 10-20 drops every 2 hours, to be taken in warm water.
Product licence: No. PL0298/5492.
Constituents: per 100 ml angelica (*Archangelica*) root 1.1 %, cinnamon (*Cinnamomum verum*) 1.5 %, clove (*Syzygium aromaticum*) 0.65 %, coriander (*Coriandrum sativum*)0.75 %, lemon (*Citrus limon*) oil 0.06 %, lemon balm (*Melissa*) leaf 4.5 %, nutmeg (*Myristica fragrans*) 2.3 %, aqua cherry laurel (*Laurocerasus*) 11 ml, nominal ethanol content 55 % v/v.
Uses: the relief of irritating coughs.
Special notes:
Caution: do not exceed the stated dose. Not recommended for children or during pregnancy or breastfeeding. May antidote any homoeopathic remedies you are taking.

Cranesbill
(Gerard House)

Dose: 1-2 tablets when necessary 3 times a day with water; children 12 years and over 1 tablet twice a day with water.
Product licence: No. 1661/5004R.
Constituents: wild cranesbill (*Geranium maculatum*) 270 mg, sugar 100 mg, talc 12 mg, magnesium stearate 3 mg, sodium starch glycollate 5 mg, lactose 50 mg, malto-dextrin 80 mg.
Uses: short-term relief of diarrhoea.
Special notes: vegetarian, yeast free.
Caution: not recommended for children under 12 years. Not to be used in pregnancy without practitioner supervision.

Digest
(Modern Health)

Dose: 2 tablets to be taken 3 times a day before meals.
Product licence: No. PL1146/5009R.

Constituents: parsley (*Petroselinum crispum*) 80 mg, centaury (*Centaurium erythraea*) 70 mg, marshmallow root (*Althaea officinalis*) 70 mg, excipients.
Uses: stimulates appetite, reduces flatulence, soothes the stomach, relieves spasm, aids digestion, tonic, relieves inflammation of mouth and stomach.
Special notes: not tested on animals.
Caution: not recommended for children under 12 years nor during pregnancy or breastfeeding unless prescribed.

Diuretabs
(Potters)

Dose: 2 tablets 3 times a day.
Product licence: No. 0250/5167R.
Constituents: buchu leaf (*Agathosma betulina*), juniper (*Juniperus communis*) berry oil, parsley piert (*Aphanes arvensis*), uva ursi (*Arctostaphylos uva-ursi*), excipients.
Uses: diuretic, astringent, soothing, to aid water retention and premenstrual tension.
Special notes:
Caution: not intended for use in more serious conditions caused by poor heart function. The elderly should not use this product for more than a month at a time.

Dual-Lax Extra Strong

As below, but contains 10 mg of aloin powder instead of aloes. This is a crystalline extract of aloes which is more readily absorbed and thus has a stronger action.

Dual-Lax Normal
(Lanes)

Dose: adults 1-3 tablets at night; children (7-14 years) 1 tablet at night.

Product licence: No. 1074/5014R.

Constituents: senna leaf powder B.P. 32 mg, aloes 33 mg, cascara sagrada (*Rhamnus purshiana*) extract 130 mg, calcium phosphate, corn starch, stearic acid, colloidal anhydrous silica, magnesium stearate, sodium starch glycollate, IMS, opaseal, sugar, calcium carbonate, talc, acacia, titanium dioxide, white dispersion, wax polish.

Uses: relief of temporary constipation.

Special notes: vegetarian, yeast free.

Caution: not recommended during pregnancy or breastfeeding nor for children under 7 years. May cause alkaline urine to turn red.

Echinacea
(Gerard House)

Dose: 1-2 tablets 3 times a day after meals.

Product licence: No. 1661/5006R.

Constituents: coneflower (*Echinacea angustifolia*)150 mg, purple coneflower (*Echinacea purpurea*) 52.5 mg, malto-dextrin 117.5 mg, sodium starch glycollate 2.5 mg, magnesium stearate 2.5 mg, talc 5 mg, iron oxide as coating.

Uses: antiseptic, useful for acne, spots, poor skin texture, mild eczema, boils, abscesses, sore throats, tonsillitis.

Special notes: vegan, yeast free.

Caution: not recommended for children under 12 years. Not to be used in pregnancy without practitioner supervision.

Elderflower and Peppermint with Composition Essence
(Potters)

Dose: adults: 2 5 ml teaspoonsful 3 times a day in a third of a cupful of warm water; children over 5 years half the adult dose.

Product licence: P/L0250/5094R.

Constituents: bayberry bark (*Myrica cerifera*), hemlock spruce (*Tsuga canadensis*), elderflowers (*Sambucus*), peppermint

(*Mentha piperita*) oil, syrup.

Uses: stimulant, diaphoretic (encourages perspiration). Elderflowers and peppermint have antiviral and antibacterial properties. Elderflower is anticatarrhal and expectorant, to relieve the symptoms of colds, chills, and sore throats.

Special notes:

Caution: shake the bottle before use. Not recommended for children under 5 years. Peppermint may antidote any homoeopathic remedies you are taking. Do not exceed the stated dose. Bayberry may cause nausea and flatulence in high doses.

Elixir of Damiana and Saw Palmetto
(Potters)

Dose: 2 5 ml teaspoonsful 3 times a day for 1 week, then 1 5 ml teaspoonful 3 times a day.

Product licence: P/L0250/5071R.

Constituents: cornsilk (*Zea mays*), damiana (*Turnera diffusa*), saw palmetto (*Serenoa repens*), excipients.

Uses: tonic and restorative, nutritive, mild stimulant, laxative.

Special notes:

Caution: shake the bottle before use. Not recommended for children. Damiana has a slightly irritant effect on the genito-urinary mucosa. Not recommended in pregnancy or breastfeeding without practitioner supervision.

Epogam
(Scotia)

Dose: 4-6 capsules twice a day; children over 1 year 2-4 capsules twice a day.

Product licence: No. PL4382/0005

Constituents: oil from the pressed seeds of the evening primrose (*Oenothera biennis*) plant supplying GLA 40 mg, gelatin capsule.

Uses: Epogam is licensed as a medicine for the symptomatic relief of atopic eczema.

Possible uses under practitioner prescription/supervision only: a rich source of the essential fatty acid GLA (gamma linolenic acid) which belongs to the Omega-6 group. Therapeutic effect will depend on there being an existing deficiency of GLA. Studies suggest that evening primrose oil may reduce high cholesterol levels, reduce high blood pressure, may help prevent high blood pressure during pregnancy, help with auto-immune diseases, inhibit tumour growth, reduce itching and severity of eczema, reduce allergic response, reduce premenstrual tension including breast tenderness and swelling, help mastalgia, reduce inflammatory response, may help patients with lupus, help multiple sclerosis, may aid weight loss in those who are more than 10 per cent above ideal body weight, reduce Parkinsonian tremor, help Raynaud's syndrome, help rheumatoid arthritis, help scleroderma, in alcoholism may help prevent damage to liver and neurological system and aid withdrawal.

Special notes:

Caution: some patients may experience nausea, diarrhoea or headaches on high doses. Not to be taken by epileptic patients without medical supervision. Not recommended for children under 1 year. GLA can prolong bleeding time in high doses so should be avoided by haemophiliacs and people taking anticoagulants.

Fenulin
(Gerard House)

Dose: 2 tablets after meals 3 times a day.
Product licence: No. 1661/5008R
Constituents: fenugreek (*Trigonella foenum-graecum*) 275 mg, slippery elm (*Ulmus rubra*) 30 mg, golden seal (*Hydrastis*) 5 mg, malto-dextrin 139 mg, talc 16 mg, magnesium stearate 4 mg, sugar 50mg.
Uses: digestive upsets, dyspepsia, soothes irritated tissue.
Special notes: vegan, yeast free.

Caution: Hydrastis is not to be used in pregnancy or breastfeeding. Not recommended for children.

Fragador Tablets
(Weleda)

Dose: 2 tablets 3 times a day.
Product licence: No. PL0298/5512.
Constituents: scurvy grass (*Cochlearia officinalis*) 0.2 mg, conchae 4 mg, wild strawberry (*Fragaria vesca*) fruit 2 mg, glycogen 10x 2 mg, lovage (*Levisticum*) root 5 mg, mel 1x 1 mg, natrum carbonicum 1x 2 mg, aniseed (*Pimpinella anisum*) fruit 3 mg, sage (*Salvia officinalis*) 2 mg, wheat germ 50 mg, stinging nettle (*Urtica dioica*) 10 mg, ferrum phosphoricum 4x 2 mg, excipients.
Uses: to relieve occasional nerviness and edginess brought on by everyday stress and strain.
Special notes:
Caution: not recommended during pregnancy or breastfeeding.

Gardolex
(Modern Health)

Dose: 1 tablet 3 times a day; children 5-12 years 1 tablet before going to bed.
Product licence: No. 1146/5001R.
Constituents: garlic oil 22 mg, marshmallow (*Althaea officinalis*) root 125 mg, parsley (*Petroselinum crispum*) 25 mg, excipients.
Uses: antibacterial, anti-inflammatory, expectorant, for colds, catarrh, and chest infections. See also notes under Garlic Preparations.
Caution: not be used in pregnancy or breastfeeding unless prescribed by a practitioner.

GARLIC PREPARATIONS
Opinions differ regarding the value of fresh garlic compared with that of supplements. It is commonly held that fresh garlic is

the finest and most therapeutic form to take and that the supplements make it convenient to take daily and to reduce odour. There is also some evidence to suggest that too much fresh garlic may irritate or damage the lining of the digestive tract or cause anaemia.

Constituents: oil or powder from garlic (*Allium sativum*) plant.
Uses: garlic is licensed as an over-the-counter medicine to treat the symptoms of colds and catarrh.
Possible uses under practitioner prescription/supervision only: may lower blood pressure; studies suggest significant reduction of cholesterol and triglyceride levels during supplementation. Studies also suggest decreased tendency to thrombosis (formation of blood clots) and increased ability for the body to dissolve existing clots; may help protect against arteriosclerosis, expectorant, helps protect against colds, cleanser, antispasmodic, antibacterial. Studies demonstrate activity against 17 strains of fungus, and high efficacy against pathogenic yeasts, intestinal antiseptic; may help protect against amoebic dysentery and typhoid. Studies suggest possibility of inhibiting tumour growth.
Caution: Gerard House recommends that garlic supplements are not given to young children owing to a possible toxic hazard.

Gardolex
(Modern Health)

See separate entry.

Garlic Perles
(Gerard House)

Capsules of garlic oil 0.972 mg, soya bean oil 411 mg, gelatin 103 mg, glycerin 48mg.
Product licence: No. 1661/5030R.

Garlic Tablets
(Gerard House)

Pulverized garlic 198 mg, garlic oil 60 mg, sugar 55 mg, lactose 50 mg, tricalcium phosphate 10 mg, starch 9 mg, talc 4.5 mg, povidone 3 mg, coating: titanium dioxide 1.5 mg, iron oxide, kaolin, gum Arabic, syrup.
Product licence: No. 1661/5009R.

Garlic Tablets
(Potters)

Garlic powder and garlic oil
Product licence: No. 0250/5228R.

Lusty's Garlic Perles
(Lanes)

Essential oil of garlic 0.66 mg, soya bean oil, gelatin, glycerin.
Product licence: No. 1074/5041R.

Gerard 99
(Gerard House)

Dose: 2 tablets after meals 3 times a day.
Product licence: No. PL1661/5010R.
Constituents: hops (*Humulus lupulus*) 45 mg, passionflower (*Passiflora*) 100 mg, valerian (*Valeriana officinalis*) extract 20 mg, gentian (*Gentiana lutea*) extract 30 mg, malto-dextrin 87.50 mg, sugar 40 mg, talc 4 mg, magnesium stearate 1 mg, sodium starch glycollate 2.5 mg. iron oxide and syrup as coating.
Uses: mild sedative, antispasmodic, to help with restlessness, irritability, nervousness, anxiety, tenseness.
Special notes: vegan, yeast free.
Caution: not to be used in pregnancy. Not recommended for

children under 12 years. May cause drowsiness.

Gladlax
(Gerard House)

Dose: 1-2 tablets as required, to be taken at bedtime.
Product licence: 1661/5011R
Constituents: Cape aloes 50 mg, fennel (*Foeniculum vulgare*) 15 mg, valerian 30 mg, holy thistle (*Cnicus benedictus*) 60 mg, myrrh (*Commiphora molmol*) 15 mg, malto-dextrin 90 mg, sodium starch glycollate 12.5 mg, talc 3 mg, sugar 40 mg, lactose 20 mg, magnesium stearate 1.5 mg, starch 3mg.
Uses: occasional or non-persistent constipation. Aloes acts as a laxative and stool softener, valerian is to reduce and to prevent griping, fennel is anti-inflammatory, holy thistle is to stimulate and aid digestion.
Special notes: vegetarian, yeast free.
Caution: not to be taken with other laxatives, during pregnancy or breastfeeding, or by children under 12 years.

Golden Seal Compound
(Gerard House)

Dose: 2 tablets 3 times a day between meals.
Product licence: No. 1661/5005R.
Constituents: marshmallow (*Althaea officinalis*) root 100 mg, golden seal (*Hydrastis*) 10 mg, cranesbill (*Geranium maculatum*) 30 mg, dandelion root (*Taraxacum officinale*) 60 mg, malto-dextrin 130 mg, talc 5 mg, magnesium stearate 2.50 mg, sodium starch glycollate 2.5 mg, sugar 60 mg, ethyl cellulose as coating.
Uses: indigestion, heartburn, flatulence, nausea, gastric irritation.
Special notes: vegan, yeast free.
Caution: not to be used in pregnancy or breastfeeding. Not recommended for children under 12 years.

Helonias Compound
(Gerard House)

Dose: 1 tablet 3 times a day after meals.
Product licence: No. 1661/5017R.
Constituents: unicorn root (*Helonias*) 120 mg, parsley 60 mg, black cohosh (*Cimicifuga racemosa*) 30 mg, raspberry leaf extract 16.7 mg, chlorophyllin 0.10 mg, malto-dextrin 100 mg, sugar 63.20 mg, talc 6 mg, magnesium stearate 1.5 mg, sodium starch glycollate 2.5 mg, ethyl cellulose as coating.
Uses: diuretic, uterine tonic, to help premenstrual tension with fluid retention, abdominal bloating and tenderness.
Special notes: vegan, yeast free.
Caution: not to be used during pregnancy or breastfeeding. Not to be used for children or for the elderly.

Herbal Powder No. 8
(Gerard House)

Dose: half-a-teaspoon 3 times a day after meals.
Product licence: 1661/5018R.
Constituents: half-a-teaspoonful will deliver approximately dandelion (*Taraxacum officinale*) 528 mg, uva ursi 132 mg, couch grass (*Agopyron repens*) 132 mg, buchu (*Agathosma betulina*) 88 mg.
Uses: diuretic, antiseptic, to relieve fluid retention, cystitis.
Special notes: vegan, yeast free.
Caution: not recommended for children under 12 years. Not to be used in pregnancy without practitioner supervision.

Horehound and Aniseed Cough Mixture
(Potters)

Dose: adults 2 5 ml teaspoonsful 3 times a day; children over 5 years 1 5 ml teaspoonful 3 times a day.
Product licence: P/L0250/5096R.

Constituents: pleurisy root (*Asclepias tuberosa*), elecampane (*Inula helenium*), horehound (*Marrubium vulgare*), skunk cabbage (*Symplocarpus foetidus*), lobelia (*Lobelia inflata*), syrup.
Uses: to relieve coughs.
Special notes:
Caution: not recommended during pregnancy or breastfeeding nor for children under 5 years. Do not exceed the stated dose.

Iceland Moss Compound
(Gerard House)

Dose: 1-2 tablets as necessary every 4 hours; children (5-12 years) 1 tablet each morning and night.
Product licence: No. 1661/5013R.
Constituents: Iceland moss (*Cetraria islandica*) 250 mg, liquorice (*Glycyrrhiza glabra*) 30 mg, lobelia (*Lobelia inflata*) 20 mg, malto-dextrin 100 mg, lactose 100 mg, talc 16 mg, magnesium stearate 4 mg.
Uses: relief of congestion in the respiratory tract, chesty coughs, colds.
Special notes: vegetarian, yeast free.
Caution: not recommended for children under 5 years. Not to be used during pregnancy without practitioner supervision. Do not exceed the stated dose.

Indian Brandee
(Potters)

Dose: 1 5 ml teaspoonful in or with a little water. Repeat once or twice if necessary.
Product licence: P/L0250/5098R.
Constituents: capsicum tincture, strong ginger (*Zingiber officinale*) tincture, compound rhubarb tincture.
Uses: a warming remedy which helps relieve nausea and digestive discomfort.

Special notes:
Caution: not recommended for children or during pregnancy.

Indigestion and Flatulence Naturtabs
(Larkhall)
'Cantassium'

Dose: 1-2 tablets to be taken after meals.
Product licence: No. PL/0912/5997R.
Constituents: capsicin B.P. 30 mg, valerian (*Valeriana officinalis*) extract 14 mg, fennel (*Foeniculum vulgare*) 14 mg, myrrh (*Commiphora molmol*) 19 mg, papain B.P.C. 1 mg, excipients.
Uses: to aid digestive discomfort.
Special notes: vegan, yeast free, hypoallergenic.
Caution: not recommended for children or during pregnancy or breastfeeding.

Indigestion and Flatulence Tablets
(Booker)
'Heath & Heather'

Dose: 2 tablets to be taken with water 3 times a day after meals.
Product licence: No. PL1713/5064R.
Constituents: peppermint (*Mentha piperita*) oil 0.01 ml, fennel (*Foeniculum vulgare*) oil 0.005 ml, capsicum oleoresin 0.1 mg, dicalcium phosphate, microcrystalline cellulose, silica, magnesium stearate, stearic acid.
Uses: to relieve the symptoms of indigestion and flatulence.
Special notes: vegan, yeast free.
Caution: not to be taken during early pregnancy without practitioner supervision. Not recommended for children. May antidote any homoeopathic remedies you are taking. Susceptible individuals may be sensitive to the menthol content of peppermint oil.

Indigestion Mixture
(Potters)

Dose: 1 5 ml teaspoonful after meals 3-4 times a day.
Product licence: No. PL0250/5065R.
Constituents: meadowsweet (*Filipendula ulmaria*) extract, concentrated compound gentian infusion, spindle tree (*Euonymus*) tincture.
Uses: to relieve the symptoms of indigestion, heartburn, and flatulence. Meadowsweet is the herbalist's antacid, gentian and *Euonymus* tone the liver and improve digestive function.
Special notes:
Caution: not recommended for children or during pregnancy or breastfeeding.

Indigestion Naturtabs
(Larkhall)
'Cantassium'.

Dose: 1-2 tablets to be taken after meals.
Product licence: No. PL0912/7313R.
Constituents: myrrh (*Commiphora molmol*) 20 mg, fennel (*Foeniculum vulgare*)15 mg, valerian (*Valeriana officinalis*) extract 4 mg, papain 1.5 mg, capsicin 0.3 mg, calcium carbonate, calcium sulphate dihydrate, sago flour, calcium phosphate tribasic, vegetable fatty acid, magnesium trisilicate.
Uses: to relieve indigestion.
Special notes: vegan, yeast free, hypoallergenic.
Caution: not recommended for children or during pregnancy or breastfeeding.

Inner Fresh Tablets
(Booker)
'Heath & Heather'

Dose: 1-2 tablets to be taken before going to bed.

Product licence: No. P/L1713/5031R.
Constituents: alder buckthorn bark (*Rhamnus frangula*) extract equivalent to total glucofrangulins 20 mg, dicalcium phosphate, microcrystalline cellulose, stearic acid, magnesium stearate, coating: hypromellose, polyethylene glycol, vegetable carbon, titanium dioxide.
Uses: a stimulant laxative for the relief of occasional constipation.
Special notes: vegan, yeast free.
Caution: may cause griping pain in susceptible individuals. Not recommended for children or during pregnancy. Discoloration of the urine, which may occur, is harmless.

Jamaican Sarsaparilla
(Potters)

Dose: 2 5 ml teaspoonsful in water 3 times a day.
Product licence: No. P/L0250/5093R.
Constituents: sarsaparilla (*Smilax reqelii*) root extract, syrup.
Uses: to relieve minor skin complaints, blemishes, and rashes.
Special notes:
Caution: not to be used for children or during pregnancy or breastfeeding without practitioner supervision.

Kalms
(Lanes)

Dose: 2 tablets twice a day after meals and 2 more at bedtime.
Product licence: No. 1074/5045R.
Constituents: valerian (*Valeriana officinalis*) extract 33.75 mg (equivalent to valerian 135 mg), hops (*Humulus lupulus*) 45 mg, gentian (*Gentiana lutea*) extract 22.5 mg (equivalent to gentian 90 mg), corn starch, gum acacia, sugar, sodium starch glycollate, magnesium stearate, vegetable stearic acid, silica, shellac, industrial methylated spirit, calcium carbonate, talc, titanium dioxide, white dispersion, wax polish.
Uses: anxiety, irritability, insomnia, flushing and cold sweats of

Caution: not recommended for children.

Apis mellifica (Apis mel.)
(Weleda 6c, 30c; Nelsons 6c)

Prepared from honey bee venom.

Uses: burning stinging pains, cystitis with constant desire to urinate, arthritis with red, swollen, shiny joints, hot red swelling anywhere in body, swollen ankles, swollen lower eyelids, bites and stings which become red and swollen, allergic reactions (if the reaction is severe or there is difficult breathing, seek medical help immediately), urticaria, symptoms tend to affect the right side of the body most, thirstlessness, burning sore throat.
Suited to: busy, restless people who may become ill after emotional upset.
Symptoms better for: cold bathing, open air.
Symptoms worse for: heat, touch, after sleep, fright, anger, grief, bad news.
Low time: mid-afternoon.

Appetiser Mixture (formerly Tonic and Nervine Essence)
(Potters)

Dose: 1 5 ml teaspoonful 3 times a day in a little water before meals.
Product licence: No. P/L0250/5106R.
Constituents: camomile (*Chamaemelum nobile*), calumba (*Jateorhiza palmata*) root, gentian (*Gentiana lutea*), excipients.
Uses: tonic, to promote appetite and relieve symptoms of flatulence.
Special notes:
Caution: not recommended during pregnancy or breastfeeding, nor for children.

Aproten
(Ultrapharm)

Low-protein, gluten-free preparation supplied as anellini, ditalini, rigatoni, tagliatelle, biscuits, crispbread, flour, bread mix, and cake mix. It is used for patients suffering from phenylketonuria, kidney and liver failure, cirrhosis of the liver, and gastro-enteritic diseases where sensitivity to gluten is present.

Aquasept
(Hough, Hoseason)

A solution used as a disinfectant for skin and body cleansing and disinfecting.

Dose: use as a soap.
Side effects:
Caution: keep out of the eyes.
Not to be used for:
Not to be used with:
Contains: triclosan.
Other preparations:

Aradolene
(Fisons)

A cream used as an analgesic rub to treat rheumatic conditions.

Dose: massage into the affected area 2-3 times a day.
Side effects: may be irritant
Caution:
Not to be used for: areas such as near the eyes, on broken or inflamed skin, or on membranes (such as the mouth).
Not to be used with:
Contains: diethylamine salicylate, capsicum oleoresin, camphor oil, menthol.

Other preparations:

Argentum nitricum (Argent nit.)
(Weleda 6c, 30c; Nelsons 6c)

Prepared from silver nitrate.

Uses: nervousness, anticipatory fear, heartburn, acidity, flatulence, headache relieved by pressure, mental strain, vertigo with buzzing in the ears, tremor, agoraphobia, claustrophobia, nervous diarrhoea, hoarseness.
Suited to: hurried, fidgety, impulsive, nervous people who suffer from anticipatory fear.
Symptoms better for: open air, cold bathing.
Symptoms worse for: anticipatory fear, overwork, overstudy, sugar, ice-cream, warmth.
Low time: night.

Arnica
(Weleda 6x, 6c, 30c; Nelsons 6c)

Prepared from entire *Arnica montana* plant (mountain tobacco).

Uses: after physical shock or injury; bruises, sprains, exhaustion, jet lag, aching muscles; body feeling sore and bruised all over, concussion, haemorrhages, compound fractures.
Symptoms better for: lying down with head low.
Symptoms worse for: touch, movement, cold, damp.
Low time:

Arnica Lotion
(Weleda)

Dose: dilute one dessertspoonful in ½ pint of water and bathe the affected part, or apply as a compress. A tablespoonful in a

warm bath will help relieve aching muscles after exercise.
Product licence: No. PL0298/5685.
Constituents: arnica (*Arnica montana*) ethanolic extract (1=5), nominal ethanol content 30 %.
Uses: to relieve muscular pain, stiffness, sprains, bruises, immediate application will help prevent bruising.
Caution: shake the bottle before use; do not apply to broken skin.

Arnica Massage Balm
(Weleda)

Dose: massage into affected part 3-4 times a day as required.
Product licence: No. PL0298/5528.
Constituents: per 100 ml: *Arnica* flowers 3 g, birch (*Betula verrucosa*) leaves 3 g, rosemary (*Rosmarinus officinalis*) oil 4 ml, lavender (*Lavendula angustifolia*) oil 2 ml, base.
Uses: bruising, stiffness, backache, sciatica, fibrositis, rheumatic pain; when used daily from the second month of pregnancy it can help prevent stretch marks.
Caution: do not apply to broken skin.

Arnica Ointment
(Weleda)

Dose: apply sparingly to the affected part as soon as possible after the injury; repeat 3-4 times a day or as required.
Constituents: per 100g: arnica (*Arnica montana*) tincture (1=2) 10 ml, lanolin, beeswax, vegetable oils.
Uses: bruises, sprains, strains, muscular pain, swelling, stiffness.
Caution: do not apply to broken skin. Some individuals may be sensitive to lanolin.

Arret
(Janssen)

A capsule used to treat diarrhoea.

Dose: up to 8 capsules daily.
Availability;
Side effects: rashes
Caution: in severe colitis.
Not to be used for: children.
Not to be used with:
Contains: loperamide.
Other preparations: Imodium capsules and syrup on prescription.

Arsenicum album (Arsen. alb.)
(Weleda 6c, 30c; Nelsons 6c)

Prepared from the white oxide of metallic arsenic.

Uses: food poisoning, holiday stomach upsets, sudden violent vomiting and diarrhoea, restlessness, icy chills, burning pains especially throat or stomach, anxiety, fear, insomnia with overactive mind and anxious dreams.
Suited to: patients who are tidy, fastidious, precise, and anxious.
Symptoms better for: heat, cool air around head.
Symptoms worse for: cold, cold food and drinks.
Low time: after midnight.

Artichoke Formula
(Bio-Strath: imported by Cedar Health Ltd)

Dose: 20 drops (0.6 ml) in a little water 3 times a day before meals.
Product licence: No. PL4210/0004.

Constituents: artichoke (*Cynara scolymus*) leaf extract 22.5 %, thistle seed (*Carduus marianus*) extract 22.5 %, peppermint (*Mentha piperita*) leaf extract 5 %, *Torula utilis* yeast plasmolysate 50 %, (ethanol content 38 % v/v approx.).
Uses: to relieve the symptoms of indigestion after eating fatty foods
Special notes:
Caution: may antidote any homoeopathic remedies which you are taking.

Ascabiol
(M & B)

An emulsion used as an insect-destroying preparation to treat scabies, pediculosis.

Dose:
Side effects: irritation.
Caution: keep out of the eyes.
Not to be used for:
Not to be used with:
Contains: benzyl benzoate.
Other preparations:

Asilone
(Rorer)

A white liquid used as an antacid, anti-wind preparation to treat gastritis, ulcers, dyspepsia, wind.

Dose: adults 5-10 ml before meals and at bedtime; children use infant suspension or half adult dose.
Side effects: few; occasionally constipation.
Caution:
Not to be used for: infants.
Not to be used with:

Contains: activated dimethicone, aluminium hydroxide gel, magnesium oxide.
Other preparations: Asilone Gel, Asilone Infant Suspension, Asilone Tablets; Infacol (Pharmax); Polycrol Gel and Tablets, Polycrol Forte Gel (Nicholas); Unigest (Unigreg) — private prescription and over the counter only; Siloxyl (Martindale) — private prescription and over the counter only.

Aspellin
(Fisons)

A liniment or a spray used as a topical analgesic to treat muscular rheumatism, sciatica, lumbago, fibrositis, chilblains.

Dose: massage gently into the affected area every 3-4 hours.
Side effects: may be irritant.
Caution:
Not to be used for: areas near the eyes, or where the skin is broken or inflamed, or on membranes (such as the mouth).
Not to be used with:
Contains: aspirin, menthol, camphor, methyl salicylate.
Other preparations:

---

aspirin

A white tablet supplied at a strength of 300 mg and used as an analgesic to relieve pain and reduce fever.

Dose: 1-3 tablets every 4-6 hours as needed to a maximum of 12 tablets a day.
Side effects: stomach upsets, allergy, asthma.
Caution: in pregnant women, the elderly, or in patients with a history of allergy to aspirin, asthma, impaired kidney or liver function, indigestion.
Not to be used for: children, nursing mothers, or for patients suffering from haemophilia or ulcers.

Not to be used with: anticoagulants (blood-thinning drugs), some antidiabetic drugs, anti-inflammatory agents, methotrexate, spironolactone, steroids, some antacids, some uric-acid lowering drugs.
Contains:
Other preparations: dispersible aspirin.

AT 10
(Sterling Research Laboratories)

A solution used as a source of vitamin D to treat vitamin D deficiency.

Dose: 1-7 ml taken by mouth each week.
Side effects: loss of appetite, listlessness, vertigo, stupor, nausea, urgent need to urinate.
Caution: in nursing mothers. Your doctor may advise that your calcium levels should be checked regularly.
Not to be used for: children.
Not to be used with:
Contains: dihydrotachysterol.
Other preparations:

Athera
(Modern Health)

Dose: 2-3 tablets to be taken 3 times a day after meals.
Product licence: No. 2452/5001R.
Constituents: parsley (*Petroselinum crispum*) 60 mg, vervain (*Verbena officinalus*) 10 mg, vervain extract 90 mg, clivers (*Galium aparine*) extract 60 mg, senna leaf 4 mg, senna extract 10 mg, excipients.
Uses: for menopausal symptoms, to ease fluid retention, soothe the stomach, relax, increase vitality, tone the system, maintain healthy bowel action.
Special notes: not tested on animals.

Caution: may occasionally cause diarrhoea, not recommended for children or during pregnancy or breastfeeding. Senna is not to be used in colitis or spastic colon. Senna may harmlessly colour the urine or stools.

Audax
(Napp Consumer)

Drops used as an analgesic to relieve pain associated with acute inflammation of the outer or middle ear..

Dose: fill the ear with the liquid and plug it.
Side effects:
Caution:
Not to be used for:
Not to be used with:
Contains: choline salicylate.
Other preparations:

Auralgicin
(Fisons)

A liquid used as an antibacterial treatment for inflammation of the middle ear.

Dose: fill the ear with the liquid every hour and plug until the pain is relieved, and then treat every 3 hours for 24 hours.
Side effects:
Caution:
Not to be used for:
Not to be used with:
Contains: ephedrine hydrochloride, benzocaine, chlorbutol, potassium hydroxyquinolone sulphate, phenazone, glycerin.
Other preparations:

Auraltone
(Fisons)

Drops used as an analgesic, local anaesthetic treatment for acute inflammation of the eardrum or inner ear.

Dose: fill the ear with the drops and plug lightly, repeating every hour if needed.
Side effects: skin eruptions.
Caution:
Not to be used for:
Not to be used with:
Contains: phenazone, benzocaine.
Other preparations:

Avena Sativa Comp.
(Weleda)

Dose: 10-20 drops to be taken in water half an hour before going to bed. If necessary this dose may be repeated; children: half the adult dose.
Product licence: No. PL0298/5473.
Constituents: per 100 ml: oats (*Avena sativa*) tincture 25 ml, hops (*Humulus lupulus*) 1x 4 ml, passionflower (*Passiflora incarnata*) tincture 7.5 ml, valerian (*Valeriana officinalis*) tincture 30 ml, *Coffea tosta* 60x 15 ml, nominal ethanol content 45 % v/v.
Uses: to aid relaxation at the end of the day.
Special notes:
Caution: may cause sleepiness. Not recommended during pregnancy or breastfeeding.

Avomine
(Wellcome)

A white, scored tablet supplied at a strength of 25 mg and used

as an antihistamine treatment for travel sickness, nausea, vomiting, vertigo.

Dose: adults travel sickness 1 tablet at bedtime before long journeys or 1-2 hours before short journeys, nausea 1 tablet 1-3 times a day; children 5-10 years half adult dose.
Side effects: drowsiness, reduced reactions, rarely skin eruptions.
Caution: in patients suffering from liver or kidney disease.
Not to be used for: children under 5 years.
Not to be used with: alcohol, sedatives, some antidepressants (MAOIs).
Contains: promethazine, theoclate.
Other preparations:

Backache Tablets
(Potters)

Dose: 2 tablets 3 times a day.
Product licence: No. 0250/5182R
Constituents: gravel root (*Eupatorium purpureum*), hydrangea (*Hydrangea arborescens*) root, buchu (*Agathosma betulina*), uva ursi (*Arctostaphylos uva-ursi*), excipients.
Uses: relief of backache; this formula arises from the herbalist's view that the urinary system must also be toned effectively to deal with backache.
Special notes:
Caution: not recommended during pregnancy nor for children.

Bacticlens
(S & N)

A solution in a sachet used as a disinfectant to clean the skin, wounds, or broken skin.

Dose: use as needed.

Side effects: throw away any remaining solution straight away after use.
Caution:
Not to be used for:
Not to be used with:
Contains: chlorhexidine gluconate.
Other preparations:

Balm of Gilead
(Potters)

Dose: adults: 2 5 ml teaspoonsful 3-4 times a day; children over 5 years 1 5 ml teaspoonful, which may be diluted with water if necessary, 3-4 times a day.
Product licence: No. P/L0250/5085R.
Constituents: acetum scillae (squill vinegar), lobelia (*Lobelia inflata*) tincture, balm of Gilead (*Populus candicans*), lungwort, (*Pulmonaria officinalis*), excipients.
Uses: expectorant, to relieve symptoms of coughs and colds.
Special notes: sugar-free base — concentrated apple juice is used as sweetener.
Caution: shake bottle before use. Not recommended during pregnancy or breastfeeding nor for children under 5 years. Do not exceed the stated dose — high doses of *Lobelia* may cause nausea and vomiting.

Balm of Gilead Cough Mixture
(Booker)
'Heath & Heather'

Dose: 2 5 ml teaspoonsful 3 times a day.
Product licence: No. PL1713/5083R.
Constituents: per 10 ml balm of Gilead (*Populus candicans*) liquid extract 0.8 ml, squill (*Drimia maritima*) tincture 0.25 ml, lobelia (*Lobelia inflata*) tincture 0.2 ml, sugar syrup, xanthum gum, nipastat sodium.

Uses: to relieve symptoms of coughs and catarrh.
Special notes: vegan, yeast free.
Caution: shake before use. Not recommended during pregnancy or breastfeeding nor for children. Do not exceed the stated dose — high doses of *Lobelia* may cause nausea and vomiting.

Balm of Gilead Cough Pastilles
(Booker)
'Heath & Heather'

Dose: allow a pastille to dissolve in the mouth when needed. Not more than 12 to be taken in 24 hours.
Product licence: No. P/L1713/5084R.
Constituents: balm of Gilead (*Populus candicans*) buds 8 %, squill (*Drimia maritima*) tincture 2.5 %, lobelia (*Lobelia inflata*) tincture 2 %, sugar, liquid glucose, gelatin, liquorice (*Glycyrrhiza glabra*), beetroot red as colouring, anise oil as flavouring, peppermint oil, caramel, vegetable fat.
Uses: to relieve the symptoms of coughs and catarrh.
Special notes: yeast free.
Caution: not recommended for children or during pregnancy or breastfeeding. Do not exceed the stated dose — high doses of *Lobelia* may cause nausea and vomiting. May antidote any homoeopathic remedies you are taking.

Balmosa
(Pharmax)

A cream used as an analgesic rub to treat muscular rheumatism, fibrositis, lumbago, sciatica, unbroken chilblains.

Dose: massage into the affected area as needed.
Side effects: may be irritant
Caution:
Not to be used for: areas near the eyes, on broken or inflamed

skin, or on membranes (such as the mouth).
Not to be used with:
Contains: menthol, camphor, methyl salicylate, capsicum oleoresin.
Other preparations:

Balneum with Tar
(Merck)

A bath oil used as an emollient and antipsoriatic to treat eczema, itchy or thickening skin disorders, psoriasis.

Dose: adults add 4 5 ml teaspoonsful to the bath water; children over 2 years add 2 teaspoonsful and use for a maximum of 6 weeks.
Side effects:
Caution:
Not to be used for: children under 2 years or for patients suffering from wet or weeping skin problems or where the skin is badly broken.
Not to be used with:
Contains: coal tar, soya oil.
Other preparations:

Balsamicum Ointment
(Weleda)

Dose: apply directly to the affected part or on a dry dressing several times a day.
Product licence: No. PL0298/5474.
Constituents: per 100 g: marigold (*Calendula officinalis*) ethanolic extract from 3 g of herb, dog's mercury (*Mercurialis perennis*) ethanolic extract from 5 g of herb, balsam of Peru B.P.C. 0.7 g, Stibium Metallicum Praeparatum 0.05 g, lanolin, beeswax, vegetable oils, yellow soft paraffin.
Uses: to aid healing of abrasions, boils, nappy rash, minor

wounds.
Caution: some individuals may be sensitive to lanolin.

Baltar
(Merck)

A liquid used as an antipsoriatic treatment for psoriasis, dandruff, eczema, dermatoses of the scalp.

Dose: shampoo the hair with the liquid 1-3 times a week.
Side effects:
Caution: keep out of the eyes.
Not to be used for: children under 2 years or for patients suffering from wet or weeping dermatoses or where the skin is badly broken.
Not to be used with:
Contains: coal tar.
Other preparations:

Balto Foot Balm
(Lanes)

Dose: massage into feet after bathing; use morning and evening as required.
Product licence: No. PLO1074/5003R.
Constituents: sulphur 3.0 %, camphor 0.5 %, menthol 0.2 %, zinc oxide 0.47 %, pine oil, seaweed extract, chlorbutol, emulsifying wax, white soft paraffin, lanolin, glycerin, sodium lauryl ether sulphate, chlorophyll, industrial methylated spirit.
Uses: soothes tired aching feet, curbs excessive perspiration, softens hard skin.
Caution: may antidote any homoeopathic remedies you are taking. Avoid contact with silver or other jewellery. Some individuals may be sensitive to lanolin.

Banocide
(Wellcome)

A white, scored tablet supplied at a strength of 50 mg and used as an anti-worm agent to treat worms in the blood and lymph channels.

Dose: as advised by the physician.
Side effects: itchy skin, eye disorders.
Caution: your doctor may advise regular eye tests.
Not to be used for: pregnant women.
Not to be used with:
Contains: diethylcarbamazine.
Other preparations:

Bayolin
(Bayer)

A cream used as an analgesic rub to treat rheumatism, fibrositis, lumbago, sciatica.

Dose: massage gently into the affected area 2-3 times a day.
Side effects: may be irritant.
Caution:
Not to be used for: areas near the eyes, broken or inflamed skin, or on membranes (such as the mouth).
Not to be used with:
Contains: heparinoid, glycol salicylate, benzyl nicotinate.
Other preparations:

BC 500
(Wyeth)

An orange, oblong tablet used as a multivitamin preparation to treat vitamin B and vitamin C deficiencies, and to aid recovery from illness, long-term alcoholism, long-term antibiotic treatment.

Dose: 1 tablet a day.
Side effects:
Caution:
Not to be used for: children.
Not to be used with: levodopa.
Contains: thiamine mononitrate, riboflavine, pyridoxine hydrochloride, nicotinamide, calcium pantothenate, ascorbic acid, cyanocoblamin.
Other preparations:

BC 500 with Iron
(Wyeth)

A red tablet used as a vitamin and iron supplement to treat iron deficiency anaemia.

Dose: 1 tablet a day.
Side effects: nausea, constipation.
Caution:
Not to be used for: children.
Not to be used with: tetracyclines, levodopa.
Contains: ferrous fumarate, thiamine mononitrate, riboflavine, pyridoxine hydrochloride, nicotinamide, calcium pantothenate, ascorbic acid.
Other preparations:

Becalm
(Heath & Heather)

Dose: 1 tablet 3 times a day with water.
Product licence: P/L1713/500R.
Constituents: valerian (*Valeriana officinalis*) extract equivalent to 160 mg, hops (*Humulus lupulus*) extract equivalent to 200 mg, passionflower (*Passiflora*) extract equivalent to 130 mg, dicalcium phosphate, microcrystalline cellulose, stearic acid, magnesium stearate; coating titanium dioxide, iron oxide,

polyethylene glycol.
Uses: sedative, to aid relaxation and calm.
Special notes: vegan, yeast free.
Caution: not recommended for children or during pregnancy or breastfeeding. May cause drowsiness, if affected do not drive or operate machinery and avoid alcohol.

Becosym
(Roche)

A brown tablet used as a source of B vitamins to treat vitamin B deficiencies.

Dose: adults 1-3 tablets a day; children use syrup.
Side effects:
Caution:
Not to be used for:
Not to be used with: levodopa.
Contains: thiamine, riboflavine, pyridoxine, nicotinamide.
Other preparations: Becosym Syrup (not available on NHS), Becosym Forte Tablets (not available on NHS).

Beecham's Powders

Beecham's Powders contain aspirin and caffeine; powder capsules have paracetamol, caffeine, and phenylephrine. Beecham's Hot Lemon is paracetamol with ascorbic acid (vitamin C). The main caution is to observe total daily dose of asprin or paracetamol.

Belladonna
(Weleda 6c, 30c; Nelsons 6c)

Prepared from entire *Atropa belladonna* (deadly nightshade) plant when beginning to flower.

Uses: severe throbbing headache, sudden fevers with flushed face and dilated pupils, excitability during fever, skin is dry hot and burning, sunstroke, throbbing earache, acne, acute local inflammations which are red and throbbing; symptoms tend to be on right side of body.

Suited to: lively, cheerful, excitable children or adults who become restless and agitated when ill.

Symptoms better for: warmth, sitting upright.

Symptoms worse for: touch, movement, noise, sun.

Low time: mid-afternoon.

Bellocarb
(Sinclair)

A beige tablet used as an antacid and anti-spasm treatment for bowel spasm, ulcers, dyspepsia.

Dose: 1-2 tablets 4 times a day.

Side effects: few; occasional constipation.

Caution: in patients suffering from enlarge prostate, heart, kidney, or liver problems.

Not to be used for: patients suffereing from glaucoma.

Not to be used with:

Contains: belladonna, magnesium trisilicate, magnesium carbonate.

Other preparations:

Benerva
(Roche)

A white tablet supplied in strengths of 25 mg, 50 mg, 100 mg and used as a source of vitamin B_1 to treat beri-beri, neuritis.

Dose: 25-50 mg a day.

Side effects:

Caution:

Not to be used for:
Not to be used with: levodopa.
Contains: thiamine hydrochloride.
Other preparations: Benerva Compound.

Benoxyl 5
(Stiefel)

A cream used as an antibacterial and skin softener to treat acne.

Dose: wash and dry the affected area, then apply once a day.
Side effects: irritation, peeling.
Caution: keep out of the eyes, nose, and mouth.
Not to be used for:
Not to be used with:
Contains: benzoyl peroxide.
Other preparations: Benoxyl 5 with Sulphur, Benoxyll 10, Benoxyl 10 with Sulphur.

Benylin Day and Night

Benylin Day and Night contains paracetamol and is a useful tablet preparation for treating the common cold.

Side effects: drowsiness, reduced reactions.
Caution: in patients suffering from liver or kidney disease.

Benylin Expectorant
(Warner-Lambert)

A syrup used as an antihistamine, expectorant, and sputum softener to treat cough, bronchial congestion.

Dose: adults 1-2 5 ml teaspoonsful every 2-3 hours; children 1-5 years ½ teaspoonful every 3-4 hours, 6-12 years 1 teaspoon-

ful every 3-4 hours.
Side effects:
Caution:
Not to be used for: children under 1 year.
Not to be used with:
Contains: diphenhydramine hydrochloride, ammonium chloride, sodium citrate, menthol.
Other preparations: Benylin Paediatric, Benylin Decongestant, Benylin with Codeine.

Benzagel
(Bioglan)

A white gel used as an antibacterial and skin softener to treat acne.

Dose: wash and dry the affected area, then apply 1-2 times a day.
Side effects: irritation, peeling.
Caution: keep out of the eyes, nose, and mouth.
Not to be used for:
Not to be used with:
Contains: benzoyl peroxide.
Other preparations:

Betadine
(Cilag)

A pessary and applicator supplied at a strength of 200 mg and used as an antiseptic to treat inflammation of the vagina.

Dose: 1 pessary to be inserted into the vagina night and morning for at least 14 days.
Side effects: irritation and sensitivity.
Caution:
Not to be used for: children.

Not to be used with:
Contains: povidone-iodine.
Other preparations: Betadine Vaginal Gel, Betadine VC Kit.

Betadine Gargle and Mouthwash
(Napp)

A solution used as an antiseptic to treat inflammation of the mouth and pharynx brought on by thrush and other bacterial infections.

Dose: wash out the mouth or gargle with the diluted or undiluted solution every 2-4 hours.
Side effects: rarely local irritation and sensitivity.
Caution:
Not to be used for:
Not to be used with:
Contains: povidone-iodine.
Other preparations:

Betadine Ointment
(Napp)

An ointment used as an antiseptic to treat ulcers.

Dose: apply to the affected area and cover once a day.
Side effects: rarely irritation.
Caution: in patients sensitive to iodine.
Not to be used for:
Not to be used with:
Contains: povidone-iodine.
Other preparations:

Betadine Scalp and Skin Cleanser
(Napp)

A solution used as an antiseptic and detergent to treat acne, seborrhoeic scalp and skin disorders.

Dose: use as a shampoo or apply directly to the skin and then cleanse properly.
Side effects: rarely irritation or sensitivity.
Caution:
Not to be used for:
Not to be used with:
Contains: povidone-iodine.
Other preparations: Betadine Skin Cleanser, Betadine Shampoo.

Betadine Spray
(Napp)

A spray used as an antiseptic to treat infected cuts, wounds, and burns.

Dose: spray on to the affected area once a day or as needed, and cover.
Side effects:
Caution: keep out of the eyes.
Not to be used for: patients suffering from non-toxic colloid goitre
Not to be used with:
Contains: povidone-iodine.
Other preparations: Betadine Dry Powder, Betadine Antiseptic Paint, Betadine Antiseptic Solution, Betadine Alcoholic Solution, Betadine Surgical Scrub.

Bi-Aglut
(Ultrapharm)

Gluten-free preparation supplied as a biscuit. It is used for patients suffering from gastro-enteritic diseases where sensitivity to gluten is present.

Other preparations: Bi-Aglut Cracker Toast.

Biobalm Powder
(Modern Health)

Dose: 1-2 level teaspoons to be taken up to 4 times a day; children 5-12 years half the above dosage.
Product licence: No. 1146/5004R.
Constituents: Per 100 g slippery elm bark (*Ulmus rubra*) 13 g, marshmallow root (*Althaea officinalis*) 8 g, Irish moss (*Chondrus crispus*) 6 g, camomile, barley flour, excipients.
Uses: indigestion, flatulence, soothes gastro-intestinal lining.
Special notes: vegetarian.
Caution:

Biophyllin
(Gerard House)

Dose: 2 tablets after meals 3 times a day.
Product licence: No. 1661/5000R.
Constituents: valerian (*Valeriana officinalis*) 150 mg, scullcap (*Scutellaria lateriflora*)108 mg, Jamaican dogwood (*Piscidia erythrina*) 9 mg, black cohosh (*Cimicifuga racemosa*) 30 mg, cayenne (*Capsicum frutescens*) 3 mg, malto-dextrin 140 mg, calcium phosphate 50 mg, sugar 40 mg, sodium starch glycollate 20 mg, magnesium stearate 2 mg, talc 8 mg.
Uses: nervousness, tension, restlessness, irritability.
Special notes: vegan, yeast free.
Caution: not to be used during pregnancy or breastfeeding, not recommended for children under 12 years.

Biophylline
(Delandale)

A syrup used as a bronchodilator to treat bronchial spasm.

Dose: adults 1-2 5 ml teaspoonsful every 6-8 hours; children 2-6 years ½ 5 ml teaspoonsful every 6-8 hours, 6-12 years ½-1 5 ml teaspoonful every 6-8 hours.
Side effects: rapid heart rate, stomach upset, headache, sleeplessness, nausea, abnormal rhythms.
Caution: in the elderly, pregnant women, nursing mothers, and in patients suffering from heart or liver disease or peptic ulcer.
Not to be used for:
Not to be used with: cimetidine, erythromycin, ciprofloxacin, interferon.
Contains: theophylline hydrate.
Other preparations:

Bioral
(Winthrop)

A gel used as a cell-surface protector to treat mouth ulcers.

Dose: apply after meals and at bed time.
Side effects:
Caution:
Not to be used for:
Not to be used with:
Contains: carbenoxolone sodium.
Other preparations:

Blue Flag Root Compound
(Gerard House)

Dose: 1 tablet after meals 3 times a day.
Product licence: No. 1661/5002R.
Constituents: blue flag (flag lily) (*Iris versicolor*) 90 mg, burdock (*Arctium lappa*) extract 46 mg, sarsaparilla (*Smilax ornata*) extract 35 mg, sugar 100 mg, lactose 40 mg, sodium starch

glycollate 10 mg, talc 3.8 mg, magnesium stearate 0.9 mg, starch 1500 2.8 mg.
Uses: minor acne, eczema, dermatitis.
Special notes: vegetarian, yeast free.
Caution: not recommended for children under 12 years, not to be used in pregnancy.

Bocasan
(Oral-B)

A sachet of white granules used as a disinfectant to treat gingivitis and mouth infections.

Dose: dissolve a sachet of granules in warm water and rinse out the mouth 3 times a day after meals.
Side effects:
Caution:
Not to be used for: patients suffering from kidney disease.
Not to be used with:
Contains: sodium perborate monohydrate, sodium hydrogen tartrate.
Other preparations:

Boldo Herbal Aid for Slimmers
(Larkhall)
'Cantassium'

Dose: 1-2 tablets 3 times a day after meals.
Product licence: No. PLO912/7342R.
Constituents: boldo (*Peumus boldus*) extract 64.8 mg, clivers (*Galium aparine*) extract 24.4 mg, dandelion (*Taraxacum officinale*) root 24.4 mg, uva ursi (*Arctostaphylos uva-ursi*) extract 32.4 mg, bladderwrack (*Fucus vesiculosus*) 45.8 mg, dicalcium phosphate 0.2358 g, magnesium stearate 1.6 mg, stearic acid (palm oil) 1.6 mg, potato starch 15 mg, talc 5 mg.
Uses: for women who experience water retention.

Special notes: vegan, yeast free, hypoallergenic.
Caution: not to be used in pregnancy or breastfeeding without practitioner supervision. Not recommended for children. Do not exceed the stated dose, large doses of boldo cause vomiting.

Boldo Herbal Aid to Slimming
(Potters)

Dose: 1-2 tablets 3 times a day; elderly: 1 tablet 3-4 times a day.
Product licence: No. 0250/5200R.
Constituents: dandelion root (*Taraxacum officinale*), butternut bark (*Juglans cinerea*), boldo (*Peumus boldus*), bladderwrack (*Fucus*), excipients.
Uses: increases the activity of the digestive organs, diuretic, use as an aid to slimming in conjunction with a calorie controlled diet.
Special notes:
Caution: do not exceed the stated dose. Large doses of boldo cause vomiting. Not recommended for children.

Bonjela

Bonjela is a mouth ointment which contains choline salicylate (related to aspirin), chloride, menthol, alcohol, and glycerin. It is useful for mouth ulcers and teething problems. Small quantities should be applied every four hours because large quantities may deliver too much aspirin, especially to children.

Bradosol
(Ciba)

A white lozenge supplied at a strength of 0.5 mg and used as a disinfectant to treat infections of the mouth and throat.

Dose: 1 lozenge to be sucked every 2-3 hours.

Side effects: rarely local irritation and sensitivity.
Caution:
Not to be used for:
Not to be used with:
Contains: domiphen bromide.
Other preparations: Bradosol Plus.

Brasivol
(Stiefel)

A paste used as an abrasive to treat acne.

Dose: wet the area, then rub in vigorously for 15-20 seconds, rinse and repeat 1-3 times a day.
Side effects:
Caution:
Not to be used for: patients suffering from visible superficial arteries or veins on the skin.
Not to be used with:
Contains: aluminium oxide.
Other preparations:

Brolene Eye Drops
(Fisons)

These contain propamidine isethionate 0.1%, benzalkonium chloride 0.1%. An ointment is also available. These substances disinfect the eye and reduce redness. They may cause some local stinging and should not be used if redness of the eye persists or worsens. Allergies often in the eyes, particularly hay fever, cosmetic and dust allergies.

Brovon
(Torbet)

A solution used as a bronchodilator to treat bronchial spasm brought on by chronic bronchitis, bronchial asthma, emphysema.

Dose: inhale 1-2 times a day and once at night.
Side effects: nervousness, tremor, dry mouth, abnormal heart rhythms.
Caution: in patients suffering from diabetes.
Not to be used for: children or for patients suffering from heart disease, high blood pressure, overactive thyroid gland.
Not to be used with: sympathomimetics.
Contains: adrenaline, atropine methonitrate, papaverine hydrochloride.
Other preparations:

Bryonia
(Weleda 6c, 30c; Nelsons 6c)

Prepared from root of *Bryonia alba* plant (white bryony).

Uses: dry, painful, irritating cough, dry mucous membranes, dry lips, fevers which develop slowly over a few days, irritability, mastitis, arthritis, sharp stitching pains; headache accompanies many acute complaints and patient will often be very thirsty.
Suited to: lean, dark-haired people.
Symptoms better for: keeping absolutely still, lying on painful side, pressure, fresh air, cold, cold food and drinks.
Symptoms worse for: movement, touch, warmth.
Low time: mid-evening.

Buchu Compound
(Gerard House)

Dose: 2 tablets with water 3 times a day.
Product licence: No. 1661/5015R.

Constituents: dandelion root (*Taraxacum officinale*) 60 mg, buchu extract (*Agathosma betulina*) 20 mg, uva ursi (*Arctostaphylos uva-ursi*) extract 20 mg, clivers (*Galium aparine*) extract 4 mg, cayenne (*Capsicum frutescens*) 15 mg, sugar 45 mg, sodium starch glycollate 9 mg, magnesium stearate 1 mg, lactose 52 mg, talc 4 mg, iron oxide as a coating.
Uses: diuretic; buchu acts as an antiseptic to the urinary tract — helpful for recurring cystitis and fluid retention.
Special notes: vegetarian, yeast free.
Caution: not recommended for children. Not to be used in pregnancy or breastfeeding without practitioner supervision.

Cafadol
(Typharm)

A yellow, scored tablet used as an analgesic to relieve pain including period pain.

Dose: adults 2 tablets every 3-4 hours; children 5-12 years half adult dose.
Side effects:
Caution: in patients with liver or kidney disease.
Not to be used for: children under 5 years.
Not to be used with:
Contains: paracetamol, caffeine.
Other preparations:

Caladryl see **Calamine lotion**

Calamine lotion

Calamine lotion is a zinc-containing pink solution which is especially useful in chicken pox to reduce itch. It can also be used in other irritating skin conditions. Other preparations of calamine include Caladryl (also contains an antihistamine and camphor) and Eczederm.

Calcarea carbonica (Calc. Carb.)
(Weleda 6c, 30c; Nelsons 6c)

Prepared from calcium carbonate from middle layer of oyster shell.

Uses: obesity, cold extremities, cracked itching skin, profuse sour perspiration especially on head, vertigo, anxiety, indigestion, poor assimilation of nutrients, swollen glands, premenstrual tension, insomnia, menses early, profuse, painful, and protracted, constipation; children — difficult and delayed dentition, head sweats, slow closure of fontanelles, poor calcium absorption.
Suited to: fair-haired, timid patients who tend to put on weight easily.
Symptoms better for: dry weather, lying on painful side.
Symptoms worse for: cold, damp, draughts, teething, drinking milk, exertion, standing.
Low time:

Calcarea fluorica (Calc. fluor.)
(New Era 6x; Weleda 6c, 30c; Nelsons 6c)

Prepared from calcium fluoride.

Uses: promotes elasticity of tissues; varicose veins, stretch marks, arthritis, prevention of adhesions after surgery, haemorrhoids, croup, head colds with discharge, catarrh, deficient enamel of teeth.
Symptoms better for: movement, warmth.
Symptoms worse for: rest, damp.
Low time:

Calcarea phosphorica (Calc. phos.)
(New Era 6x; Weleda 6c, 30c; Nelsons 6c)

Prepared from tricalcic phosphate.

Uses: adolescents lacking energy and concentration, emaciation, cough with yellow mucus, stomach pains after eating,
acne, enlarged adenoids, headache from overstudying, swollen glands, chronic catarrh, non-union of fractures, debility
remaining after acute disease.
Suited to: general debility with discontent.
Symptoms better for: summer, lying down.
Symptoms worse for: cold, damp, draughts, wet weather,
fresh air, mental exertion.
Low time:

Calcarea sulphurica (Calc. Sulph.)
(New Era 6x)

Prepared from calcium sulphate.

Uses: blood purifier, helps rid the body of toxins, aids healing
of abcesses after they have begun to discharge, acne, catarrh,
boils, wounds which won't heal.
Symptoms better for: open air, bathing, eating, heat to the
affected part.
Symptoms worse for: hot stuffy rooms, touch, draughts.
Low time:

Calcichew
(Shire)

A white, chewable tablet supplied at a strength of 500 mg and
used as a calcium supplement to treat calcium deficiency.

Dose: 1 tablet chewed 3 times a day.

Side effects: constipation, wind.
Caution:
Not to be used for: children, or for patients suffering from overactive parathyroid glands, severe kidney disease, decalcifying tumours.
Not to be used with: tetracyclines.
Contains: calcium carbonate.
Other preparations:

Calcimax
(Wallace)

A brown syrup used as a calcium and vitamin supplement to treat calcium deficiency where vitamins are also needed.

Dose: adults 4 5 ml teaspoonsful 2-3 times a day; children 1-2 5 ml teaspoonsful 3 times a day.
Side effects:
Caution:
Not to be used for: children, or for patients suffering from overactive parathyroid glands, severe kidney disease, decalcifying tumours.
Not to be used with:
Contains: calcium glycine hydrochloride, calciferol, thiamine, riboflavine, pyridoxine, cyanocobalamin, calcium panthothenate.
Other preparations:

Calcisorb
(3M Riker)

A powder in a sachet of 4.7 g and used as an ion-exchange compound to treat raised calcium levels in the urine, recurring kidney stones, osteoporosis.

Dose: adults 1 sachet dispersed in water with meals or sprinkled on to food 3 times a day; children 2 sachets a day in 3

divided doses with food.
Side effects: diarrhoea.
Caution: treatment of children should be monitored, and the treatments should be accompanied by a low-calcium diet with foods rich in oxalates.
Not to be used for: pregnant women, nursing mothers, or for patients suffering from kidney disease, congestive heart disease, or any other conditions in which a low-sodium diet is needed.
Not to be used with:
Contains: sodium cellulose phosphate.
Other preparations:

Calcium Resonium
(Winthrop)

A powder used as an ion-exchange resin to treat raised potassium levels.

Dose: adults 15 g 3-4 times a day; children 1 g per kg body weight a day in divided doses.
Side effects: hyper calcaemia (raised calcium levels).
Caution: potassium and calcium levels should be checked.
Not to be used for: patients suffering from overactive parathyroid glands, multiple myeloma (a bone marrow tumour), sarcoidosis (a disease causing raised calcium levels), certain forms of cancer with kidney failure and hypercalcaemia.
Not to be used with:
Contains: calcium polystyrene sulphonate.
Other preparations:

Calendolon Ointment
(Weleda)

Dose: apply 2-3 times a day directly to area or on a dry dressing; use after each nappy change; apply sparingly after breastfeeding.

Constituents: per 100 g: marigold (*Calendula officinalis*) tincture (1=2), lanolin, beeswax, vegetable oils.
Uses: antiseptic, anti-inflammatory, for cuts, minor wounds, abrasions, nappy rash, sore nipples.
Caution: consult your doctor before using this product during pregnancy. If redness or itching occurs discontinue use. Some individuals may be sensitive to the lanolin content.
Not to be used for: patients where a deep infection is present because *Calendula* promotes surface healing and may seal in sepsis.

Calendula Lotion
(Weleda)

Dose: 1 teaspoonful to a glass of cool boiled water to cleanse wounds or as a compress. 1 teaspoonful to ½ glass of lukewarm boiled water as a mouthwash.
Product licence: No. PL0298/5777.
Constituents: marigold (*Calendula officinalis*) ethanolic extract (1=5), nominal ethanol content 46 % v/v.
Uses: to aid healing of cuts, abrasions, minor wounds, skin infection, sore gums.
Caution: shake bottle before use.
Not to be used for: patients where a deep infection is present because *Calendula* promotes surface healing and may seal in sepsis.

Callusolve
(Dermal)

A paint used as a skin softener to treat warts.

Dose: apply 4-5 drops of the paint to the wart, cover for 24 hours, rub away the treated part, and repeat the process.
Side effects:
Caution: apply only to warts and avoid healthy skin.

Not to be used for: treating warts on the face or anal and genital areas
Not to be used with:
Contains: benzalkonium chloride-bromine.
Other preparations:

Calming Tablets (previously known as Nerve Tablets)
(Seven Seas)

Dose: 2 tablets to be taken 3 times a day with meals.
Product licence: No. PL2210/5066.
Constituents: asafoetida BPC (*Ferula foetida*) oleoresin 24 mg, valerian (*Valerian officinalis*) root 3.02 mg, *Teucrium canadense* 2.16 mg, gentian (*Gentian lutea*) root 1.51 mg, plus aqueous extractives from: scullcap 28 mg, gentian 19 mg, valerian 31.4 mg. Excipients dicalcium phosphate, maize starch, hydroxypropylmethylcellulose, magnesium stearate, talc, silica, ethylcellulose, titanium dioxide, iron oxides, glycerol.
Uses: to reduce anxiety, worry, and nervous tension.
Special notes:
Caution: may cause drowsiness, if affected do not drive or operate machinery. Avoid alcoholic drinks. Should not be taken with other sedatives. If you are already receiving medical treatment, tell your doctor you are taking this product. Not to be used for children or during pregnancy or breastfeeding.

Calm Night (previously known as Restful Night)
(Seven Seas)

Dose: 1 tablet to be taken 3 times daily after food, plus 3 tablets before going to bed, or 3 tablets with the evening meal and 3 tablets before going to bed.
Product licence: No. PL1907/5015.
Constituents: wild lettuce (*Lactuca virosa*) 10 mg, passion-flower (*Passiflora incarnata*) 90 mg, Jamaica dogwood (*Piscidia erythrina*) bark 45 mg, hops (*Humulus lupulus*) 30 mg, aqueous

extractives from wild lettuce 90 mg, dicalcium phosphate, maize starch, hydroxypropylmethylcellulose, talc, silica, ethylcellulose, titanium dioxide, iron oxide, glycerol.

Uses: insomnia.

Special notes:

Caution: may cause drowsiness, if affected do not drive or operate machinery. Avoid alcoholic drinks. Should not be taken with other sedatives without consulting medical advice. Those patients with a known hypersensitivity to the Compositae family of plants should exercise caution taking these tablets. Not to be used for children or during pregnancy or lactation.

Calogen
(S.H.S.)

A low-electrolyte emulsion of arachis oil in water. It is used for patients suffering from kidney failure and other conditions where a diet high in energy but low in fluid and electrolytes is needed.

Caloreen
(Roussel)

A low-electrolyte, protein-, gluten-, lactose-, sucrose-, galactose-, and fructose-free glucose polymer powder. It is used for patients suffering from chronic kidney failure, amino acid disorders, hypoglycaemia, and other conditions where a high-energy, low-fluid, and low-electrolyte diet is needed.

Cam
(Rybar)

A syrup used as a bronchodilator to treat bronchial spasm.

Dose: adults 4 5 ml teaspoonsful 3-4 times a day; children

under 2 years ½ 5 ml teaspoonsful 3-4 times a day, 2-4 years 1 5 ml teaspoonful 3-4 times a day, over 4 years 2 5 ml teaspoonsful 3-4 times a day.
Side effects: nervousness, sleeplessness, restlessness, dry mouth, cold hands and feet, abnormal heart rhythms.
Caution: in patients suffering from diabetes.
Not to be used for: patients suffering from heart disease, high blood pressure, overactive thyroid gland.
Not to be used with: MAOIs.
Contains: ephedrine hydrochloride, butethamate citrate.
Other preparations:

Canesten
(Baypharm)

A solution used as an antifungal treatment for fungal inflammation and infection of the outer ear, skin, and nails.

Dose: 2-3 applications a day until 14 days.after the symptoms have gone.
Side effects: local irritation.
Caution:
Not to be used for:
Not to be used with:
Contains: clotrimazole, polyethylene glycol solution.
Other preparations: Canesten Spray, Canesten Powder.

Cantharis
(Weleda 6c, 30c; Nelsons 6c)

Prepared from the *Cantharis vesicatoria* beetle.

Uses: cystitis with burning pains before and after urination, constant urge to urinate, severe difficulty urinating and with scalding sensation, burning pains; second degree burns and scalds before blisters form or where blistering is present, sunburn.

Symptoms better for: warmth, rest; pain of burns is better for cold compresses.

Symptoms worse for: urination, touch, coffee, drinking cold water.

Low time:

Capitol
(Dermal)

A gel used as an antibacterial treatment for dandruff and other similar scalp disorders.

Dose: use as a shampoo.
Side effects:
Caution: in patients sensitive to iodine.
Not to be used for:
Not to be used with:
Contains: benzalkonium chloride.
Other preparations:

Caprin
(Sinclair)

A pink tablet supplied at a strength of 324 mg and used as an analgesic to treat rheumatic and associated conditions.

Dose: 3 tablets 3-4 times a day.
Side effects: stomach upsets, allergy, asthma.
Caution: in pregnant women, the elderly, and in patients with a history of allergy to aspirin, asthma, impaired kidney or liver function, indigestion.
Not to be used for: children, nursing mothers, or for patients suffering from haemophilia or ulcers.
Not to be used with: anticoagulants (blood-thinning drugs), some antidiabetic drugs, anti-inflammatory agents,

methotrexate, spironolactone, steroids, some antacids, some uric-acid lowering drugs.
Contains: aspirin.
Other preparations:

Carbel Instant
(Cow & Gate)

An instant carob bean gum preparation used for patients suffering from persistent vomiting and regurgitation of food.

Carbellon
(Torbet)

A black tablet used as an anti-spasm, anti-wind, antacid preparation to treat acidity, ulcers, food poisoning.

Dose: adults 2-4 tablets 3 times a day; children 1-3 tablets a day.
Side effects: few; occasionally constipation.
Caution:
Not to be used for: patients suffering from glaucoma, pyloric stenosis, enlarged prostate.
Not to be used with:
Contains: belladonna, magnesium hydroxide, charcoal, peppermint oil.
Other preparations:

Carbo-Dome
(Lagap)

A cream used as an antipsoriatic treatment for psoriasis.

Dose: apply to the affected area 2-3 times a day.
Side effects: irritation, sensitivity to light.

Carbomix
(Penn)

Granules used as an adsorbent to treat acute poisoning, overdose of drugs.

Dose: adults dissolve the contents of the bottle in water and take by mouth as soon as possible after poisoning; children usually take half adult dose.
Side effects:
Caution: your doctor may advise additional treatment for certain overdoses.
Not to be used for:
Not to be used with: antidotes or emetics taken by mouth.
Contains: activated charcoal.
Other preparations:

Carbo vegetabilis (Carbo veg.)
(Weleda 6c, 30c; Nelsons 6c)

Prepared from vegetable charcoal.

Uses: indigestion with excessive flatulence, bloated abdomen with rumbling, sluggish venous circulation, shivering but with a desire for open window, cold limbs at night, violent racking cough, hoarseness, loss of voice, tinnitus with nausea and vertigo.
Symptoms better for: eructations, being fanned.
Symptoms worse for: fatty foods, warm damp weather.
Low time: evening, night.

Carylderm
(Napp Consumer)

A lotion used as a pediculicide to treat lice in the head and pubic areas.

Dose: rub into the hair and allow to dry, then shampoo.
Side effects:
Caution: keep out of the eyes.
Not to be used for:
Not to be used with:
Contains: carbaryl.
Other preparations: Carylderm Liquid Shampoo.

Cascade
(Modern Health)

Dose: 2 tablets to be taken 3 times a day before meals.
Product licence: No. 1146/5005R.
Constituents: burdock root (*Arctium lappa*) 50 mg, uva ursi (*Arctostaphylos uva-ursi*) 75 mg, clivers (*Galium aparine*) 75mg.
Uses: diuretic, antiseptic, soothes, strengthens, and tones urinary tract, for premenstrual water retention, cystitis.
Special notes: not tested on animals.
Caution: prolonged use of uva ursi may cause constipation. Not recommended for children under 12 years or during pregnancy or breastfeeding unless prescribed.

Casilan
(Farley)

A powder used as a low-electrolyte, gluten-free protein for patients suffering from hypoproteinaemia.

Catarrh Cream
(Weleda)

Dose: a small quantity to be inserted into each nostril as desired.

Product licence: PL0298/7748.

Constituents: per 100 g: aesculin 0.1 g, alcoholic extracts from barberry (*Berberis*) fruct. 1 g, blackthorn (*Prunus spinosa*) fruct. 1 g, *Bryonia* 3x 10 g, camphor (*Cinnamomum camphora*) 0.012 g, purple coneflower (*Echinacea purpurea*) (1:3) 4 g, *Mercurius sulphuratus ruber* 5x 10 g, eucalyptus (*Eucalyptus globulus*) oil 0.388 g, peppermint (*Mentha piperita*) oil 0.388 g, thyme (*Thymus vulgaris*) oil 0.012 g.

Uses: to relieve catarrhal congestion and inflammation of nasal mucosa.

Caution: not recommended during pregnancy. May antidote any other homoeopathic remedies you are taking.

Availability: pharmacies only.

Catarrh Mixture
(Potters)

Dose: adults 1 5 ml teaspoonful 3 times a day;
children over 7 years 1 5 ml teaspoonful morning and evening.

Product licence: No. P/L0250/5051R.

Constituents: boneset (*Eupatorium perfoliatum*), blue flag (*Iris versicolor*), burdock root (*Arctium lappa*), hyssop (*Hyssopus officinalis*), capsicum, excipients.

Uses: to relieve the symptoms of nasal catarrh and catarrh of the throat.

Special notes: sugar free.

Caution:

Catarrh Naturtabs
(Larkhall)
'Cantassium'

Dose: 1-2 tablets 3 times a day with water, preferably after a meal.
Product licence: No. PL0912/7178R.
Constituents: Yarrow (*Achillea millefolium*) extract 6 mg, vervain (*Verbena officinalis*) extract 5 mg, white horehound extract (*Marrubium vulgare*) 6 mg, sage (*Salvia officinalis*) extract 4 mg, calcium phosphate tribasic, calcium sulphate dihydrate, potato starch, vegetable fatty acid.
Uses: upper respiratory tract discomfort and catarrh, especially in winter.
Special notes: vegan, yeast free, hypoallergenic.
Caution: not to be taken by pregnant women, or by anyone being treated for high blood pressure.

Catarrh Pastilles
(Booker)
'Heath & Heather'

Dose: allow a pastille to dissolve in the mouth when needed. Not more than 12 to be taken in 24 hours.
Product licence: P/L1713/5088R.
Constituents: squill (*Drimia maritima*) vinegar 9.4 %, pumilio pine (*Pinus mugo*) oil 0.6 %, eucalyptus (*Eucalyptus globulus*) oil 0.5 %, sugar, liquid glucose, crystal gum, menthol, beetroot red as colouring, caramel, vegetable fat.
Uses: expectorant, decongestant, to relieve the symptoms of coughs, colds, sore throats, and catarrh.
Special notes: vegan, yeast free.
Caution: not recommended for children. May antidote any homoeopathic remedies you are taking.

Catarrh Tablets
(Booker)
'Heath & Heather'

Dose: 1 tablet 3 times a day.
Product licence: No. P/L1713/509R.
Constituents: white horehound extract (*Marrubium vulgare*) 500 mg, squill (*Drimia maritima*) 30 mg, dicalcium phosphate, microcrystalline cellulose, stearic acid, magnesium stearate; coating: hypromellose, polyethylene glycol, copper chlorophyllin, titanium dioxide.
Uses: to relieve the symptoms of coughs and catarrh.
Special notes: vegan, yeast free.
Caution: not to be taken during pregnancy without practitioner supervision.

Catarrh Tablets
(Seven Seas)

Dose: 2 tablets 3 times a day with meals.
Product licence: No. PL2210/5020.
Constituents: lobelia (*Lobelia inflata*) 31.7 mg, yarrow (*Achillea millefolium*) 3.17 mg, red sage (*Salvia officinalis*) 3.17 mg, boneset (*Eupatorium perfoliatum*) 3.17 mg, white horehound (*Marrubium vulgare*) 3.17 mg, capsicum minimum oleoresin BPC 0.5 mg; plus aqueous extractives from: yarrow 33 mg, vervain (*Verbena officinalis*) 33 mg, red sage 33 mg, boneset 33 mg, white horehound 28.5 mg; excipients dicalcium phosphate, maize starch, hydroxypropylmethylcellulose, talc, silica, ethyl cellulose, titanium dioxide, iron oxides, glycerol.
Uses: the relief of sinus obstruction and catarrh, particulary associated with hayfever.
Special notes:
Caution: do not exceed the stated dose. Should not be used in the presence of any cardiac disease or gastric hyperacidity. Individuals with a known hypersensitivity to yarrow or other members of the Compositae family should exercise caution

when taking the tablets, although no instances of a reaction have been reported. Should not be used during pregnancy or breastfeeding. Not recommended for children.

Causticum
(Weleda 6c)

Prepared from potassium hydrate.

Uses: sore throat with raw burning pain, hoarseness, hollow spasmodic cough which is constant and exhausting, chemical burns and third degree burns (seek medical help immediately), to relieve soreness in the site of old burns, constipation with ineffectual urging, cystitis with frequent urging but difficulty passing urine, retention of urine, incontinence of urine on coughing, raw sore pains.
Suited to: patients who are lean, dark haired, and sensitive.
Symptoms better for: mild wet weather, cold drinks.
Symptoms worse for: dry cold or raw air, winds, drafts, grief.
Low time: evening.

Caved-S
(Tillotts)

A brown tablet used as a cell-surface protector and antacid to treat peptic ulcer.

Dose: adults 2 tablets chewed between meals; children 10-14 years half adult dose.
Side effects: few; occasionally constipation.
Caution:
Not to be used for: infants.
Not to be used with: tetracycline antibiotics.
Contains: liquorice extract, aluminium hydroxide, magnesium carbonate, sodium bicarbonate.
Other preparations: Rabro (Sinclair).

Ceanel Concentrate
(Quinoderm)

A liquid used as an antibacterial, antifungal treatment for psoriasis, seborrhoeic inflammation of the scalp.

Dose: use as a shampoo 3 times a week at first and then twice a week, or apply directly to other areas of the skin as needed.
Side effects:
Caution: keep out of the eyes.
Not to be used for:
Not to be used with:
Contains: phenylethyl alcohol.
Other preparations:

Ce-Cobalin
(Paines & Byrne)

A syrup used as a multivitamin preparation to treat anorexia, recovery from long-term illness.

Dose: adults 1-2 5 ml teaspoonsful 3 times a day; children 1 teaspoonful 3 times a day.
Side effects:
Caution:
Not to be used for:
Not to be used with:
Contains: cyanocoblamin.
Other preparations:

Cedocard
(Tillotts)

A blue, scored tablet or a green, scored tablet according to strengths of 20 mg, 40 mg and used as a nitrate treatment for severe congestive heart failure.

Dose: 10-40 mg 3-4 times a day.
Side effects: headache, flushes, dizziness.
Caution:
Not to be used for: children, or for patients suffering from severe low blood pressure, heart shock, severe anaemia, brain haemorrhage.
Not to be used with:
Contains: isosorbide dinitrate.
Other preparations: Cedocard I.V.

Celery Seed Tablets
(Booker)
'Heath & Heather'

Dose: 1 tablet 3 times a day.
Product licence: No. P/L1713/5026R.
Constituents: celery seed (*Apium graveolens*) extract 600 mg, microcrystalline cellulose, dicalcium phosphate, stearic acid, magnesium stearate; coating hypromellose, glycerin, copper chlorophyllin, curcumin, iron oxide, titanium dioxide.
Uses: relief of rheumatic pain, lumbago, and fibrositis.
Special notes: vegan, yeast free.
Caution: not to be taken in pregnancy without practitioner supervision.

Cerumol
(LAB)

Drops used as a wax softener to remove wax from the ears.
Dose: 5 drops into the ear twice a day for 3 days may enable syringing to be avoided.
Side effects:
Caution:
Not to be used for: inflammation of the outer ear, dermatitis, eczema.
Not to be used with:

Calcarea carbonica (Calc. Carb.)
(Weleda 6c, 30c; Nelsons 6c)

Prepared from calcium carbonate from middle layer of oyster shell.

Uses: obesity, cold extremities, cracked itching skin, profuse sour perspiration especially on head, vertigo, anxiety, indigestion, poor assimilation of nutrients, swollen glands, premenstrual tension, insomnia, menses early, profuse, painful, and protracted, constipation; children — difficult and delayed dentition, head sweats, slow closure of fontanelles, poor calcium absorption.
Suited to: fair-haired, timid patients who tend to put on weight easily.
Symptoms better for: dry weather, lying on painful side.
Symptoms worse for: cold, damp, draughts, teething, drinking milk, exertion, standing.
Low time:

Calcarea fluorica (Calc. fluor.)
(New Era 6x; Weleda 6c, 30c; Nelsons 6c)

Prepared from calcium fluoride.

Uses: promotes elasticity of tissues; varicose veins, stretch marks, arthritis, prevention of adhesions after surgery, haemorrhoids, croup, head colds with discharge, catarrh, deficient enamel of teeth.
Symptoms better for: movement, warmth.
Symptoms worse for: rest, damp.
Low time:

Calcarea phosphorica (Calc. phos.)
(New Era 6x; Weleda 6c, 30c; Nelsons 6c)

Prepared from tricalcic phosphate.

Uses: adolescents lacking energy and concentration, emaciation, cough with yellow mucus, stomach pains after eating, acne, enlarged adenoids, headache from overstudying, swollen glands, chronic catarrh, non-union of fractures, debility remaining after acute disease.
Suited to: general debility with discontent.
Symptoms better for: summer, lying down.
Symptoms worse for: cold, damp, draughts, wet weather, fresh air, mental exertion.
Low time:

Calcarea sulphurica (Calc. Sulph.)
(New Era 6x)

Prepared from calcium sulphate.

Uses: blood purifier, helps rid the body of toxins, aids healing of abcesses after they have begun to discharge, acne, catarrh, boils, wounds which won't heal.
Symptoms better for: open air, bathing, eating, heat to the affected part.
Symptoms worse for: hot stuffy rooms, touch, draughts.
Low time:

Cantharis
(Weleda 6c, 30c; Nelsons 6c)

Prepared from the *Cantharis vesicatoria* beetle.

Uses: cystitis with burning pains before and after urination, constant urge to urinate, severe difficulty urinating and with

scalding sensation, burning pains; second degree burns and scalds before blisters form or where blistering is present, sunburn.
Symptoms better for: warmth, rest; pain of burns is better for cold compresses.
Symptoms worse for: urination, touch, coffee, drinking cold water.
Low time:

Carbo vegetabilis (Carbo veg.)
(Weleda 6c, 30c; Nelsons 6c)

Prepared from vegetable charcoal.

Uses: indigestion with excessive flatulence, bloated abdomen with rumbling, sluggish venous circulation, shivering but with a desire for open window, cold limbs at night, violent racking cough, hoarseness, loss of voice, tinnitus with nausea and vertigo.
Symptoms better for: eructations, being fanned.
Symptoms worse for: fatty foods, warm damp weather.
Low time: evening, night.

Causticum
(Weleda 6c)

Prepared from potassium hydrate.

Uses: sore throat with raw burning pain, hoarseness, hollow spasmodic cough which is constant and exhausting, chemical burns and third degree burns (seek medical help immediately), to relieve soreness in the site of old burns, constipation with ineffectual urging, cystitis with frequent urging but difficulty passing urine, retention of urine, incontinence of urine on coughing, raw sore pains.
Suited to: patients who are lean, dark haired, and sensitive.

Symptoms better for: mild wet weather, cold drinks.
Symptoms worse for: dry cold or raw air, winds, drafts, grief.
Low time: evening.

Chamomilla
(Weleda 3x, 30c; also available from Weleda in 3x drops)

Prepared from entire plant *Chamomilla recutita* (German camomile — formerly known as *Matricaria chamomilla*).

Uses: severe pains, irritability, toothache which is worse for warm drinks, oversensitivity to unpleasant stimuli, period pains which worsen after anger, sleeplessness from pain, anger, or too much coffee; children — babies who cry constantly and are quiet only when carried, teething remedy, colic, green diarrhoea especially during teething, earache.
Suited to: children who are irritable and restless when ill and want to be carried all the time.
Symptoms better for: being carried.
Symptoms worse for: teething, anger, coffee.
Low time: morning, evening, night.

Cina
(Weleda 6c)

Prepared from the unexpanded flower heads of *Artemisia maritima* (sea wormwood).

Uses: children very irritable, petulant, capricious, want to be rocked but not touched or carried, digestive problems, extreme hunger, refuses mother's milk, grinding teeth or crying out during sleep, intestinal worms.
Symptoms better for: lying on abdomen, rocking, movement.
Symptoms worse for: touch, during sleep.
Low time: morning, night.

Cocculus
(Weleda 6c)

Prepared from powdered seeds of *Cocculus indicus* plant.

Uses: travel sickness, loss of sleep, jet lag especially after long-haul flights, effects of crossing time zones, vertigo with sensation as if at sea, nausea, vomiting, weakness and great pain with menses which are early and profuse.
Suited to: patients who are fair haired and sensitive.
Symptoms better for: sitting, lying on side.
Symptoms worse for: motion of cars, boats; swimming, touch, emotion, open air, noise, eating, menses.
Low time:

Coffea
(Weleda 6c)

Prepared from raw coffee berries.

Uses: sleeplessness from mental activity, excessive sensitivity to noise and pain, agitation, toothache with shooting pains which is better for holding ice-cold water in the mouth, one-sided nervous headache.
Suited to: patients who are tall, dark haired, and cheerful.
Symptoms better for: sleep, warmth, lying down.
Symptoms worse for: noise, touch, odours, open air, mental exertion, excitement, emotion, overeating, alcohol.
Low time: night.

Cold and Influenza (Prevention Tablets)
(Nelsons)

Prepared from: 30c influenza virus (Asian) 1957, 30c influenza virus A 1954, 30c influenza virus B 1954, 30c *Bacillus influenza* 1918 30c Bacillinum, 30c influenza virus A (Hong Kong) 1968,

30c influenza virus B (Hong Kong) 5/72, 30c influenza virus A (England) 42/72, 30c influenza virus A (Port Chalmers) 1/73.

Uses: to help prevent colds and influenza.

Colocynthis (Colocynth.)
(Weleda 6c)

Prepared from pulp of *Citrullus colocynth* fruit (bitter cucumber).

Uses: abdominal colic, cramps and spasms, diarrhoea, vomiting from pain, neuralgic pains, sciatica, trigeminal neuralgia, vertigo from turning the head quickly, cramp in calves.
Symptoms better for: heat, pressure, doubling up.
Symptoms worse for: anger, lying on painless side.
Low time:

Combination A
(New Era)

Combination of Ferr. Phos. 6x, Kali. Phos. 6x, Mag. Phos. 6x.

Uses: sciatica, neuralgia, neuritis.

Combination B
(New Era)

Combination of Calc. Phos. 6x, Kali. Phos. 6x, Ferr. Phos 6x.

Uses: general debility, edginess, nervous exhaustion, convalescence.

Combination C
(New Era)

Combination of Mag. Phos. 6x, Nat. Phos. 6x, Nat. Sulph. 6x, Silica 6x.

Uses: acidity, heartburn, dyspepsia.

Combination D
(New Era)

Combination of Kali. Mur. 6x, Kali. Sulph. 6x, Calc. Sulph. 6x, Silica 6x.

Uses: minor skin ailments.

Combination E
(New Era)

Combination of Calc. Phos. 6x, Mag. Phos. 6x, Nat. Phos. 6x, Nat Sulph. 6x.

Uses: flatulence, colic, indigestion.

Combination F
(New Era)

Combination of Kali. Phos. 6x, Mag. Phos. 6x, Nat. Mur. 6x, Silica 6x.

Uses: migraine, headaches from emotional upset.

Combination G
(New Era)

Combination of Calc. Fluor. 6x, Calc. Phos. 6x, Kali. Phos. 6x, Nat. Mur. 6x.

Uses: backache, lumbar pain.

Combination H
(New Era)

Combination of Mag. Phos. 6x, Nat. Mur. 6x, Silica 6x.

Uses: hayfever, allergic rhinitis.

Combination I
(New Era)

Combination of Ferr. Phos. 6x, Kali. Sulph. 6x, Mag. Phos. 6x.

Uses: fibrositis, muscular pain, stiffness.

Combination J
(New Era)

Combination of Ferr. Phos. 6x, Kali. Mur. 6x, Nat. Mur. 6x.

Uses: coughs, colds, chestiness.

Combination K
(New Era)

Combination of Kali. Sulph. 6x, Nat. Mur. 6x, Silica 6x.

Uses: brittle nails, falling hair.

Combination L
(New Era)

Combination of Calc. Fluor. 6x, Ferr. Phos. 6x, Nat. Mur. 6x.

Uses: varicose veins, circulatory disorders.

Combination M
(New Era)

Combination of Nat. Phos. 6x, Nat. Sulph. 6x, Kali. Mur. 6x, Calc. Phos. 6x.

Uses: rheumatic pain.

Combination N
(New Era)

Combination of Calc. Phos. 6x, Kali. Mur. 6x, Kali. Phos. 6x, Mag. Phos. 6x.

Uses: menstrual pain.

Combination P
(New Era)

Combination of Calc. Fluor. 6x, Calc. Phos. 6x, Kali. Phos. 6x, Mag. Phos. 6x.

Uses: aching legs and feet.

Combination Q
(New Era)

Combination of Ferr. Phos. 6x, Kali. Mur. 6x, Kali. Sulph. 6x, Nat. Mur. 6x.

Uses: catarrh, sinus disorders.

Combination R
(New Era)

Combination of Calc. Fluor. 6x, Calc. Phos. 6x, Ferr. Phos. 6x, Mag. Phos. 6x, Silica 6x.

Uses: infants' teething pains.

Combination S
(New Era)

Combination of Kali. Mur. 6x, Nat. Phos. 6x, Nat. Sulph. 6x.

Uses: stomach upsets, sick headaches, biliousness.

Cuprum metallicum (Cuprum met.)
(Weleda 6c, 30c; Nelsons 6c)

Prepared from copper.

Uses: cramps and spasms, cramp in fingers, legs, or toes, nausea and vomiting with abdominal cramps, diarrhoea, metallic taste in mouth, spasmodic cough with shortness of breath and vomiting, cold hands and feet, bluish face and lips.
Symptoms better for: cold drinks.
Symptoms worse for: cold air, touch, before menstruation, coughing, after vomiting.
Low time: evening, night.

Drosera
(Weleda 6c, 30c; Nelsons 6c)

Prepared from *Drosera rotundifolia* (round-leaved sundew) plant.

Uses: constant tickling cough, violent attacks of coughing which may end in vomiting, deep, hoarse, barking cough with retching, sore throat which is worse for swallowing, laryngitis with a dry throat making speech difficult.
Symptoms better for: open air.
Symptoms worse for: talking, laughing, drinking, lying down, warmth.
Low time: after midnight.

Elasto
(New Era)

Combination of Calc. Fluor. 6x, Calc. Phos. 6x, Ferr. Phos. 6x, Mag. Phos. 6x.

Uses: promotes the formation of elastin which is responsible for the repair and maintenance of the elastic tissues in the body; for varicose veins, aching legs.

Euphrasia
(Weleda 6c, 30c; Nelsons 6c)

Prepared from entire plant *Euphrasia officinalis* (eyebright).

Uses: colds with watering eyes and streaming nose, hayfever, conjunctivitis with burning tears, photophobia, cough which comes only during the day and has copious mucus.
Symptoms better for: dim light, cold applications.
Symptoms worse for: sunlight, warmth, being indoors.
Low time: evening.

Ferrum Phosphoricum (Ferr. Phos.)
(Weleda 6c, 30c; New Era 6x; Nelsons 6c)

Prepared from white phosphate of iron.

Uses: early stages of colds (after Aconite), early stages of fever and inflammation before exudation begins, anaemia, sluggish venous circulation, hammering congestive headaches, nosebleeds, rheumatism.
Suited to: pale, delicate people who flush easily on exertion.
Symptoms better for: cold applications, summer.
Symptoms worse for: touch, noise, cold.
Low time: night.

Feverfew
(Weleda 6x)

Prepared from feverfew plant (*Chrysanthemum parthenium*).

Uses: to reduce frequency and severity of migraine attacks. The indications for homoeopathic feverfew are the same as for taking it as a herbal remedy. The potentized form has been prepared because some patients were complaining of mouth ulcers after taking the herbal form (which is not licensed as a medicine).

Gelsemium
(Weleda 6c, 30c; Nelsons 6c)

Prepared from bark of the root of *Gelsemium sempervirens* (yellow jasmine).

Uses: Influenza and its after-effects, fatigue, aching, trembling, weakness, heaviness, sneezing, sore throat, difficulty swallowing, headache, chills up and down the spine, vertigo, drooping eyelids, anticipatory fear.

Suited to: excitable, sensitive people who suffer from anticipatory fear.
Symptoms better for: urination, sweating.
Symptoms worse for: humidity, heat of sun, receiving bad news, shocks, anticipation, tobacco.
Low time: mid-morning.

Graphites
(Weleda 6c, 30c; Nelsons 6c)

Prepared from amorphous carbon.

Uses: eczema which cracks and weeps, thickening and hardening of skin, cracks and fissures, wounds which tend to suppurate, styes, overweight, constipation, anal fissures, tinnitus, hot flushes, dandruff.
Suited to: cautious, indecisive people who tend to put on weight.
Symptoms better for: touch, more clothing, eating.
Symptoms worse for: during and after menstruation, cold, light.
Low time: night.

Hamamelis
(Weleda 6c, 30c; Nelsons 6c)

Prepared from fresh bark of twigs and roots of *Hamamelis virginica* (witch hazel).

Uses: varicose veins, haemorrhoids, bruised soreness, chilblains with bluish colour, nosebleeds, venous congestion.
Symptoms better for:
Symptoms worse for: injuries, bruises, day, touch, pressure, humidity.
Low time: night.

Hayfever
(Nelsons)

Combination of 6c *Allium cepa*, 6c *Euphrasia officinalis*, 6c *Sabadilla officinarum*.

Uses: relief of hayfever.

Hepar Sulphuris (Hepar Sulph.)
(Weleda 6c, 30c; Nelsons 6c)

Prepared from a sulphide of calcium made by burning the white interior of oyster shells and sulphur together.

Uses: hypersensitivity, irritability, intolerance of pain, skin highly sensitive to touch, eczema, acne, intense chilliness, croup, cough brought on by exposure to cold air, wheezing, sensation of splinter at back of throat, tonsillitis, earache; all wounds tend to suppurate; will hasten abcesses; establishes suppuration around and removes foreign body.
Symptoms better for: warmth, humidity.
Symptoms worse for: cold dry air, winter, drafts, touch, noise, exertion.
Low time: night.

Hypericum
(Weleda 6c, 30c; Nelsons 6c)

Prepared from entire plant *Hypericum perforatum* (perforate St John's wort).

Uses: painful injuries to parts rich in nerve endings especially fingers and toes, lacerated wounds involving nerve endings, violent shooting pains, falls injuring spine especially coccyx, blows or crush injuries to fingers or toes, headache after blow to the occiput.

Symptoms better for: bending backwards, rubbing.
Symptoms worse for: shock, touch, movement, cold damp.
Low time:

Ignatia
(Weleda 6c, 30c; Nelson 6c)

Prepared from the seeds of the *Ignatia amara* tree.

Uses: grief, fright, bereavement, exhaustion from prolonged grief, sighing, spasms, sensation of lump in throat, sore throat which is better for swallowing, piercing headache, haemorrhoids which are better when walking, croup, irritating cough which worsens with coughing, constipation.
Suited to: sensitive, emotional people who prefer to be alone.
Symptoms better for: being alone, eating.
Symptoms worse for: emotion, worry, coffee, tobacco smoke.
Low time: morning.

Ipecacuanha (Ipecac.)
(Weleda 6c, 30c: Nelsons 6c)

Prepared from dried root of *Cephaelis ipecacuanha* plant.

Uses: nausea, vomiting, morning sickness, travel sickness, gastric upset with clean tongue, bronchitis, loose coarse rattle in chest without expectoration, nausea and shortness of breath accompany most complaints.
Symptoms better for: open air, rest, closing eyes, cold drinks, pressure.
Symptoms worse for: warmth, overeating, change of weather, vomiting, motion.
Low time:

Kalium Bichromicum (Kali. Bich.)
(Weleda 6c, 30c: Nelsons 6c)

Prepared from potassium bichromate.

Uses: catarrh which is stringy and tenacious, hard cough with plugs of mucus, pain in small spots (can be covered with point of finger), sore throat, migraine with blurred vision preceding the attack.
Suited to: reserved, conscientious people with a tendency to put on weight.
Symptoms better for: movement, pressure.
Symptoms worse for: alcohol, hot weather.
Low time: morning, 2-3 am.

Kalium Muriaticum (Kali. Mur.)
(New Era 6x)

Prepared from potassium chloride.

Uses: a blood purifier and cleanser, may help prevent blood from clotting too easily; white or greyish-white coated tongue and throat, sore throat, swollen glands, tonsillitis, thick white sticky catarrh, deafness from catarrh and blocked eustachian tubes, indigestion from fatty food, rheumatic swellings.
Symptoms better for: cold drinks, rubbing.
Symptoms worse for: open air, menstruation, movement, dampness, rich food.
Low time:

Kalium Phosphoricum (Kali. Phos.)
(Weleda 6c, 30c; New Era 6x; Nelsons 6c)

Prepared from potassium phosphate.

Uses: nervous exhaustion, nervousness, insomnia, depres-

sion, anxiety, vertigo, headache with humming in the ears, shingles, nervous asthma, hoarseness, dry tongue; night fears in children.
Symptoms better for: sleep, eating, gentle movement.
Symptoms worse for: worry, excitement, touch, pain, overwork.
Low time:

Kalium Sulphuricum (Kali. Sulph.)
(New Era 6x)

Prepared from potassium sulphate.

Uses: skin problems with scaling, psoriasis, athlete's foot, brittle nails, yellow slimy coating on the tongue, yellow catarrh, rheumatism which moves from joint to joint.
Symptoms better for: cool open air, walking.
Symptoms worse for: warmth of room, noise.
Low time: evening.

Lachesis
(Weleda 6c)

Prepared from venom of *Trigonocephalus lachesis* snake (surukuku).

Uses: throbbing headache with head feeling hot and heavy, hot flushes, hot perspiration, menopause, intolerance of touch, pressure of clothing aggravates, symptoms occur more on left side of body or travel from left to right, poor circulation with bluish mottled appearance, sore throat extending to ear — better for swallowing solids but worse for liquids, tonsillitis.
Suited to: talkative excitable people.
Symptoms better for: open air, cold drinks, menstruation.
Symptoms worse for: sleep, heat, spring, summer, sun, touch, pressure, alcohol, hot drinks.
Low time: morning.

Ledum
(Weleda 6c)

Prepared from entire plant *Ledum palustre*.

Uses: puncture wounds, insect bites, bee stings, bruised or bloodshot eyes, cold blue swellings, chilliness, rheumatic or arthritic conditions which start in the lower limbs and ascend, gout.
Symptoms better for: cold applications, resting.
Symptoms worse for: warmth, movement, alcohol.
Low time: night.

Lycopodium
(Weleda 6c, 30c; Nelsons 6c)

Prepared from *Lycopodium clavatum* plant (common club moss).

Uses: abdominal bloating and flatulence, excessive hunger but a few mouthfuls satiate, loud rumbling especially in lower abdomen, craving sweets although they aggravate, symptoms are mainly on the right side of body or moving from right to left, ailments from anticipation, fear of failure, cystitis, gout.
Suited to: people who may appear proud or argumentative but are lacking in self-confidence.
Symptoms better for: warm drinks, movement, eructations.
Symptoms worse for: pressure of clothes, eating, sleep, bread, onions, cabbage, wine, coffee, smoking.
Low time: late afternoon to mid-evening.

Magnesia Phosphorica (Mag. Phos.)
(New Era 6x)

Prepared from magnesium phosphate.

Uses: colic, cramps, spasms, neuralgic pains, right-sided com-

plaints, sharp lightning-like pains, writer's cramp, menstrual cramp, facial neuralgia, headache relieved by warmth, sciatica.
Suited to: dark-haired, thin, nervous people.
Symptoms better for: warmth, hot bathing, pressure, rubbing, doubling up.
Symptoms worse for: cold, being uncovered.
Low time: night.

Mercurius Solubilis (Merc. Sol.)
Weleda 6c, 30c, Nelsons 6c.

Prepared from dimercurous ammonium nitrate.

Uses: suppuration, abcesses, mouth ulcers, sore throat, tonsillitis, excessive saliva, metallic taste in mouth, bad breath, tongue swollen and flabby showing imprint of teeth, profuse sweats, feverish head cold with offensive green/yellow catarrh, earache, diarrhoea with straining, tremor.
Suited to: those who are hurried and impulsive.
Symptoms better for: even temperature, rest.
Symptoms worse for: temperature changes.
Low time: night.

Mixed Pollen
(Weleda 30c)

Prepared from the following pollens: grasses — bent, brome, cocksfoot, crested dogtail, false oat, fescue, meadowgrass, rye grass, timothy grass, vernal, Yorkshire fog; trees — alder, ash, beech, silver birch, elm, hazel, oak, plane, poplar, willow; flowering plants — heather, nettle, plantain, fat hen, mugwort, borage, rape.

Uses: the relief of hayfever resulting from the above pollens.

Natrum Muriaticum (Nat. Mur.)
(Weleda 6c, 30c; New Era 6x; Nelsons 6c)

Prepared from sodium chloride.

Uses: excessive moisture or dryness in any part of the system, profuse watery colds, hayfever, severe headache, migraine, vertigo, pain in eyes from reading, effects of longstanding grief, depression, dry skin, eczema, cold sores, warts, menstrual pain, constipation, incontinence.
Suited to: thin, pale, reserved people who, though emotionally sensitive, dislike consolation.
Symptoms better for: open air, cool bathing.
Symptoms worse for: sun, emotion, consolation, touch, noise, music, salt, seaside.
Low time: mid- to late morning

Natrum Phosphoricum (Nat. Phos.)
(New Era 6x)

Prepared from sodium phosphate.

Uses: an acid neutralizer; helps remove excesses of lactic and uric acid from the body and thus aids digestive and rheumatic disorders, sour vomiting, yellow creamy coating at base of tongue, dyspepsia, tightness of muscles and tendons, gout.
Symptoms better for: cold.
Symptoms worse for: sugar, milk, fatty food.
Low time: evening.

Natrum Sulphuricum (Nat. Sulph.)
(New Era 6x)

Prepared from sodium sulphate.

Uses: regulates density of intercellular fluids by eliminating excess water; aids the healthy functioning of the liver, biliousness, bitter taste in mouth, brown tongue, yellow diarrhoea, painful flatulence, rumbling abdomen, photophobia, inflammation of nailbed.

Symptoms better for: open air, changing position.
Symptoms worse for: all forms of damp, night air, music.
Low time: morning.

Nervone
(New Era)

Combination of Calc. Phos. 6x, Kali. Mur. 6x, Kali. Phos. 6x, Mag. Phos. 6x.

Uses: nervous debility, nerve pains and allied conditions.

Noctura
(Nelsons)

Combination of Kali. Brom. 6c, *Coffea* 6c, *Passiflora* 6c, *Avena sativa* 6c, valerian 6c.

Uses: to encourage restful sleep.

Nux vomica (Nux vom.)
(Weleda 6c, 30c; Nelsons 6c)

Prepared from seeds of *Strychnos nux-vomica* (strychnine) tree.

Uses: hypersensitivity to external stimuli, irritability, effects of overwork, effects of overeating, hangover, headache with nausea or dizziness, dyspepsia, nausea, vomiting, travel sickness, hiccough, raw sore throat, colds, hayfever, violent cough, spasms, menstrual cramps, colic, constipation with ineffectual

urging, itching haemorrhoids.
Suited to: solid, compact, muscular people who are inclined to be impatient, irritable, and fastidious.
Symptoms better for: warmth, evening, resting.
Symptoms worse for: cold, alcohol, coffee, noise, light, odours, music, mental exertion, vexation.
Low time: early morning.

Phosphorus
(Weleda 6c, 30c; Nelsons 6c)

Prepared from red amorphous phosphorus.

Uses: cough with difficult rapid breathing, bronchitis, painful hoarseness, laryngitis, vomiting, diarrhoea, heartburn, burning sensations in small areas, need to eat often, anxiety, oversensitivity, vertigo, exhaustion with weakness and trembling, tendency to bleed or bruise easily.
Suited to: tall, slender, fine-boned, sensitive people.
Symptoms better for: cold food, ices, sleep.
Symptoms worse for: cold, thunderstorms, emotional upset, warm food, mental fatigue, lying on left side.
Low time: evening.

Phytolacca
(Weleda 6c)

Prepared from roots, berries and leaves of *Phytolacca decandra* plant (Virginian pokeweed).

Uses: mastitis, breast abscess, sore throat with intense burning and dryness, tonsillitis, rheumatism, shooting pains like shocks through the body, teething pains which are better when infant bites on something.
Symptoms better for: lying on abdomen, rest.
Symptoms worse for: movement, menstruation, cold damp,

swallowing hot drinks.
Low time:

Pulsatilla
(Weleda 6c, 30c; Nelsons 6c)

Prepared from entire flowering *Pulsatilla nigricans* plant (wind anemone).

Uses: changeability of symptoms and of mood, pains which move and change, menstrual irregularities, menstrual pain, colds with thick bland yellow catarrh, thick coated white tongue, stomach upsets from rich fatty foods, thirstless even though mouth is dry, weepy, yielding, babies who are quiet only when carried, styes, arthritis, cystitis, poor circulation, varicose veins.
Suited to: affectionate, emotional people easily moved to laughter or tears, fair haired, tend to put on weight easily.
Symptoms better for: open air, slow movement, consolation.
Symptoms worse for: rich foods, stuffy rooms.
Low time: evening.

Rhus toxicodendron (Rhus tox.)
(Weleda 6c 30c; Nelsons, 6c)

Prepared from leaves of *Rhus toxicodendron* plant (oakleaf poison ivy) gathered at sunset just before flowering.

Uses: strains, sprains, overexertion, strains of muscles and tendons, pain in ligaments, rheumatism, stiffness, arthritis, sciatica, shooting pains, cold sores, herpes, eczema, tickling cough, restlessness.
Symptoms better for: continued movement, heat, hot bathing, rubbing, stretching, warm dry weather.
Symptoms worse for: first movement, cold, wet, drafts, before storms.
Low time: after midnight.

Ruta graveolens (Ruta grav.)
(Weleda 6c, 30c; Nelson 6c)

Prepared from entire *Ruta graveolens* plant (rue).

Uses: bruised bones, injuries to periosteum (membrane covering the bone), strains and sprains where Rhus tox. is ineffective, bruised sore aching with restlessness, synovitis, rheumatism, tennis elbow, eye strain.
Symptoms better for: warmth, movement, rubbing.
Symptoms worse for: overexertion, cold, menstruation.
Low time: evening.

Sepia
(Weleda 6c, 30c; Nelsons 6c)

Prepared from the ink of *Sepia officinalis* (common cuttlefish).

Uses: depression, indifference to loved ones, menopause, hot flushes, hot sweats, hair loss, irregular periods, premenstrual tension, uterine pain with bearing down sensation, loss of sex drive, headache comes in shocks, sluggish irregular circulation, sudden tiredness.
Suited to: those who become depressed easily and lose interest in work, pleasure, loved ones, and sex.
Symptoms better for: exercise, dancing, hot applications.
Symptoms worse for: cold air, rest.
Low time: afternoon, evening.

Shock and Distress Relief
(Nelsons)

Combination of Arnica 6c, Hypericum 6c, Rhus tox. 6c, Ruta grav. 6c, Symphytum 6c.

Uses: to relieve the effects of physical shock and trauma.

Silica
(Weleda 6c, 30c; New Era 6x; Nelsons 6c)

Prepared from flint.

Uses: abcesses, boils, expulsion of foreign bodies, acne, fungal infections, athlete's foot, tendency to suppurate, whitlow, offensive sweats particularly of the feet, persistent colds, hayfever, chilliness, swollen glands, migraine, poor assimilation of nutrients, brittle unhealthy nails, white spots on nails, constipation.
Suited to: delicate, pale, fair-haired people who are both timid and obstinate.
Symptoms better for: warmth, summer, humidity.
Symptoms worse for: cold, drafts, noise, touch, alcohol.
Low time: morning.

Sulphur
(New Era 6c, 30c; Nelsons 6c)

Prepared from sublimated sulphur.

Uses: skin eruptions which are hot and burning, redness, eczema, acne, burning pains, excoriating discharges, itching, mid-morning hunger, early morning diarrhoea, unrefreshing sleep, flushes of heat, burning soles of feet, burning itching haemorrhoids, insomnia.
Suited to: intellectual, self-absorbed, and untidy people.
Symptoms better for: open air, walking, movement.
Symptoms worse for: bathing, becoming overheated, standing, eating sweets, atmospheric changes.
Low time: late morning

Symphytum
(Weleda 6c)

Prepared from *Symphytum officinale* plant (comfrey).

Uses: facilitates union of fractured bones (do not take unless you know the bones are in good alignment), pricking stitching pains, cartilage injuries, painful old injuries, blows to the eye from blunt objects.
Symptoms worse for: touch.
Symptoms better for:
Low time:

Thuja
(Weleda 6c, 30c; Nelsons 6c)

Prepared from fresh green twigs of *Thuja occidentalis* tree (American arbor vitae, northern white cedar).

Uses: warts, catarrh, stabbing headaches, migraine, vertigo when closing the eyes, tooth decay at roots, ear inflammations, cystitis, insomnia, rumbling and flatulence in abdomen.
Suited to: dark-haired, dark-skinned, reserved and perhaps inflexible people.
Symptoms better for: warmth, movement, sneezing, rubbing.
Symptoms worse for: cold, damp, menstruation, tea, coffee, sweets, onions, bright light, sun.
Low time: mid-afternoon, night.

Travel Sickness
(Nelsons)

Combination of *Apomorphium* 6c, *Staphisagria* 6c, *Cocculus indicus* 6c, Nux vom. 6c, petroleum 6c, *Tabacum* 6c, *Theridion* 6c.

Uses: the relief of travel sickness.

Urtica Urens
(Weleda 6c)

Prepared from the flowering *Urtica urens* plant (nettle).

Uses: skin rashes and irritations especially from heat or allergy, stinging and burning pains, urticaria, itchy red raised blotches, minor burns which do not blister, sunburn, insufficient breast milk, gout.
Symptoms better for:
Symptoms worse for: cool bathing, cool moist air, touch.
Low time:

Zeif
(New Era)

Combination of Ferr. Phos. 6x, Nat. Phos. 6x, Nat. Sulph. 6x, Silica 6x.

Uses: rheumatic pain and allied conditions.

PART 3

ALPHABETICAL LISTING

AAA Spray
(Rorer)

An aerosol used as an antibacterial and local anaesthetic to treat sore throat, minor infections of the nose and throat.

Dose: 2 sprays every 2-3 hours up to a maximum of 16 sprays in 24 hours; children over 6 years half adult dose.
Side effects:
Caution:
Not to be used for: children under 6 years.
Not to be used with:
Contains: benzocaine, cetalkonium chloride.
Other preparations:

Abidec
(Warner-Lambert)

Drops used as a multivitamin preparation to treat vitamin deficiencies.

Dose: adults and children over 1 year 0.6 ml a day; infants under 1 year half adult dose.
Side effects:
Caution:
Not to be used for:
Not to be used with: levodopa.
Contains: calciferol, thiamine hydrochloride, riboflavine, pyridoxine hydrochloride, nicotinamide, ascorbic acid.
Other preparations: Abidec Capsules (not available on NHS).

Acetoxyl
(Stiefel)

A gel used as an antibacterial and skin softener to treat acne.
Dose: wash and dry the affected area and apply the gel once

a day.
Side effects: irritation, peeling.
Caution: keep out of the eyes, nose, and mouth; children should use the weaker gel.
Not to be used for:
Not to be used with:
Contains: benzoyl peroxide.
Other preparations:

Acidosis
(Potters)

Dose: 2 tablets 3 times a day after meals.
Product licence: No. 0250/5190R.
Constituents: meadowsweet (*Filipendula ulmaria*), vegetable charcoal, rhubarb (*Rheum officinale*), aniseed oil (*Pimpinella anisum*), caraway oil (*Carum carvi*), cardamom (*Elettaria cardamom*), cinnamon (*Cinnamomum verum*), excipients.
Uses: indigestion, hyperacidity, heartburn.
Special notes:
Caution: not recommended for children.

Aci-Jel
(Cilag)

A jelly with applicator used as an antiseptic to treat non-specific vaginal infection.

Dose: 1 application into the vagina twice a day.
Side effects: irritation and inflammation.
Caution:
Not to be used for: children.
Not to be used with:
Contains: acetic acid.
Other preparations:

Acnegel
(Stiefel)

A gel used as an antibacterial and skin softener to treat acne.

Dose: wash and dry the affected area and apply the gel once a day.
Side effects: irritation, peeling.
Caution: keep out of the eyes, nose, and mouth.
Not to be used for:
Not to be used with:
Contains: benzoyl peroxide.
Other preparations: Acnegel Forte.

Acnidazil
(Janssen)

A cream used as an antibacterial and skin softener to treat acne.

Dose: wash and dry the affected area and apply the cream once a day for the first week, then twice a day for the next 4-8 weeks.
Side effects: irritation, peeling.
Caution: keep out of the eyes, nose, and mouth.
Not to be used for:
Not to be used with:
Contains: miconazole nitrate, benzoyl peroxide.
Other preparations:

Aconite
(Weleda 6c, 30c; Nelsons 6c)

Prepared from entire plant *Aconitum napellus* (wolfbane).

Uses: emotional shock, panic attacks, intense fear, anxiety, restlessness; useful in the first stages of a cold or fever — up to 48 hours from onset, complaints come on suddenly and patient may have hot red cheeks and be thirsty for cold drinks although everything tastes bitter; sudden high fevers with intense thirst and dry skin, burning sore throat, intolerable pain, toothache or earache after exposure to cold dry wind; croup, dry suffocating barking cough, insomnia with anxious dreams.

Suited to: patients suffering from illness following fright or shock.

Symptoms better for: open air, reduced covering.

Symptoms worse for: fright, shock, bad news, warm room, heat of sun, cold dry winds, lying on affected side, tobacco smoke, music.

Low time: midnight.

Acriflex

Acriflex is a cream containing chlorhexidine gluconate as a disinfectant. It may be useful to soothe burns and to prevent secondary infection.

Actaea racemosa (Actaea rac.)
(Weleda 6c, 30c; Nelsons 6c)

Prepared from root of *Cimicifuga racemosa* plant (black cohosh).

Uses: depression, claustrophobia, irritability, headaches with severe pains which start at the back of the head and spread upwards and which are relieved by cool fresh air, neuralgia, stiff neck, tinnitus, painful muscles after exercise, rheumatic pains in back and neck, heavy exhausting menstruation, chilliness.

Suited to: patients who are sensitive, nervous, excitable, and talkative and who may also become despondent.

Symptoms better for: warmth, eating.

Symptoms worse for: cold, damp, motion, menstruation.

Low time: morning.

Actal
(Winthrop)

A white tablet supplied at a strength of 360 mg and used as an antacid to treat indigestion, dyspepsia.

Dose: 1-2 tablets when needed.
Side effects: few; sodium overload is possible.
Caution:
Not to be used for: children.
Not to be used with: tetracycline antibiotics.
Contains: alexitol sodium.
Other preparations: Actal Suspension.

Actidil
(Wellcome)

A white, scored tablet supplied at a strength of 2.5 mg and used as an antihistamine to treat allergies.

Dose: adults 1-2 tablets 3 times a day; children use elixir.
Side effects: drowsiness, reduced reactions, rarely skin eruptions.
Caution: in patients suffering from liver or kidney disease.
Not to be used for:
Not to be used with: alcohol, sedatives, some antidepressants (MAOIs).
Contains: triprolidine hydrochloride.
Other preparations:

Actifed Compound
(Wellcome)

A linctus used as an antihistamine to treat cough, congestion.

Dose: adults 2 5 ml teaspoonsful 3 times a day; children 2-5 years ½

teaspoonful 3 times a day, 6-12 years 1 teaspoonful 3 times a day..
Side effects: drowsiness, reduced reactions.
Caution: in patients suffering from liver or kidney disease.
Not to be used for: children under 2 years
Not to be used with: alcohol, sedatives, some antidepressants (MAOIs).
Contains: triprolidine hydrochloride, pseudoephedrine hydrochloride, dextromethorphan hydrobromide.
Other preparations: Actifed Expectorant, Actifed Tablets, Actifed Syrup.

Actonorm
(Wallace)

A white liquid supplied in 200 ml bottles and used as an antacid to treat indigestion, wind.

Dose: 5-20 ml after meals.
Side effects: few; occasionally constipation or diarrhoea.
Caution:
Not to be used for: children.
Not to be used with: tetracycline antibiotics.
Contains: aluminium hydroxide, magnesium hydroxide, activated dimethicone.
Other preparations:

Adiantine
(Potters)

Dose: use night and morning, massage gently into the scalp.
Product licence: No. PL0250/5081R.
Constituents: southernwood (*Artemisia abrotanum*) extract, bay (*Laurus nobilis*) oil, rosemary (*Rosmarinus officinalis*) oil, witch hazel (*Hamamelis*) water.
Uses: to improve hair condition and eliminate dandruff.
Caution: shake the bottle before use.

Afrazine
(Kirby-Warrick)

A spray or nasal drops used as a sympathomimetic treatment for blocked nose.

Dose: adults and children over 5 years 2-3 sprays or drops in each nostril 2-3 times a day; children under 5 years use Paediatric drops.
Side effects: itching nose, headache, sleeplessness, rapid heart rate.
Caution: in patients suffering from overactive thyroid gland, diabetes, coronary disease. Do not use for extended periods.
Not to be used for:
Not to be used with: MAOIs.
Contains: oxymetazoline hydrochloride.
Other preparations: Afrazine Paediatric.

Agarol
(Warner-Lambert)

An emulsion used as a lubricant and stimulant to treat constipation.
Dose: adults 5-15 ml at bedtime; children 5-12 years 5 ml at bedtime.
Side effects: allergies to phenolphthalein, blood or protein in the urine.
Caution:
Not to be used for: children under 5 years.
Not to be used with:
Contains: liquid paraffin, phenolphthalein, agar.
Other preparations:

Aglutella
(Nutricia)

Gluten-, sucrose-, and lactose-free protein which is low in

sodium and potassium. It is supplied as macaroni, pasta spirals, spaghetti, spaghetti rings, tagliatelle, and semolina. It is used for patients suffering from phenylketonuria, chronic kidney failure, cirrhosis of the liver, and diseases of the digestive tract where there is sensitivity to gluten.

Other preparations: Aglutella Azeta

Al 110
(Nestle)

Gluten-, and sucrose-free powder containing fat, protein, carbohydrate, vitamins, and minerals. It is used for patients suffering from an intolerance to lactose, and galactosaemia, galactokinase.

Albumaid
(S.H.S.)

Beef serum hydrolysate containing amino acids, carbohydrate, minerals, vitamins, and trace elements. It is used for patients suffering from tyrosinosis and tyrosinaemia.

Other preparations: Albumaid XP, Albumaid XP Concentrate, Albumaid Methionine Low, Albumaid RVHB Complete.

Alcopar
(Wellcome)

Dispersible granules in a sachet of 2.5 g used as an anti-worm treatment.

Dose: adults and children over 2 years 1 sachet dispersed in water; children under 2 years half adult dose.
Side effects: stomach upset.

Caution:
Not to be used for: patients who are continuously vomiting.
Not to be used with:
Contains: bephenium hydroxy-naphthoate.
Other preparations:

Alembicol D
(Alembic)

A liquid containing mainly fatty acids from coconut oil. It is used in diluted form for patients suffering from impaired ability to absorb fats.

Alfare
(Nestle)

A powder containing fat, protein, carbohydrate, vitamins, and minerals. It is used for patients suffering from an intolerance to protein.

Algesal
(Duphar)

A cream used as an analgesic rub to treat rheumatic conditions.

Dose: massage into the affected area 3 times a day.
Side effects:
Caution:
Not to be used for: children under 6 years.
Not to be used with:
Contains: diethylamine salicylate.
Other preparations:

Algicon
(Rorer)

A white tablet used as an antacid to treat heartburn, hiatus hernia indigestion.

Dose: 1-2 tablets 4 times a day after meals and at night.
Side effects: few; constipation or diarrhoea.
Caution: in patients suffering from diabetes because of sucrose content.
Not to be used for: children, or in patients suffering from kidney failure or severe debilitation.
Not to be used with: tetracycline antibiotics.
Contains: magnesium alginate, aluminium hydroxide/magnesium carbonate, magnesium carbonate, potassium bicarbonate.
Other preparations: Algicon Suspension.

Alka Seltzer
(Bayer)

Alka Seltzer contains aspirin, citric acid, and sodium bicarbonate. Although the sodium bicarbonate is an alkali, the combination with aspirin means that this preparation is not suitable for those with ulcer disease, because aspirin makes ulcers bleed. Alka Seltzer can be used for mild headache and indigestion combined, for example in those with a hangover.

Allbee with C
(Robins)

A green/yellow capsule used as a multivitamin treatment for vitamin B and vitamin C deficiencies.

Dose: adults 1-3 capsules a day; children 1 capsule a day.
Side effects:

Allium cepa
(Weleda 6c)

Prepared from entire *Allium cepa* plant (red onion).

Uses: hayfever, catarrh, inflammation of mucous membranes, colds with profuse burning watery discharge, eyes watering burning, and smarting, laryngitis.
Symptoms better for: cold room, open air.
Symptoms worse for: warm room.
Low time: evening.

Alophen
(Warner-Lambert)

A brown pill used as a stimulant and anticholinergic to treat constipation.

Dose: 1-3 pills at bedtime.
Side effects: allergies to phenolphthalein, skin rash, protein in the urine.
Caution:
Not to be used for: children or for patients suffering from glaucoma or inflammatory bowel disease.
Not to be used with:
Contains: aloin, phenolphthalein, ipecacuanha, belladonna extract.
Other preparations:

Alphosyl
(Stafford Miller)

A cream used as an anti-psoriatic to treat psoriasis.

Dose: massage thoroughly into the affected area 2-4 times a day.
Side effects: irritation, sensitivity to light.
Caution:
Not to be used for: patients suffering from acute psoriasis.
Not to be used with:
Contains: coal tar extract, allantoin.
Other preparations: Alphosyl Lotion, Alphosyl Shampoo.

Altacite Plus
(Roussel)

A white liquid supplied in 500 ml bottles and used as an antacid and anti-wind preparation to treat wind, indigestion, dyspepsia, and gastric ulcers.

Dose: adults 10 ml between meals and at bedtime; children 8-12 years half adult dose.
Side effects: few; occasional diarrhoea and constipation.
Caution:
Not to be used for: children under 8 years.
Not to be used with: tetracycline antibiotics.
Contains: hydrotalcite, activated dimethicone.
Other preparations: higher-strength suspension.and tablets.

Alu-Cap
(3M Riker)

A green/red capsule supplied at a strength of 475 mg and used as an antacid to treat hyperacidity.

Dose: 1 capsule 4 times a day and at bedtime.
Side effects: few; occasional bowel disorder such as constipation.
Caution:
Not to be used for: children.
Not to be used with: tetracycline antibiotics.
Contains: aluminium hydroxide gel.
Other preparations:

Aluhyde
(Sinclair)

A white scored tablet used as an antispasmodic and antacid to treat hyperacidity and intestinal spasm.

Dose: 2 tablets after meals.
Side effects: occasionally constipation and blurred vision.
Caution: in patients suffering from prostate enlargement.
Not to be used for: children or for patients suffering from glaucoma.
Not to be used with: tetracycline antibiotics.
Contains: aluminium hydroxide gel, magnesium trisilicate, belladonna liquid extract.
Other preparations:

Aluminium-free Indigestion Tablets
(Larkhall)
'Cantassium'

Dose: 1-4 tablets to be taken as required after meals.
Product licence: No. PL0912/5238R.
Constituents: calcium carbonate 75 mg, cinnamon (*Cinnamomum verum*) 30 mg, nutmeg (*Myristica*) 24 mg, clove (*Caryophyllin*) 12 mg, cardamom (*Elettaria cardamom*) seed 9 mg, mannitol 20 mg, calcium sulphate dihydrate 0.4 g, potato starch 40 mg, stearic acid (palm oil) 3 mg, gum acacia.

Uses: indigestion relief without risk from aluminium.
Special notes: vegan, hypoallergenic.
Caution: not recommended during pregnancy or breastfeeding without practitioner supervision. May antidote any homoeopathic remedies which you are taking.

Aminex
(Cow & Gate)

Sucrose- and lactose-free biscuit which is low in protein, sodium, phenylalanine, and potassium. It is used for patients suffering from phenylketonuria, chronic kidney failure, cirrhosis of the liver, and lactose with sucrose intolerance.

Aminogran
(UCB)
Phenylalanine-free powder supplying essential and non-essential amino acids. It is used for patients suffering from phenylketonuria.

Other preparations: Aminogran Mineral Mixture.

Anaflex
(Geistlich)

A white lozenge supplied at a strength of 30 mg and used as an antibacterial and antifungal treatment for thrush and other bacterial infections of the mouth and throat.

Dose: adults 6-10 lozenges a day; children over 6 years half adult dose.
Side effects:
Caution:
Not to be used for: children under 6 years.
Not to be used with:

Contains: polynoxylin.
Other preparations: Anaflex Cream, Anaflex Paste, Anaflex Powder.

Anaflex Cream
(Geistlich)

A cream used as an antibacterial and antifungal treatment for skin infections.

Dose: apply the cream to the affected area 1-2 times a day.
Side effects:
Caution:
Not to be used for:
Not to be used with:
Contains: polynoxylin.
Other preparations: Anaflex, Anaflex Paste, Anaflex Powder, Anaflex Aerosol.

Analog
(S.H.S.)

Phenylalanine-free powder supplying proteins, fats, vitamins, minerals, and trace elements. It is used for infants suffering from phenylketonuria.

Other preparations: Analog MSUD; Analog RVHB; Analog XPHEN TYR; Analog XMET, THRE, VAL, ISOLEU.

Anased Pain Relief Tablets
(Potters)

Dose: 1-2 tablets 3 times daily and 2 at bedtime.
Product licence: No. 0250/5223R.
Constituents: hops (*Humulus lupulus*), Jamaica dogwood

(*Piscidia erythrina*), wild lettuce (*Lactuca virosa*), passionflower (*Passiflora*), wind anemone (*Pulsatilla*), excipients.
Uses: sedative, analgesic, relief of minor aches, tension headaches, insomnia, irritability.
Special notes:
Caution: not recommended during pregnancy or breastfeeding, nor for children.

Andrew's see **ENO**

Andrew's Answer see **ENO**

Andursil
(Geigy)

A white liquid supplied in 100 ml bottles and used as an antacid and anti-wind preparation to treat dyspepsia, heartburn, peptic ulcer.

Dose: 5-10 ml 3 times a day and at bedtime.
Side effects: few; possibly constipation or diarrhoea.
Caution:
Not to be used for: children.
Not to be used with: tetracycline antibiotics.
Contains: aluminium oxide, magnesium hydroxide, aluminium hydroxide/magnesium carbonate, activated dimethicone.
Other preparations: Andursil Tablets.

Antepar
(Wellcome)

An elixir used as an anti-worm treatment.

Dose: adults up to 30 ml as a single dose; children reduced doses.

Side effects: stomach upset, changes in the central nervous system, hypersensitivity, bruising, blood changes, liver disorder.

Caution: in nursing mothers and in patients suffering from nervous disorders.

Not to be used for: patients suffering from epilepsy, or kidney or liver disease.

Not to be used with:

Contains: piperazine hydrate, piperazine citrate.

Other preparations:

Anthisan
(Fisons)

Anthisan is a topical antihistamine cream containing mepyramine maleate 2 %. It is used for the treatment of allergic skin reactions and allergies.

Antibron Tablets
(Potters)

Dose: 2 tablets 3 times a day; children over 7 years 1 tablet 3 times a day.

Product licence: No. 0250/5177R.

Constituents: lobelia (*Lobelia inflata*), wild lettuce (*Lactuca virosa*) extracts, coltsfoot (*Tussilago farfara*), euphorbia (*Euphorbia hirta*), pleurisy root (*Asclepias tuberosa*), snake root (*Polygala senega*), liquorice (*Glycyrrhiza glabra*), capsicum, excipients.

Uses: expectorant, antispasmodic, anti-asthmatic, sedative, to relieve coughs.

Special notes:

Caution: do not exceed the stated dose — *Lobelia* may cause nausea and vomiting in high doses.

Antifect
(Potters)

Dose: 2 tablets 3 times a day; children over 8 years half the adult dose.
Product licence: No. 0250/5222R.
Constituents: garlic (*Allium sativum*), garlic oil, coneflower (*Echinacea angustifoilia*) extract, vegetable charcoal, excipients.
Uses: expectorant, antibiotic, antibacterial, antiviral, for catarrh, rhinitis, nasal congestion, sinusitis, hayfever.
Special notes:
Caution:

Antiglan Tablets
(Potters)

Dose: elderly males 2 tablets 3 times a day, in severe cases 3 tablets 3 times a day.
Product licence: No. 0250/5076R.
Constituents: kava (*Piper methysticum*), saw palmetto (*Serenoa repens*), horsetail (*Equisetum*), hydrangea (*Hydrangea arborescens*), excipients.
Uses: short-term relief of mild bladder discomfort; may help with enlarged prostate glands — holding the condition and, in some cases, edging it back — helpful for those waiting for a prostate operation.
Special notes:
Caution:

Anti-smoking
(Larkhall)
'Cantassium'

Dose: 1 tablet to be swallowed with water when craving a smoke. Do not take more than 9 tablets in 24 hours.
Product licence: No. PL/0912/5977R.

Constituents: kolanuts (*Cola acuminata*) 20 mg, lobelia (*Lobelia inflata*) 65 mg, dicalcium phosphate 0.55 g, icing sugar 95 mg, magnesium trisilicate 30 mg, quassia (*Picrasma excelsa*) powder 25 mg, sago flour 20.3 mg, talc 3 mg, industrial methylated spirits 0.05 ml, stearic acid (palm oil) 2 mg.
Uses: a smoking deterrent preparation.
Special notes: vegan, hypoallergenic.
Caution: not to be taken during pregnancy or breastfeeding. Do not exceed the stated dose — higher doses may produce nausea and vomiting.

Antismoking Tablets
(Potters)

Dose: 1 tablet to be taken every hour all day; each tablet should be sucked for half-a-minute, then swallowed whole.
Product licence: No. PL/0250/5178.
Constituents: lobelia (*Lobelia inflata*), excipients.
Uses: to reduce addiction to tobacco smoking.
Special notes:
Caution: do not exceed the stated dose; higher doses may produce nausea and vomiting. Not to be taken during pregnancy or breastfeeding.

Antitis Tablets
(Potters)

Dose: 2 tablets 3 times a day.
Product licence: No. 0250/5224R.
Constituents: buchu (*Agathosma betulina*), clivers (*Galium aparine*), couchgrass (*Agropyron repens*), horsetail (*Equisetum*), shepherd's purse (*Capsella bursa-pastoris*), uva ursi (*Arctostaphylos uva-ursi*), excipients.
Uses: diuretic, antiseptic, to relieve cystitis.
Special notes: Potter's recommend increasing fluid intake, and that drinks containing bicarbonate of soda are especially useful.

Caution: not recommended for children.

Apis mellifica (Apis mel.)
(Weleda 6c, 30c; Nelsons 6c)

Prepared from honey bee venom.

Uses: burning stinging pains, cystitis with constant desire to urinate, arthritis with red, swollen, shiny joints, hot red swelling anywhere in body, swollen ankles, swollen lower eyelids, bites and stings which become red and swollen, allergic reactions (if the reaction is severe or there is difficult breathing, seek medical help immediately), urticaria, symptoms tend to affect the right side of the body most, thirstlessness, burning sore throat.
Suited to: busy, restless people who may become ill after emotional upset.
Symptoms better for: cold bathing, open air.
Symptoms worse for: heat, touch, after sleep, fright, anger, grief, bad news.
Low time: mid-afternoon.

Appetiser Mixture (formerly Tonic and Nervine Essence)
(Potters)

Dose: 1 5 ml teaspoonful 3 times a day in a little water before meals.
Product licence: No. P/L0250/5106R.
Constituents: camomile (*Chamaemelum nobile*), calumba (*Jateorhiza palmata*) root, gentian (*Gentiana lutea*), excipients.
Uses: tonic, to promote appetite and relieve symptoms of flatulence.
Special notes:
Caution: not recommended during pregnancy or breastfeeding, nor for children.

Aproten
(Ultrapharm)

Low-protein, gluten-free preparation supplied as anellini, ditalini, rigatoni, tagliatelle, biscuits, crispbread, flour, bread mix, and cake mix. It is used for patients suffering from phenylketonuria, kidney and liver failure, cirrhosis of the liver, and gastro-enteritic diseases where sensitivity to gluten is present.

Aquasept
(Hough, Hoseason)

A solution used as a disinfectant for skin and body cleansing and disinfecting.

Dose: use as a soap.
Side effects:
Caution: keep out of the eyes.
Not to be used for:
Not to be used with:
Contains: triclosan.
Other preparations:

Aradolene
(Fisons)

A cream used as an analgesic rub to treat rheumatic conditions.

Dose: massage into the affected area 2-3 times a day.
Side effects: may be irritant
Caution:
Not to be used for: areas such as near the eyes, on broken or inflamed skin, or on membranes (such as the mouth).
Not to be used with:
Contains: diethylamine salicylate, capsicum oleoresin, camphor oil, menthol.

Other preparations:

Argentum nitricum (Argent nit.)
(Weleda 6c, 30c; Nelsons 6c)

Prepared from silver nitrate.

Uses: nervousness, anticipatory fear, heartburn, acidity, flatulence, headache relieved by pressure, mental strain, vertigo with buzzing in the ears, tremor, agoraphobia, claustrophobia, nervous diarrhoea, hoarseness.
Suited to: hurried, fidgety, impulsive, nervous people who suffer from anticipatory fear.
Symptoms better for: open air, cold bathing.
Symptoms worse for: anticipatory fear, overwork, overstudy, sugar, ice-cream, warmth.
Low time: night.

Arnica
(Weleda 6x, 6c, 30c; Nelsons 6c)

Prepared from entire *Arnica montana* plant (mountain tobacco).

Uses: after physical shock or injury; bruises, sprains, exhaustion, jet lag, aching muscles; body feeling sore and bruised all over, concussion, haemorrhages, compound fractures.
Symptoms better for: lying down with head low.
Symptoms worse for: touch, movement, cold, damp.
Low time:

Arnica Lotion
(Weleda)

Dose: dilute one dessertspoonful in ½ pint of water and bathe the affected part, or apply as a compress. A tablespoonful in a

warm bath will help relieve aching muscles after exercise.
Product licence: No. PL0298/5685.
Constituents: arnica (*Arnica montana*) ethanolic extract (1=5), nominal ethanol content 30 %.
Uses: to relieve muscular pain, stiffness, sprains, bruises, immediate application will help prevent bruising.
Caution: shake the bottle before use; do not apply to broken skin.

Arnica Massage Balm
(Weleda)

Dose: massage into affected part 3-4 times a day as required.
Product licence: No. PL0298/5528.
Constituents: per 100 ml: *Arnica* flowers 3 g, birch (*Betula verrucosa*) leaves 3 g, rosemary (*Rosmarinus officinalis*) oil 4 ml, lavender (*Lavendula angustifolia*) oil 2 ml, base.
Uses: bruising, stiffness, backache, sciatica, fibrositis, rheumatic pain; when used daily from the second month of pregnancy it can help prevent stretch marks.
Caution: do not apply to broken skin.

Arnica Ointment
(Weleda)

Dose: apply sparingly to the affected part as soon as possible after the injury; repeat 3-4 times a day or as required.
Constituents: per 100g: arnica (*Arnica montana*) tincture (1=2) 10 ml, lanolin, beeswax, vegetable oils.
Uses: bruises, sprains, strains, muscular pain, swelling, stiffness.
Caution: do not apply to broken skin. Some individuals may be sensitive to lanolin.

Arret
(Janssen)

A capsule used to treat diarrhoea.

Dose: up to 8 capsules daily.
Availability;
Side effects: rashes
Caution: in severe colitis.
Not to be used for: children.
Not to be used with:
Contains: loperamide.
Other preparations: Imodium capsules and syrup on prescription.

Arsenicum album (Arsen. alb.)
(Weleda 6c, 30c; Nelsons 6c)

Prepared from the white oxide of metallic arsenic.

Uses: food poisoning, holiday stomach upsets, sudden violent vomiting and diarrhoea, restlessness, icy chills, burning pains especially throat or stomach, anxiety, fear, insomnia with overactive mind and anxious dreams.
Suited to: patients who are tidy, fastidious, precise, and anxious.
Symptoms better for: heat, cool air around head.
Symptoms worse for: cold, cold food and drinks.
Low time: after midnight.

Artichoke Formula
(Bio-Strath: imported by Cedar Health Ltd)

Dose: 20 drops (0.6 ml) in a little water 3 times a day before meals.
Product licence: No. PL4210/0004.

Constituents: artichoke (*Cynara scolymus*) leaf extract 22.5 %, thistle seed (*Carduus marianus*) extract 22.5 %, peppermint (*Mentha piperita*) leaf extract 5 %, *Torula utilis* yeast plasmolysate 50 %, (ethanol content 38 % v/v approx.).
Uses: to relieve the symptoms of indigestion after eating fatty foods
Special notes:
Caution: may antidote any homoeopathic remedies which you are taking.

Ascabiol
(M & B)

An emulsion used as an insect-destroying preparation to treat scabies, pediculosis.

Dose:
Side effects: irritation.
Caution: keep out of the eyes.
Not to be used for:
Not to be used with:
Contains: benzyl benzoate.
Other preparations:

Asilone
(Rorer)

A white liquid used as an antacid, anti-wind preparation to treat gastritis, ulcers, dyspepsia, wind.

Dose: adults 5-10 ml before meals and at bedtime; children use infant suspension or half adult dose.
Side effects: few; occasionally constipation.
Caution:
Not to be used for: infants.
Not to be used with:

Contains: activated dimethicone, aluminium hydroxide gel, magnesium oxide.
Other preparations: Asilone Gel, Asilone Infant Suspension, Asilone Tablets; Infacol (Pharmax); Polycrol Gel and Tablets, Polycrol Forte Gel (Nicholas); Unigest (Unigreg) — private prescription and over the counter only; Siloxyl (Martindale) — private prescription and over the counter only.

Aspellin
(Fisons)

A liniment or a spray used as a topical analgesic to treat muscular rheumatism, sciatica, lumbago, fibrositis, chilblains.

Dose: massage gently into the affected area every 3-4 hours.
Side effects: may be irritant.
Caution:
Not to be used for: areas near the eyes, or where the skin is broken or inflamed, or on membranes (such as the mouth).
Not to be used with:
Contains: aspirin, menthol, camphor, methyl salicylate.
Other preparations:

---

aspirin

A white tablet supplied at a strength of 300 mg and used as an analgesic to relieve pain and reduce fever.

Dose: 1-3 tablets every 4-6 hours as needed to a maximum of 12 tablets a day.
Side effects: stomach upsets, allergy, asthma.
Caution: in pregnant women, the elderly, or in patients with a history of allergy to aspirin, asthma, impaired kidney or liver function, indigestion.
Not to be used for: children, nursing mothers, or for patients suffering from haemophilia or ulcers.

Not to be used with: anticoagulants (blood-thinning drugs), some antidiabetic drugs, anti-inflammatory agents, methotrexate, spironolactone, steroids, some antacids, some uric-acid lowering drugs.
Contains:
Other preparations: dispersible aspirin.

AT 10
(Sterling Research Laboratories)

A solution used as a source of vitamin D to treat vitamin D deficiency.

Dose: 1-7 ml taken by mouth each week.
Side effects: loss of appetite, listlessness, vertigo, stupor, nausea, urgent need to urinate.
Caution: in nursing mothers. Your doctor may advise that your calcium levels should be checked regularly.
Not to be used for: children.
Not to be used with:
Contains: dihydrotachysterol.
Other preparations:

Athera
(Modern Health)

Dose: 2-3 tablets to be taken 3 times a day after meals.
Product licence: No. 2452/5001R.
Constituents: parsley (*Petroselinum crispum*) 60 mg, vervain (*Verbena officinalus*) 10 mg, vervain extract 90 mg, clivers (*Galium aparine*) extract 60 mg, senna leaf 4 mg, senna extract 10 mg, excipients.
Uses: for menopausal symptoms, to ease fluid retention, soothe the stomach, relax, increase vitality, tone the system, maintain healthy bowel action.
Special notes: not tested on animals.

Caution: may occasionally cause diarrhoea, not recommended for children or during pregnancy or breastfeeding. Senna is not to be used in colitis or spastic colon. Senna may harmlessly colour the urine or stools.

Audax
(Napp Consumer)

Drops used as an analgesic to relieve pain associated with acute inflammation of the outer or middle ear..

Dose: fill the ear with the liquid and plug it.
Side effects:
Caution:
Not to be used for:
Not to be used with:
Contains: choline salicylate.
Other preparations:

Auralgicin
(Fisons)

A liquid used as an antibacterial treatment for inflammation of the middle ear.

Dose: fill the ear with the liquid every hour and plug until the pain is relieved, and then treat every 3 hours for 24 hours.
Side effects:
Caution:
Not to be used for:
Not to be used with:
Contains: ephedrine hydrochloride, benzocaine, chlorbutol, potassium hydroxyquinolone sulphate, phenazone, glycerin.
Other preparations:

Auraltone
(Fisons)

Drops used as an analgesic, local anaesthetic treatment for acute inflammation of the eardrum or inner ear.

Dose: fill the ear with the drops and plug lightly, repeating every hour if needed.
Side effects: skin eruptions.
Caution:
Not to be used for:
Not to be used with:
Contains: phenazone, benzocaine.
Other preparations:

Avena Sativa Comp.
(Weleda)

Dose: 10-20 drops to be taken in water half an hour before going to bed. If necessary this dose may be repeated; children: half the adult dose.
Product licence: No. PL0298/5473.
Constituents: per 100 ml: oats (*Avena sativa*) tincture 25 ml, hops (*Humulus lupulus*) 1x 4 ml, passionflower (*Passiflora incarnata*) tincture 7.5 ml, valerian (*Valeriana officinalis*) tincture 30 ml, *Coffea tosta* 60x 15 ml, nominal ethanol content 45 % v/v.
Uses: to aid relaxation at the end of the day.
Special notes:
Caution: may cause sleepiness. Not recommended during pregnancy or breastfeeding.

Avomine
(Wellcome)

A white, scored tablet supplied at a strength of 25 mg and used

as an antihistamine treatment for travel sickness, nausea, vomiting, vertigo.

Dose: adults travel sickness 1 tablet at bedtime before long journeys or 1-2 hours before short journeys, nausea 1 tablet 1-3 times a day; children 5-10 years half adult dose.
Side effects: drowsiness, reduced reactions, rarely skin eruptions.
Caution: in patients suffering from liver or kidney disease.
Not to be used for: children under 5 years.
Not to be used with: alcohol, sedatives, some antidepressants (MAOIs).
Contains: promethazine, theoclate.
Other preparations:

Backache Tablets
(Potters)

Dose: 2 tablets 3 times a day.
Product licence: No. 0250/5182R
Constituents: gravel root (*Eupatorium purpureum*), hydrangea (*Hydrangea arborescens*) root, buchu (*Agathosma betulina*), uva ursi (*Arctostaphylos uva-ursi*), excipients.
Uses: relief of backache; this formula arises from the herbalist's view that the urinary system must also be toned effectively to deal with backache.
Special notes:
Caution: not recommended during pregnancy nor for children.

Bacticlens
(S & N)

A solution in a sachet used as a disinfectant to clean the skin, wounds, or broken skin.

Dose: use as needed.

Side effects: throw away any remaining solution straight away after use.
Caution:
Not to be used for:
Not to be used with:
Contains: chlorhexidine gluconate.
Other preparations:

Balm of Gilead
(Potters)

Dose: adults: 2 5 ml teaspoonsful 3-4 times a day; children over 5 years 1 5 ml teaspoonful, which may be diluted with water if necessary, 3-4 times a day.
Product licence: No. P/L0250/5085R.
Constituents: acetum scillae (squill vinegar), lobelia (*Lobelia inflata*) tincture, balm of Gilead (*Populus candicans*), lungwort, (*Pulmonaria officinalis*), excipients.
Uses: expectorant, to relieve symptoms of coughs and colds.
Special notes: sugar-free base — concentrated apple juice is used as sweetener.
Caution: shake bottle before use. Not recommended during pregnancy or breastfeeding nor for children under 5 years. Do not exceed the stated dose — high doses of *Lobelia* may cause nausea and vomiting.

Balm of Gilead Cough Mixture
(Booker)
'Heath & Heather'

Dose: 2 5 ml teaspoonsful 3 times a day.
Product licence: No. PL1713/5083R.
Constituents: per 10 ml balm of Gilead (*Populus candicans*) liquid extract 0.8 ml, squill (*Drimia maritima*) tincture 0.25 ml, lobelia (*Lobelia inflata*) tincture 0.2 ml, sugar syrup, xanthum gum, nipastat sodium.

Uses: to relieve symptoms of coughs and catarrh.
Special notes: vegan, yeast free.
Caution: shake before use. Not recommended during pregnancy or breastfeeding nor for children. Do not exceed the stated dose — high doses of *Lobelia* may cause nausea and vomiting.

Balm of Gilead Cough Pastilles
(Booker)
'Heath & Heather'

Dose: allow a pastille to dissolve in the mouth when needed. Not more than 12 to be taken in 24 hours.
Product licence: No. P/L1713/5084R.
Constituents: balm of Gilead (*Populus candicans*) buds 8 %, squill (*Drimia maritima*) tincture 2.5 %, lobelia (*Lobelia inflata*) tincture 2 %, sugar, liquid glucose, gelatin, liquorice (*Glycyrrhiza glabra*), beetroot red as colouring, anise oil as flavouring, peppermint oil, caramel, vegetable fat.
Uses: to relieve the symptoms of coughs and catarrh.
Special notes: yeast free.
Caution: not recommended for children or during pregnancy or breastfeeding. Do not exceed the stated dose — high doses of *Lobelia* may cause nausea and vomiting. May antidote any homoeopathic remedies you are taking.

Balmosa
(Pharmax)

A cream used as an analgesic rub to treat muscular rheumatism, fibrositis, lumbago, sciatica, unbroken chilblains.

Dose: massage into the affected area as needed.
Side effects: may be irritant
Caution:
Not to be used for: areas near the eyes, on broken or inflamed

skin, or on membranes (such as the mouth).
Not to be used with:
Contains: menthol, camphor, methyl salicylate, capsicum oleoresin.
Other preparations:

Balneum with Tar
(Merck)

A bath oil used as an emollient and antipsoriatic to treat eczema, itchy or thickening skin disorders, psoriasis.

Dose: adults add 4 5 ml teaspoonsful to the bath water; children over 2 years add 2 teaspoonsful and use for a maximum of 6 weeks.
Side effects:
Caution:
Not to be used for: children under 2 years or for patients suffering from wet or weeping skin problems or where the skin is badly broken.
Not to be used with:
Contains: coal tar, soya oil.
Other preparations:

Balsamicum Ointment
(Weleda)

Dose: apply directly to the affected part or on a dry dressing several times a day.
Product licence: No. PL0298/5474.
Constituents: per 100 g: marigold (*Calendula officinalis*) ethanolic extract from 3 g of herb, dog's mercury (*Mercurialis perennis*) ethanolic extract from 5 g of herb, balsam of Peru B.P.C. 0.7 g, Stibium Metallicum Praeparatum 0.05 g, lanolin, beeswax, vegetable oils, yellow soft paraffin.
Uses: to aid healing of abrasions, boils, nappy rash, minor

wounds.
Caution: some individuals may be sensitive to lanolin.

Baltar
(Merck)

A liquid used as an antipsoriatic treatment for psoriasis, dandruff, eczema, dermatoses of the scalp.

Dose: shampoo the hair with the liquid 1-3 times a week.
Side effects:
Caution: keep out of the eyes.
Not to be used for: children under 2 years or for patients suffering from wet or weeping dermatoses or where the skin is badly broken.
Not to be used with:
Contains: coal tar.
Other preparations:

Balto Foot Balm
(Lanes)

Dose: massage into feet after bathing; use morning and evening as required.
Product licence: No. PLO1074/5003R.
Constituents: sulphur 3.0 %, camphor 0.5 %, menthol 0.2 %, zinc oxide 0.47 %, pine oil, seaweed extract, chlorbutol, emulsifying wax, white soft paraffin, lanolin, glycerin, sodium lauryl ether sulphate, chlorophyll, industrial methylated spirit.
Uses: soothes tired aching feet, curbs excessive perspiration, softens hard skin.
Caution: may antidote any homoeopathic remedies you are taking. Avoid contact with silver or other jewellery. Some individuals may be sensitive to lanolin.

Banocide
(Wellcome)

A white, scored tablet supplied at a strength of 50 mg and used as an anti-worm agent to treat worms in the blood and lymph channels.

Dose: as advised by the physician.
Side effects: itchy skin, eye disorders.
Caution: your doctor may advise regular eye tests.
Not to be used for: pregnant women.
Not to be used with:
Contains: diethylcarbamazine.
Other preparations:

Bayolin
(Bayer)

A cream used as an analgesic rub to treat rheumatism, fibrositis, lumbago, sciatica.

Dose: massage gently into the affected area 2-3 times a day.
Side effects: may be irritant.
Caution:
Not to be used for: areas near the eyes, broken or inflamed skin, or on membranes (such as the mouth).
Not to be used with:
Contains: heparinoid, glycol salicylate, benzyl nicotinate.
Other preparations:

BC 500
(Wyeth)

An orange, oblong tablet used as a multivitamin preparation to treat vitamin B and vitamin C deficiencies, and to aid recovery from illness, long-term alcoholism, long-term antibiotic treatment.

Dose: 1 tablet a day.
Side effects:
Caution:
Not to be used for: children.
Not to be used with: levodopa.
Contains: thiamine mononitrate, riboflavine, pyridoxine hydrochloride, nicotinamide, calcium pantothenate, ascorbic acid, cyanocoblamin.
Other preparations:

BC 500 with Iron
(Wyeth)

A red tablet used as a vitamin and iron supplement to treat iron deficiency anaemia.

Dose: 1 tablet a day.
Side effects: nausea, constipation.
Caution:
Not to be used for: children.
Not to be used with: tetracyclines, levodopa.
Contains: ferrous fumarate, thiamine mononitrate, riboflavine, pyridoxine hydrochloride, nicotinamide, calcium pantothenate, ascorbic acid.
Other preparations:

Becalm
(Heath & Heather)

Dose: 1 tablet 3 times a day with water.
Product licence: P/L1713/500R.
Constituents: valerian (*Valeriana officinalis*) extract equivalent to 160 mg, hops (*Humulus lupulus*) extract equivalent to 200 mg, passionflower (*Passiflora*) extract equivalent to 130 mg, dicalcium phosphate, microcrystalline cellulose, stearic acid, magnesium stearate; coating titanium dioxide, iron oxide,

polyethylene glycol.

Uses: sedative, to aid relaxation and calm.

Special notes: vegan, yeast free.

Caution: not recommended for children or during pregnancy or breastfeeding. May cause drowsiness, if affected do not drive or operate machinery and avoid alcohol.

Becosym
(Roche)

A brown tablet used as a source of B vitamins to treat vitamin B deficiencies.

Dose: adults 1-3 tablets a day; children use syrup.

Side effects:

Caution:

Not to be used for:

Not to be used with: levodopa.

Contains: thiamine, riboflavine, pyridoxine, nicotinamide.

Other preparations: Becosym Syrup (not available on NHS), Becosym Forte Tablets (not available on NHS).

Beecham's Powders

Beecham's Powders contain aspirin and caffeine; powder capsules have paracetamol, caffeine, and phenylephrine. Beecham's Hot Lemon is paracetamol with ascorbic acid (vitamin C). The main caution is to observe total daily dose of asprin or paracetamol.

Belladonna
(Weleda 6c, 30c; Nelsons 6c)

Prepared from entire *Atropa belladonna* (deadly nightshade) plant when beginning to flower.

Uses: severe throbbing headache, sudden fevers with flushed face and dilated pupils, excitability during fever, skin is dry hot and burning, sunstroke, throbbing earache, acne, acute local inflammations which are red and throbbing; symptoms tend to be on right side of body.

Suited to: lively, cheerful, excitable children or adults who become restless and agitated when ill.

Symptoms better for: warmth, sitting upright.

Symptoms worse for: touch, movement, noise, sun.

Low time: mid-afternoon.

Bellocarb
(Sinclair)

A beige tablet used as an antacid and anti-spasm treatment for bowel spasm, ulcers, dyspepsia.

Dose: 1-2 tablets 4 times a day.

Side effects: few; occasional constipation.

Caution: in patients suffering from enlarge prostate, heart, kidney, or liver problems.

Not to be used for: patients suffereing from glaucoma.

Not to be used with:

Contains: belladonna, magnesium trisilicate, magnesium carbonate.

Other preparations:

Benerva
(Roche)

A white tablet supplied in strengths of 25 mg, 50 mg, 100 mg and used as a source of vitamin B_1 to treat beri-beri, neuritis.

Dose: 25-50 mg a day.

Side effects:

Caution:

Not to be used for:
Not to be used with: levodopa.
Contains: thiamine hydrochloride.
Other preparations: Benerva Compound.

Benoxyl 5
(Stiefel)

A cream used as an antibacterial and skin softener to treat acne.

Dose: wash and dry the affected area, then apply once a day.
Side effects: irritation, peeling.
Caution: keep out of the eyes, nose, and mouth.
Not to be used for:
Not to be used with:
Contains: benzoyl peroxide.
Other preparations: Benoxyl 5 with Sulphur, Benoxyll 10, Benoxyl 10 with Sulphur.

Benylin Day and Night

Benylin Day and Night contains paracetamol and is a useful tablet preparation for treating the common cold.

Side effects: drowsiness, reduced reactions.
Caution: in patients suffering from liver or kidney disease.

Benylin Expectorant
(Warner-Lambert)

A syrup used as an antihistamine, expectorant, and sputum softener to treat cough, bronchial congestion.

Dose: adults 1-2 5 ml teaspoonsful every 2-3 hours; children 1-5 years ½ teaspoonful every 3-4 hours, 6-12 years 1 teaspoon-

ful every 3-4 hours.
Side effects:
Caution:
Not to be used for: children under 1 year.
Not to be used with:
Contains: diphenhydramine hydrochloride, ammonium chloride, sodium citrate, menthol.
Other preparations: Benylin Paediatric, Benylin Decongestant, Benylin with Codeine.

Benzagel
(Bioglan)

A white gel used as an antibacterial and skin softener to treat acne.

Dose: wash and dry the affected area, then apply 1-2 times a day.
Side effects: irritation, peeling.
Caution: keep out of the eyes, nose, and mouth.
Not to be used for:
Not to be used with:
Contains: benzoyl peroxide.
Other preparations:

Betadine
(Cilag)

A pessary and applicator supplied at a strength of 200 mg and used as an antiseptic to treat inflammation of the vagina.

Dose: 1 pessary to be inserted into the vagina night and morning for at least 14 days.
Side effects: irritation and sensitivity.
Caution:
Not to be used for: children.

Not to be used with:
Contains: povidone-iodine.
Other preparations: Betadine Vaginal Gel, Betadine VC Kit.

Betadine Gargle and Mouthwash
(Napp)

A solution used as an antiseptic to treat inflammation of the mouth and pharynx brought on by thrush and other bacterial infections.

Dose: wash out the mouth or gargle with the diluted or undiluted solution every 2-4 hours.
Side effects: rarely local irritation and sensitivity.
Caution:
Not to be used for:
Not to be used with:
Contains: povidone-iodine.
Other preparations:

Betadine Ointment
(Napp)

An ointment used as an antiseptic to treat ulcers.

Dose: apply to the affected area and cover once a day.
Side effects: rarely irritation.
Caution: in patients sensitive to iodine.
Not to be used for:
Not to be used with:
Contains: povidone-iodine.
Other preparations:

Betadine Scalp and Skin Cleanser
(Napp)

A solution used as an antiseptic and detergent to treat acne, seborrhoeic scalp and skin disorders.

Dose: use as a shampoo or apply directly to the skin and then cleanse properly.
Side effects: rarely irritation or sensitivity.
Caution:
Not to be used for:
Not to be used with:
Contains: povidone-iodine.
Other preparations: Betadine Skin Cleanser, Betadine Shampoo.

Betadine Spray
(Napp)

A spray used as an antiseptic to treat infected cuts, wounds, and burns.

Dose: spray on to the affected area once a day or as needed, and cover.
Side effects:
Caution: keep out of the eyes.
Not to be used for: patients suffering from non-toxic colloid goitre
Not to be used with:
Contains: povidone-iodine.
Other preparations: Betadine Dry Powder, Betadine Antiseptic Paint, Betadine Antiseptic Solution, Betadine Alcoholic Solution, Betadine Surgical Scrub.

Bi-Aglut
(Ultrapharm)

Gluten-free preparation supplied as a biscuit. It is used for patients suffering from gastro-enteritic diseases where sensitivity to gluten is present.

Other preparations: Bi-Aglut Cracker Toast.

Biobalm Powder
(Modern Health)

Dose: 1-2 level teaspoons to be taken up to 4 times a day; children 5-12 years half the above dosage.
Product licence: No. 1146/5004R.
Constituents: Per 100 g slippery elm bark (*Ulmus rubra*) 13 g, marshmallow root (*Althaea officinalis*) 8 g, Irish moss (*Chondrus crispus*) 6 g, camomile, barley flour, excipients.
Uses: indigestion, flatulence, soothes gastro-intestinal lining.
Special notes: vegetarian.
Caution:

Biophyllin
(Gerard House)

Dose: 2 tablets after meals 3 times a day.
Product licence: No. 1661/5000R.
Constituents: valerian (*Valeriana officinalis*) 150 mg, scullcap (*Scutellaria lateriflora*)108 mg, Jamaican dogwood (*Piscidia erythrina*) 9 mg, black cohosh (*Cimicifuga racemosa*) 30 mg, cayenne (*Capsicum frutescens*) 3 mg, malto-dextrin 140 mg, calcium phosphate 50 mg, sugar 40 mg, sodium starch glycollate 20 mg, magnesium stearate 2 mg, talc 8 mg.
Uses: nervousness, tension, restlessness, irritability.
Special notes: vegan, yeast free.
Caution: not to be used during pregnancy or breastfeeding, not recommended for children under 12 years.

Biophylline
(Delandale)

A syrup used as a bronchodilator to treat bronchial spasm.

Dose: adults 1-2 5 ml teaspoonsful every 6-8 hours; children 2-6 years ½ 5 ml teaspoonsful every 6-8 hours, 6-12 years ½-1 5 ml teaspoonful every 6-8 hours.
Side effects: rapid heart rate, stomach upset, headache, sleeplessness, nausea, abnormal rhythms.
Caution: in the elderly, pregnant women, nursing mothers, and in patients suffering from heart or liver disease or peptic ulcer.
Not to be used for:
Not to be used with: cimetidine, erythromycin, ciprofloxacin, interferon.
Contains: theophylline hydrate.
Other preparations:

Bioral
(Winthrop)

A gel used as a cell-surface protector to treat mouth ulcers.

Dose: apply after meals and at bed time.
Side effects:
Caution:
Not to be used for:
Not to be used with:
Contains: carbenoxolone sodium.
Other preparations:

Blue Flag Root Compound
(Gerard House)

Dose: 1 tablet after meals 3 times a day.
Product licence: No. 1661/5002R.
Constituents: blue flag (flag lily) (*Iris versicolor*) 90 mg, burdock (*Arctium lappa*) extract 46 mg, sarsaparilla (*Smilax ornata*) extract 35 mg, sugar 100 mg, lactose 40 mg, sodium starch

glycollate 10 mg, talc 3.8 mg, magnesium stearate 0.9 mg, starch 1500 2.8 mg.

Uses: minor acne, eczema, dermatitis.

Special notes: vegetarian, yeast free.

Caution: not recommended for children under 12 years, not to be used in pregnancy.

Bocasan
(Oral-B)

A sachet of white granules used as a disinfectant to treat gingivitis and mouth infections.

Dose: dissolve a sachet of granules in warm water and rinse out the mouth 3 times a day after meals.

Side effects:

Caution:

Not to be used for: patients suffering from kidney disease.

Not to be used with:

Contains: sodium perborate monohydrate, sodium hydrogen tartrate.

Other preparations:

Boldo Herbal Aid for Slimmers
(Larkhall)
'Cantassium'

Dose: 1-2 tablets 3 times a day after meals.

Product licence: No. PLO912/7342R.

Constituents: boldo (*Peumus boldus*) extract 64.8 mg, clivers (*Galium aparine*) extract 24.4 mg, dandelion (*Taraxacum officinale*) root 24.4 mg, uva ursi (*Arctostaphylos uva-ursi*) extract 32.4 mg, bladderwrack (*Fucus vesiculosus*) 45.8 mg, dicalcium phosphate 0.2358 g, magnesium stearate 1.6 mg, stearic acid (palm oil) 1.6 mg, potato starch 15 mg, talc 5 mg.

Uses: for women who experience water retention.

Special notes: vegan, yeast free, hypoallergenic.
Caution: not to be used in pregnancy or breastfeeding without practitioner supervision. Not recommended for children. Do not exceed the stated dose, large doses of boldo cause vomiting.

Boldo Herbal Aid to Slimming
(Potters)

Dose: 1-2 tablets 3 times a day; elderly: 1 tablet 3-4 times a day.
Product licence: No. 0250/5200R.
Constituents: dandelion root (*Taraxacum officinale*), butternut bark (*Juglans cinerea*), boldo (*Peumus boldus*), bladderwrack (*Fucus*), excipients.
Uses: increases the activity of the digestive organs, diuretic, use as an aid to slimming in conjunction with a calorie controlled diet.
Special notes:
Caution: do not exceed the stated dose. Large doses of boldo cause vomiting. Not recommended for children.

Bonjela

Bonjela is a mouth ointment which contains choline salicylate (related to aspirin), chloride, menthol, alcohol, and glycerin. It is useful for mouth ulcers and teething problems. Small quantities should be applied every four hours because large quantities may deliver too much aspirin, especially to children.

Bradosol
(Ciba)

A white lozenge supplied at a strength of 0.5 mg and used as a disinfectant to treat infections of the mouth and throat.

Dose: 1 lozenge to be sucked every 2-3 hours.

Side effects: rarely local irritation and sensitivity.
Caution:
Not to be used for:
Not to be used with:
Contains: domiphen bromide.
Other preparations: Bradosol Plus.

Brasivol
(Stiefel)

A paste used as an abrasive to treat acne.

Dose: wet the area, then rub in vigorously for 15-20 seconds, rinse and repeat 1-3 times a day.
Side effects:
Caution:
Not to be used for: patients suffering from visible superficial arteries or veins on the skin.
Not to be used with:
Contains: aluminium oxide.
Other preparations:

Brolene Eye Drops
(Fisons)

These contain propamidine isethionate 0.1%, benzalkonium chloride 0.1%. An ointment is also available. These substances disinfect the eye and reduce redness. They may cause some local stinging and should not be used if redness of the eye persists or worsens. Allergies often in the eyes, particularly hay fever, cosmetic and dust allergies.

Brovon
(Torbet)

A solution used as a bronchodilator to treat bronchial spasm brought on by chronic bronchitis, bronchial asthma, emphysema.

Dose: inhale 1-2 times a day and once at night.
Side effects: nervousness, tremor, dry mouth, abnormal heart rhythms.
Caution: in patients suffering from diabetes.
Not to be used for: children or for patients suffering from heart disease, high blood pressure, overactive thyroid gland.
Not to be used with: sympathomimetics.
Contains: adrenaline, atropine methonitrate, papaverine hydrochloride.
Other preparations:

Bryonia
(Weleda 6c, 30c; Nelsons 6c)

Prepared from root of *Bryonia alba* plant (white bryony).

Uses: dry, painful, irritating cough, dry mucous membranes, dry lips, fevers which develop slowly over a few days, irritability, mastitis, arthritis, sharp stitching pains; headache accompanies many acute complaints and patient will often be very thirsty.
Suited to: lean, dark-haired people.
Symptoms better for: keeping absolutely still, lying on painful side, pressure, fresh air, cold, cold food and drinks.
Symptoms worse for: movement, touch, warmth.
Low time: mid-evening.

Buchu Compound
(Gerard House)

Dose: 2 tablets with water 3 times a day.
Product licence: No. 1661/5015R.

Constituents: dandelion root (*Taraxacum officinale*) 60 mg, buchu extract (*Agathosma betulina*) 20 mg, uva ursi (*Arctostaphylos uva-ursi*) extract 20 mg, clivers (*Galium aparine*) extract 4 mg, cayenne (*Capsicum frutescens*) 15 mg, sugar 45 mg, sodium starch glycollate 9 mg, magnesium stearate 1 mg, lactose 52 mg, talc 4 mg, iron oxide as a coating.
Uses: diuretic; buchu acts as an antiseptic to the urinary tract — helpful for recurring cystitis and fluid retention.
Special notes: vegetarian, yeast free.
Caution: not recommended for children. Not to be used in pregnancy or breastfeeding without practitioner supervision.

Cafadol
(Typharm)

A yellow, scored tablet used as an analgesic to relieve pain including period pain.

Dose: adults 2 tablets every 3-4 hours; children 5-12 years half adult dose.
Side effects:
Caution: in patients with liver or kidney disease.
Not to be used for: children under 5 years.
Not to be used with:
Contains: paracetamol, caffeine.
Other preparations:

Caladryl see **Calamine lotion**

Calamine lotion

Calamine lotion is a zinc-containing pink solution which is especially useful in chicken pox to reduce itch. It can also be used in other irritating skin conditions. Other preparations of calamine include Caladryl (also contains an antihistamine and camphor) and Eczederm.

Calcarea carbonica (Calc. Carb.)
(Weleda 6c, 30c; Nelsons 6c)

Prepared from calcium carbonate from middle layer of oyster shell.

Uses: obesity, cold extremities, cracked itching skin, profuse sour perspiration especially on head, vertigo, anxiety, indigestion, poor assimilation of nutrients, swollen glands, premenstrual tension, insomnia, menses early, profuse, painful, and protracted, constipation; children — difficult and delayed dentition, head sweats, slow closure of fontanelles, poor calcium absorption.
Suited to: fair-haired, timid patients who tend to put on weight easily.
Symptoms better for: dry weather, lying on painful side.
Symptoms worse for: cold, damp, draughts, teething, drinking milk, exertion, standing.
Low time:

Calcarea fluorica (Calc. fluor.)
(New Era 6x; Weleda 6c, 30c; Nelsons 6c)

Prepared from calcium fluoride.

Uses: promotes elasticity of tissues; varicose veins, stretch marks, arthritis, prevention of adhesions after surgery, haemorrhoids, croup, head colds with discharge, catarrh, deficient enamel of teeth.
Symptoms better for: movement, warmth.
Symptoms worse for: rest, damp.
Low time:

Calcarea phosphorica (Calc. phos.)
(New Era 6x; Weleda 6c, 30c; Nelsons 6c)

Prepared from tricalcic phosphate.

Uses: adolescents lacking energy and concentration, emaciation, cough with yellow mucus, stomach pains after eating,
acne, enlarged adenoids, headache from overstudying, swollen glands, chronic catarrh, non-union of fractures, debility
remaining after acute disease.
Suited to: general debility with discontent.
Symptoms better for: summer, lying down.
Symptoms worse for: cold, damp, draughts, wet weather,
fresh air, mental exertion.
Low time:

Calcarea sulphurica (Calc. Sulph.)
(New Era 6x)

Prepared from calcium sulphate.

Uses: blood purifier, helps rid the body of toxins, aids healing
of abcesses after they have begun to discharge, acne, catarrh,
boils, wounds which won't heal.
Symptoms better for: open air, bathing, eating, heat to the
affected part.
Symptoms worse for: hot stuffy rooms, touch, draughts.
Low time:

Calcichew
(Shire)

A white, chewable tablet supplied at a strength of 500 mg and
used as a calcium supplement to treat calcium deficiency.

Dose: 1 tablet chewed 3 times a day.

Side effects: constipation, wind.
Caution:
Not to be used for: children, or for patients suffering from overactive parathyroid glands, severe kidney disease, decalcifying tumours.
Not to be used with: tetracyclines.
Contains: calcium carbonate.
Other preparations:

Calcimax
(Wallace)

A brown syrup used as a calcium and vitamin supplement to treat calcium deficiency where vitamins are also needed.

Dose: adults 4 5 ml teaspoonsful 2-3 times a day; children 1-2 5 ml teaspoonsful 3 times a day.
Side effects:
Caution:
Not to be used for: children, or for patients suffering from overactive parathyroid glands, severe kidney disease, decalcifying tumours.
Not to be used with:
Contains: calcium glycine hydrochloride, calciferol, thiamine, riboflavine, pyridoxine, cyanocobalamin, calcium panthothenate.
Other preparations:

Calcisorb
(3M Riker)

A powder in a sachet of 4.7 g and used as an ion-exchange compound to treat raised calcium levels in the urine, recurring kidney stones, osteoporosis.

Dose: adults 1 sachet dispersed in water with meals or sprinkled on to food 3 times a day; children 2 sachets a day in 3 divided doses with food.

Side effects: diarrhoea.

Caution: treatment of children should be monitored, and the treatments should be accompanied by a low-calcium diet with foods rich in oxalates.

Not to be used for: pregnant women, nursing mothers, or for patients suffering from kidney disease, congestive heart disease, or any other conditions in which a low-sodium diet is needed.

Not to be used with:

Contains: sodium cellulose phosphate.

Other preparations:

Calcium Resonium
(Winthrop)

A powder used as an ion-exchange resin to treat raised potassium levels.

Dose: adults 15 g 3-4 times a day; children 1 g per kg body weight a day in divided doses.

Side effects: hyper calcaemia (raised calcium levels).

Caution: potassium and calcium levels should be checked.

Not to be used for: patients suffering from overactive parathyroid glands, multiple myeloma (a bone marrow tumour), sarcoidosis (a disease causing raised calcium levels), certain forms of cancer with kidney failure and hypercalcaemia.

Not to be used with:

Contains: calcium polystyrene sulphonate.

Other preparations:

Calendolon Ointment
(Weleda)

Dose: apply 2-3 times a day directly to area or on a dry dressing; use after each nappy change; apply sparingly after breastfeeding.

Constituents: per 100 g: marigold (*Calendula officinalis*) tincture (1=2), lanolin, beeswax, vegetable oils.
Uses: antiseptic, anti-inflammatory, for cuts, minor wounds, abrasions, nappy rash, sore nipples.
Caution: consult your doctor before using this product during pregnancy. If redness or itching occurs discontinue use. Some individuals may be sensitive to the lanolin content.
Not to be used for: patients where a deep infection is present because *Calendula* promotes surface healing and may seal in sepsis.

Calendula Lotion
(Weleda)

Dose: 1 teaspoonful to a glass of cool boiled water to cleanse wounds or as a compress. 1 teaspoonful to ½ glass of lukewarm boiled water as a mouthwash.
Product licence: No. PL0298/5777.
Constituents: marigold (*Calendula officinalis*) ethanolic extract (1=5), nominal ethanol content 46 % v/v.
Uses: to aid healing of cuts, abrasions, minor wounds, skin infection, sore gums.
Caution: shake bottle before use.
Not to be used for: patients where a deep infection is present because *Calendula* promotes surface healing and may seal in sepsis.

Callusolve
(Dermal)

A paint used as a skin softener to treat warts.

Dose: apply 4-5 drops of the paint to the wart, cover for 24 hours, rub away the treated part, and repeat the process.
Side effects:
Caution: apply only to warts and avoid healthy skin.

Not to be used for: treating warts on the face or anal and genital areas
Not to be used with:
Contains: benzalkonium chloride-bromine.
Other preparations:

Calming Tablets (previously known as Nerve Tablets)
(Seven Seas)

Dose: 2 tablets to be taken 3 times a day with meals.
Product licence: No. PL2210/5066.
Constituents: asafoetida BPC (*Ferula foetida*) oleoresin 24 mg, valerian (*Valerian officinalis*) root 3.02 mg, *Teucrium canadense* 2.16 mg, gentian (*Gentian lutea*) root 1.51 mg, plus aqueous extractives from: scullcap 28 mg, gentian 19 mg, valerian 31.4 mg. Excipients dicalcium phosphate, maize starch, hydroxypropylmethylcellulose, magnesium stearate, talc, silica, ethylcellulose, titanium dioxide, iron oxides, glycerol.
Uses: to reduce anxiety, worry, and nervous tension.
Special notes:
Caution: may cause drowsiness, if affected do not drive or operate machinery. Avoid alcoholic drinks. Should not be taken with other sedatives. If you are already receiving medical treatment, tell your doctor you are taking this product. Not to be used for children or during pregnancy or breastfeeding.

Calm Night (previously known as Restful Night)
(Seven Seas)

Dose: 1 tablet to be taken 3 times daily after food, plus 3 tablets before going to bed, or 3 tablets with the evening meal and 3 tablets before going to bed.
Product licence: No. PL1907/5015.
Constituents: wild lettuce (*Lactuca virosa*) 10 mg, passion-flower (*Passiflora incarnata*) 90 mg, Jamaica dogwood (*Piscidia erythrina*) bark 45 mg, hops (*Humulus lupulus*) 30 mg, aqueous

extractives from wild lettuce 90 mg, dicalcium phosphate, maize starch, hydroxypropylmethylcellulose, talc, silica, ethylcellulose, titanium dioxide, iron oxide, glycerol.

Uses: insomnia.

Special notes:

Caution: may cause drowsiness, if affected do not drive or operate machinery. Avoid alcoholic drinks. Should not be taken with other sedatives without consulting medical advice. Those patients with a known hypersensitivity to the Compositae family of plants should exercise caution taking these tablets. Not to be used for children or during pregnancy or lactation.

Calogen
(S.H.S.)

A low-electrolyte emulsion of arachis oil in water. It is used for patients suffering from kidney failure and other conditions where a diet high in energy but low in fluid and electrolytes is needed.

Caloreen
(Roussel)

A low-electrolyte, protein-, gluten-, lactose-, sucrose-, galactose-, and fructose-free glucose polymer powder. It is used for patients suffering from chronic kidney failure, amino acid disorders, hypoglycaemia, and other conditions where a high-energy, low-fluid, and low-electrolyte diet is needed.

Cam
(Rybar)

A syrup used as a bronchodilator to treat bronchial spasm.

Dose: adults 4 5 ml teaspoonsful 3-4 times a day; children under 2 years ½ 5 ml teaspoonsful 3-4 times a day, 2-4 years 1 5 ml teaspoonful 3-4 times a day, over 4 years 2 5 ml teaspoonsful 3-4 times a day.

Side effects: nervousness, sleeplessness, restlessness, dry mouth, cold hands and feet, abnormal heart rhythms.

Caution: in patients suffering from diabetes.

Not to be used for: patients suffering from heart disease, high blood pressure, overactive thyroid gland.

Not to be used with: MAOIs.

Contains: ephedrine hydrochloride, butethamate citrate.

Other preparations:

Canesten
(Baypharm)

A solution used as an antifungal treatment for fungal inflammation and infection of the outer ear, skin, and nails.

Dose: 2-3 applications a day until 14 days.after the symptoms have gone.

Side effects: local irritation.

Caution:

Not to be used for:

Not to be used with:

Contains: clotrimazole, polyethylene glycol solution.

Other preparations: Canesten Spray, Canesten Powder.

Cantharis
(Weleda 6c, 30c; Nelsons 6c)

Prepared from the *Cantharis vesicatoria* beetle.

Uses: cystitis with burning pains before and after urination, constant urge to urinate, severe difficulty urinating and with scalding sensation, burning pains; second degree burns and scalds before blisters form or where blistering is present,

sunburn.
Symptoms better for: warmth, rest; pain of burns is better for cold compresses.
Symptoms worse for: urination, touch, coffee, drinking cold water.
Low time:

Capitol
(Dermal)

A gel used as an antibacterial treatment for dandruff and other similar scalp disorders.

Dose: use as a shampoo.
Side effects:
Caution: in patients sensitive to iodine.
Not to be used for:
Not to be used with:
Contains: benzalkonium chloride.
Other preparations:

Caprin
(Sinclair)

A pink tablet supplied at a strength of 324 mg and used as an analgesic to treat rheumatic and associated conditions.

Dose: 3 tablets 3-4 times a day.
Side effects: stomach upsets, allergy, asthma.
Caution: in pregnant women, the elderly, and in patients with a history of allergy to aspirin, asthma, impaired kidney or liver function, indigestion.
Not to be used for: children, nursing mothers, or for patients suffering from haemophilia or ulcers.
Not to be used with: anticoagulants (blood-thinning drugs), some antidiabetic drugs, anti-inflammatory agents,

methotrexate, spironolactone, steroids, some antacids, some uric-acid lowering drugs.
Contains: aspirin.
Other preparations:

Carbel Instant
(Cow & Gate)

An instant carob bean gum preparation used for patients suffering from persistent vomiting and regurgitation of food.

Carbellon
(Torbet)

A black tablet used as an anti-spasm, anti-wind, antacid preparation to treat acidity, ulcers, food poisoning.

Dose: adults 2-4 tablets 3 times a day; children 1-3 tablets a day.
Side effects: few; occasionally constipation.
Caution:
Not to be used for: patients suffering from glaucoma, pyloric stenosis, enlarged prostate.
Not to be used with:
Contains: belladonna, magnesium hydroxide, charcoal, peppermint oil.
Other preparations:

Carbo-Dome
(Lagap)

A cream used as an antipsoriatic treatment for psoriasis.

Dose: apply to the affected area 2-3 times a day.
Side effects: irritation, sensitivity to light.

Caution:
Not to be used for: patients suffering from acute psoriasis.
Not to be used with:
Contains: coal tar.
Other preparations:

Carbomix
(Penn)

Granules used as an adsorbent to treat acute poisoning, overdose of drugs.

Dose: adults dissolve the contents of the bottle in water and take by mouth as soon as possible after poisoning; children usually take half adult dose.
Side effects:
Caution: your doctor may advise additional treatment for certain overdoses.
Not to be used for:
Not to be used with: antidotes or emetics taken by mouth.
Contains: activated charcoal.
Other preparations:

Carbo vegetabilis (Carbo veg.)
(Weleda 6c, 30c; Nelsons 6c)

Prepared from vegetable charcoal.

Uses: indigestion with excessive flatulence, bloated abdomen with rumbling, sluggish venous circulation, shivering but with a desire for open window, cold limbs at night, violent racking cough, hoarseness, loss of voice, tinnitus with nausea and vertigo.
Symptoms better for: eructations, being fanned.
Symptoms worse for: fatty foods, warm damp weather.
Low time: evening, night.

Carylderm
(Napp Consumer)

A lotion used as a pediculicide to treat lice in the head and pubic areas.

Dose: rub into the hair and allow to dry, then shampoo.
Side effects:
Caution: keep out of the eyes.
Not to be used for:
Not to be used with:
Contains: carbaryl.
Other preparations: Carylderm Liquid Shampoo.

Cascade
(Modern Health)

Dose: 2 tablets to be taken 3 times a day before meals.
Product licence: No. 1146/5005R.
Constituents: burdock root (*Arctium lappa*) 50 mg, uva ursi (*Arctostaphylos uva-ursi*) 75 mg, clivers (*Galium aparine*) 75mg.
Uses: diuretic, antiseptic, soothes, strengthens, and tones urinary tract, for premenstrual water retention, cystitis.
Special notes: not tested on animals.
Caution: prolonged use of uva ursi may cause constipation. Not recommended for children under 12 years or during pregnancy or breastfeeding unless prescribed.

Casilan
(Farley)

A powder used as a low-electrolyte, gluten-free protein for patients suffering from hypoproteinaemia.

Catarrh Cream
(Weleda)

Dose: a small quantity to be inserted into each nostril as desired.
Product licence: PL0298/7748.
Constituents: per 100 g: aesculin 0.1 g, alcoholic extracts from barberry (*Berberis*) fruct. 1 g, blackthorn (*Prunus spinosa*) fruct. 1 g, *Bryonia* 3x 10 g, camphor (*Cinnamomum camphora*) 0.012 g, purple coneflower (*Echinacea purpurea*) (1:3) 4 g, *Mercurius sulphuratus ruber* 5x 10 g, eucalyptus (*Eucalyptus globulus*) oil 0.388 g, peppermint (*Mentha piperita*) oil 0.388 g, thyme (*Thymus vulgaris*) oil 0.012 g.
Uses: to relieve catarrhal congestion and inflammation of nasal mucosa.
Caution: not recommended during pregnancy. May antidote any other homoeopathic remedies you are taking.
Availability: pharmacies only.

Catarrh Mixture
(Potters)

Dose: adults 1 5 ml teaspoonful 3 times a day;
children over 7 years 1 5 ml teaspoonful morning and evening.
Product licence: No. P/L0250/5051R.
Constituents: boneset (*Eupatorium perfoliatum*), blue flag (*Iris versicolor*), burdock root (*Arctium lappa*), hyssop (*Hyssopus officinalis*), capsicum, excipients.
Uses: to relieve the symptoms of nasal catarrh and catarrh of the throat.
Special notes: sugar free.
Caution:

Catarrh Naturtabs
(Larkhall)
'Cantassium'

Dose: 1-2 tablets 3 times a day with water, preferably after a meal.
Product licence: No. PL0912/7178R.
Constituents: Yarrow (*Achillea millefolium*) extract 6 mg, vervain (*Verbena officinalis*) extract 5 mg, white horehound extract (*Marrubium vulgare*) 6 mg, sage (*Salvia officinalis*) extract 4 mg, calcium phosphate tribasic, calcium sulphate dihydrate, potato starch, vegetable fatty acid.
Uses: upper respiratory tract discomfort and catarrh, especially in winter.
Special notes: vegan, yeast free, hypoallergenic.
Caution: not to be taken by pregnant women, or by anyone being treated for high blood pressure.

Catarrh Pastilles
(Booker)
'Heath & Heather'

Dose: allow a pastille to dissolve in the mouth when needed. Not more than 12 to be taken in 24 hours.
Product licence: P/L1713/5088R.
Constituents: squill (*Drimia maritima*) vinegar 9.4 %, pumilio pine (*Pinus mugo*) oil 0.6 %, eucalyptus (*Eucalyptus globulus*) oil 0.5 %, sugar, liquid glucose, crystal gum, menthol, beetroot red as colouring, caramel, vegetable fat.
Uses: expectorant, decongestant, to relieve the symptoms of coughs, colds, sore throats, and catarrh.
Special notes: vegan, yeast free.
Caution: not recommended for children. May antidote any homoeopathic remedies you are taking.

Catarrh Tablets
(Booker)
'Heath & Heather'

Dose: 1 tablet 3 times a day.
Product licence: No. P/L1713/509R.
Constituents: white horehound extract (*Marrubium vulgare*) 500 mg, squill (*Drimia maritima*) 30 mg, dicalcium phosphate, microcrystalline cellulose, stearic acid, magnesium stearate; coating: hypromellose, polyethylene glycol, copper chlorophyllin, titanium dioxide.
Uses: to relieve the symptoms of coughs and catarrh.
Special notes: vegan, yeast free.
Caution: not to be taken during pregnancy without practitioner supervision.

Catarrh Tablets
(Seven Seas)

Dose: 2 tablets 3 times a day with meals.
Product licence: No. PL2210/5020.
Constituents: lobelia (*Lobelia inflata*) 31.7 mg, yarrow (*Achillea millefolium*) 3.17 mg, red sage (*Salvia officinalis*) 3.17 mg, boneset (*Eupatorium perfoliatum*) 3.17 mg, white horehound (*Marrubium vulgare*) 3.17 mg, capsicum minimum oleoresin BPC 0.5 mg; plus aqueous extractives from: yarrow 33 mg, vervain (*Verbena officinalis*) 33 mg, red sage 33 mg, boneset 33 mg, white horehound 28.5 mg; excipients dicalcium phosphate, maize starch, hydroxypropylmethylcellulose, talc, silica, ethyl cellulose, titanium dioxide, iron oxides, glycerol.
Uses: the relief of sinus obstruction and catarrh, particulary associated with hayfever.
Special notes:
Caution: do not exceed the stated dose. Should not be used in the presence of any cardiac disease or gastric hyperacidity. Individuals with a known hypersensitivity to yarrow or other members of the Compositae family should exercise caution

when taking the tablets, although no instances of a reaction have been reported. Should not be used during pregnancy or breastfeeding. Not recommended for children.

Causticum
(Weleda 6c)

Prepared from potassium hydrate.

Uses: sore throat with raw burning pain, hoarseness, hollow spasmodic cough which is constant and exhausting, chemical burns and third degree burns (seek medical help immediately), to relieve soreness in the site of old burns, constipation with ineffectual urging, cystitis with frequent urging but difficulty passing urine, retention of urine, incontinence of urine on coughing, raw sore pains.
Suited to: patients who are lean, dark haired, and sensitive.
Symptoms better for: mild wet weather, cold drinks.
Symptoms worse for: dry cold or raw air, winds, drafts, grief.
Low time: evening.

Caved-S
(Tillotts)

A brown tablet used as a cell-surface protector and antacid to treat peptic ulcer.

Dose: adults 2 tablets chewed between meals; children 10-14 years half adult dose.
Side effects: few; occasionally constipation.
Caution:
Not to be used for: infants.
Not to be used with: tetracycline antibiotics.
Contains: liquorice extract, aluminium hydroxide, magnesium carbonate, sodium bicarbonate.
Other preparations: Rabro (Sinclair).

Ceanel Concentrate
(Quinoderm)

A liquid used as an antibacterial, antifungal treatment for psoriasis, seborrhoeic inflammation of the scalp.

Dose: use as a shampoo 3 times a week at first and then twice a week, or apply directly to other areas of the skin as needed.
Side effects:
Caution: keep out of the eyes.
Not to be used for:
Not to be used with:
Contains: phenylethyl alcohol.
Other preparations:

Ce-Cobalin
(Paines & Byrne)

A syrup used as a multivitamin preparation to treat anorexia, recovery from long-term illness.

Dose: adults 1-2 5 ml teaspoonsful 3 times a day; children 1 teaspoonful 3 times a day.
Side effects:
Caution:
Not to be used for:
Not to be used with:
Contains: cyanocoblamin.
Other preparations:

Cedocard
(Tillotts)

A blue, scored tablet or a green, scored tablet according to strengths of 20 mg, 40 mg and used as a nitrate treatment for severe congestive heart failure.

Dose: 10-40 mg 3-4 times a day.
Side effects: headache, flushes, dizziness.
Caution:
Not to be used for: children, or for patients suffering from severe low blood pressure, heart shock, severe anaemia, brain haemorrhage.
Not to be used with:
Contains: isosorbide dinitrate.
Other preparations: Cedocard I.V.

Celery Seed Tablets
(Booker)
'Heath & Heather'

Dose: 1 tablet 3 times a day.
Product licence: No. P/L1713/5026R.
Constituents: celery seed (*Apium graveolens*) extract 600 mg, microcrystalline cellulose, dicalcium phosphate, stearic acid, magnesium stearate; coating hypromellose, glycerin, copper chlorophyllin, curcumin, iron oxide, titanium dioxide.
Uses: relief of rheumatic pain, lumbago, and fibrositis.
Special notes: vegan, yeast free.
Caution: not to be taken in pregnancy without practitioner supervision.

Cerumol
(LAB)

Drops used as a wax softener to remove wax from the ears.
Dose: 5 drops into the ear twice a day for 3 days may enable syringing to be avoided.
Side effects:
Caution:
Not to be used for: inflammation of the outer ear, dermatitis, eczema.
Not to be used with:

Contains: paradichlorobenzene, chlorbutol, arachis oil.
Other preparations:

Cetavlex
(Care)

A cream used as an antiseptic to treat minor cuts and wounds, nappy rash.

Dose: apply as needed.
Side effects: irritation, peeling.
Caution:
Not to be used for:
Not to be used with:
Contains: cetrimide.
Other preparations:

Cetavlon PC
(Care)

A liquid used as a disinfectant to treat dandruff.

Dose: use as a shampoo, diluting 1 5 ml teaspoonful in 50 ml of water, once a week or more frequently if needed.
Side effects:
Caution: keep out of the eyes.
Not to be used for:
Not to be used with:
Contains: cetrimide.
Other preparations:

Cetriclens
(S & N)

A solution in a sachet used as a disinfectant for cleansing

broken skin and dirty wounds.

Dose: use as needed.
Side effects:
Caution: throw away any unused solution straight away after use
Not to be used for:
Not to be used with:
Contains: chlorhexidine gluconate, cetrimide.
Other preparations: Cetriclens Forte.

Chamomilla
(Weleda 3x, 30c; also available from Weleda in 3x drops)

Prepared from entire plant *Chamomilla recutita* (German camomile — formerly known as *Matricaria chamomilla*).

Uses: severe pains, irritability, toothache which is worse for warm drinks, oversensitivity to unpleasant stimuli, period pains which worsen after anger, sleeplessness from pain, anger, or too much coffee; children — babies who cry constantly and are quiet only when carried, teething remedy, colic, green diarrhoea especially during teething, earache.
Suited to: children who are irritable and restless when ill and want to be carried all the time.
Symptoms better for: being carried.
Symptoms worse for: teething, anger, coffee.
Low time: morning, evening, night.

Chamomile Formula
(Bio-Strath: imported by Cedar Health Ltd)

Dose: 10-20 drops (0.3 to 0.6 ml) in a little water every 2 hours.
Product licence: No. PL04210/0001.
Constituents: German camomile flower (*Matricaria chamomilla*) extract 25 %, sage leaf (*Salvia officinalis*) extract 25 %, *Torula*

utilis yeast plasmolysate 50 %, (ethanol content 37.6 % v/v approx.).

Uses: to relieve minor acute painful conditions of the mouth and throat — ulcers, gum disorders, irritating dryness of mouth and tongue.

Special notes:

Caution: not recommended during pregnancy without practitioner supervision.

Charcoal
(Potters)

Dose: 1-4 tablets after meals; children over 5 years 1-2 tablets.

Product licence: 0250/5194R.

Constituents: medicinal vegetable charcoal (herbal source).

Uses: acts as an absorbent which is particularly useful for stomach gases; helps flatulence, indigestion, heartburn, dyspepsia.

Special notes:

Caution: may affect absorbtion of other drugs you are taking.

Chest Mixture
(Potters)

Dose: 1 5 ml teaspoonful every 3 hours.

Product licence: No. P/L0250/5000R.

Constituents: horehound (*Marrubium vulgare*), pleurisy (*Asclepias tuberosa*) root, senega (*Polygala senega*), lobelia (*Lobelia inflata*), squill (*Drimia maritima*) vinegar.

Uses: expectorant, soothing, to relieve the symptoms of coughs and catarrh of the upper respiratory tract.

Special notes:

Caution: not recommended for children or during pregnancy or breastfeeding. Do not exceed the stated dose, *Lobelia* may cause nausea and vomiting in high doses.

Chloraseptic
(Richardson-Vick)

A solution supplied with a spray and used as a disinfectant to treat sore throat, mouth ulcers, minor mouth and gum infections.

Dose: adults 5 sprays every 2 hours as needed or gargle or rinse mouth with solution diluted with equal amount of water; children 6-12 years 3 sprays every 2 hours as needed or rinse out the mouth.
Side effects: rarely local irritation and sensitivity.
Caution:
Not to be used for: children under 6 years.
Not to be used with:
Contains: phenol, sodium phenolate.
Other preparations:

Chlorasol
(Seton-Prebbles)

A solution in a sachet used as a disinfectant for cleaning and removing dead skin from ulcers.

Dose: apply to the affected areas as needed.
Side effects: irritation.
Caution: keep away from the eyes and clothes; throw away any remaining solution immediately.
Not to be used for: internal use.
Not to be used with:
Contains: sodium hypochlorite.
Other preparations:

Chlorophyll Tablets
(Potters)

Dose: 1-2 tablets 3 times a day.
Product licence: No. 0250/5126R.
Constituents: kola nut (*Cola acuminata*), chlorophyll, excipients.
Uses: Kola nut is used in the manufacture of cola-type drinks.
It contains caffeine to give extra energy and relief from temporary tiredness.
Special notes:
Caution: if tiredness persists, seek medical advice. Stimulants such as caffeine exhaust the body in prolonged use.

Chocovite
(Shire)

A buff-coloured tablet used as a calcium and vitamin D2 supplement to treat calcium deficiency.

Dose: 1-3 tablets sucked 3 times a day.
Side effects:
Caution:
Not to be used for:
Not to be used with:
Contains: calcium gluconate, calciferol.
Other preparations:

Choledyl
(Parke-Davis)

A pink tablet or a yellow tablet according to strengths of 100 mg, 200 mg and used as a bronchodilator to treat bronchial spasm brought on by chronic bronchitis or asthma.

Dose: adults 100-400 mg 4 times a day; children 3-6 years use syrup, 6-12 years 100 mg 3-4 times a day.
Side effects: rapid heart rate, stomach upset, sleeplessness, nausea, change in heart rhythms.
Caution: in pregnant women, nursing mothers, and in patients

suffering from heart or liver disease or peptic ulcer. Diabetics should avoid syrup.

Not to be used for: children under 3 years.
Not to be used with: cimetidine, erythromycin, ciprofloxacin, interferon.
Contains: choline theophyllinate.
Other preparations: Choledyl Syrup.

Chymoral Forte
(Rorer)

An orange tablet supplied at a strength of 100, 000 units and used as an enzyme to treat acute inflammatory swelling.

Dose: 1 tablet 4 times a day before meals.
Side effects: stomach disturbance.
Caution: in patients sensitive to iodine.
Not to be used for:
Not to be used with:
Contains: trypsin, chymotrypsin.
Other preparations: Chymoral.

Cina
(Weleda 6c)

Prepared from the unexpanded flower heads of *Artemisia maritima* (sea wormwood).

Uses: children very irritable, petulant, capricious, want to be rocked but not touched or carried, digestive problems, extreme hunger, refuses mother's milk, grinding teeth or crying out during sleep, intestinal worms.
Symptoms better for: lying on abdomen, rocking, movement.
Symptoms worse for: touch, during sleep.
Low time: morning, night.

Citrical
(Shire)

Orange-flavoured granules supplied in sachets of 500 mg and used as a calcium supplement to treat calcium deficiency.

Dose: 1 sachet dissolved in water 3 times a day.
Side effects: constipation, wind.
Caution:
Not to be used for: children, or for patients suffering from overactive parathyroid glands, severe kidney disease, decalcifying tumours.
Not to be used with: tetracyclines.
Contains: calcium carbonate.
Other preparations:

Cleansing Herb
(Potters)

Dose: half a level teaspoonful night and morning when required. Vary the dose as required. Place the herb in a mug. Add boiling water. Allow to stand, covered, for 15 minutes. Then drink all of it.
Product licence: No. PL0250/5143R.
Constituents: buckthorn bark (*Rhamnus catharticus*), psyllium (*Plantago ovata*) seeds light, senna leaves tinnevelly (*Cassia angustifolia*).
Uses: the relief of occasional constipation.
Special notes:
Caution: should not be used for prolonged periods without medical advice. Not recommended for children or during pregnancy or breastfeeding. Senna is not to be used in colitis or spastic colon. Senna may colour urine or stools.

Clearasil
(Proctor and Gamble)

Clearasil is available as a cream, gel, and soap. It contains triclosan and sulphur to clean and disinfect the skin, and is used in the treatment of acne.

Clinicide
(De Witt)

A liquid used as a pediculicide to treat lice in the head and pubic areas.

Dose: apply to the hair and allow to dry, then shampoo the following day.
Side effects:
Caution: keep out of the eyes.
Not to be used for:
Not to be used with:
Contains: carbaryl.
Other preparations:

Clinifeed Favour
(UCB)

A gluten- and lactose-free liquid feed used to supply protein, carbohydrate, vitamins, and minerals. It is used for patients suffering from short bowel syndrome, intractable malabsorption, inflammatory bowel disease, dysphagia, bowel fistulas, anorexia nervosa, cachexia, and for preparing undernourished patients prior to surgery or following complete gastrectomy.

Caution: unsuitable as the only source of nutrition for children under 5 years.
Not to be used for: infants under 1 year.
Other preparations: Clinifeed 400; Clinifeed Protein Rich;

Clinifeed Iso.

Clinitar Cream
(SNP)

A cream used as an antipsoriatic treatment for psoriasis, eczema.

Dose: apply to the affected area 1-2 times a day.
Side effects: sensitivity to light.
Caution:
Not to be used for: patients suffering from pustular psoriasis
Not to be used with:
Contains: coal tar extract.
Other preparations: Clinitar Gel, Clinitar Shampoo.

Cocculus
(Weleda 6c)

Prepared from powdered seeds of *Cocculus indicus* plant.

Uses: travel sickness, loss of sleep, jet lag especially after long-haul flights, effects of crossing time zones, vertigo with sensation as if at sea, nausea, vomiting, weakness and great pain with menses which are early and profuse.
Suited to: patients who are fair haired and sensitive.
Symptoms better for: sitting, lying on side.
Symptoms worse for: motion of cars, boats; swimming, touch, emotion, open air, noise, eating, menses.
Low time:

Co-Codamol

A tablet used as an analgesic to relieve pain.

Dose: adults 1-2 tablets every 4-6 hours to a maximum of 8 tablets a day; children 7-12 years ½-1 tablet every 4-6 hours to a maximum of 4 tablets a day.
Side effects:
Caution: in patients suffering from kidney or liver disease.
Not to be used for: children under 7 years.
Not to be used with:
Contains: codeine phosphate, paracetamol.
Other preparations:

Co-Codaprin Dispersible

A dispersible tablet used as an analgesic to relieve pain.

Dose: 1-2 tablets in water every 4-6 hours as needed.
Side effects: stomach upsets, allergy, asthma.
Caution: in pregnant women, the elderly, and in patients with a history of allergy to aspirin, asthma, impaired kidney or liver function, indigestion.
Not to be used for: children, nursing mothers, or for patients suffering from haemophilia or ulcers.
Not to be used with: anticoagulants (blood-thinning drugs), some antidiabetic drugs, anti-inflammatory agents, methotrexate, spironolactone, steroids, some antacids, some uric-acid lowering drugs.
Contains: aspirin, codeine phosphate.
Other preparations: Co-Codaprin.

Coffea
(Weleda 6c)

Prepared from raw coffee berries.

Uses: sleeplessness from mental activity, excessive sensitivity to noise and pain, agitation, toothache with shooting pains which is better for holding ice-cold water in the mouth, one-

sided nervous headache.
Suited to: patients who are tall, dark haired, and cheerful.
Symptoms better for: sleep, warmth, lying down.
Symptoms worse for: noise, touch, odours, open air, mental exertion, excitement, emotion, overeating, alcohol.
Low time: night.

Cold and Influenza (Prevention Tablets)
(Nelsons)

Prepared from: 30c influenza virus (Asian) 1957, 30c influenza virus A 1954, 30c influenza virus B 1954, 30c *Bacillus influenza* 1918 30c Bacillinum, 30c influenza virus A (Hong Kong) 1968, 30c influenza virus B (Hong Kong) 5/72, 30c influenza virus A (England) 42/72, 30c influenza virus A (Port Chalmers) 1/73.

Uses: to help prevent colds and influenza.

Coldrex see Lemsip

Colocynthis (Colocynth.)
(Weleda 6c)

Prepared from pulp of *Citrullus colocynth* fruit (bitter cucumber).

Uses: abdominal colic, cramps and spasms, diarrhoea, vomiting from pain, neuralgic pains, sciatica, trigeminal neuralgia, vertigo from turning the head quickly, cramp in calves.
Symptoms better for: heat, pressure, doubling up.
Symptoms worse for: anger, lying on painless side.
Low time:

Colpermin
(Tillotts)

A blue capsule used as an anti-spasm treatment for irritable bowel syndrome.

Dose: 1-2 capsules 3 times a day.
over the counter.
Side effects:
Caution:
Not to be used for: children.
Not to be used with:
Contains: peppermint oil.
Other preparations:

Combination A
(New Era)

Combination of Ferr. Phos. 6x, Kali. Phos. 6x, Mag. Phos. 6x.

Uses: sciatica, neuralgia, neuritis.

Combination B
(New Era)

Combination of Calc. Phos. 6x, Kali. Phos. 6x, Ferr. Phos 6x.

Uses: general debility, edginess, nervous exhaustion, convalescence.

Combination C
(New Era)

Combination of Mag. Phos. 6x, Nat. Phos. 6x, Nat. Sulph. 6x, Silica 6x.

Uses: acidity, heartburn, dyspepsia.

Combination D
(New Era)

Combination of Kali. Mur. 6x, Kali. Sulph. 6x, Calc. Sulph. 6x, Silica 6x.

Uses: minor skin ailments.

Combination E
(New Era)

Combination of Calc. Phos. 6x, Mag. Phos. 6x, Nat. Phos. 6x, Nat Sulph. 6x.

Uses: flatulence, colic, indigestion.

Combination F
(New Era)

Combination of Kali. Phos. 6x, Mag. Phos. 6x, Nat. Mur. 6x, Silica 6x.

Uses: migraine, headaches from emotional upset.

Combination G
(New Era)

Combination of Calc. Fluor. 6x, Calc. Phos. 6x, Kali. Phos. 6x, Nat. Mur. 6x.

Uses: backache, lumbar pain.

Combination H
(New Era)

Combination of Mag. Phos. 6x, Nat. Mur. 6x, Silica 6x.

Uses: hayfever, allergic rhinitis.

Combination I
(New Era)

Combination of Ferr. Phos. 6x, Kali. Sulph. 6x, Mag. Phos. 6x.

Uses: fibrositis, muscular pain, stiffness.

Combination J
(New Era)

Combination of Ferr. Phos. 6x, Kali. Mur. 6x, Nat. Mur. 6x.

Uses: coughs, colds, chestiness.

Combination K
(New Era)

Combination of Kali. Sulph. 6x, Nat. Mur. 6x, Silica 6x.

Uses: brittle nails, falling hair.

Combination L
(New Era)

Combination of Calc. Fluor. 6x, Ferr. Phos. 6x, Nat. Mur. 6x.

Uses: varicose veins, circulatory disorders.

Combination M
(New Era)

Combination of Nat. Phos. 6x, Nat. Sulph. 6x, Kali. Mur. 6x, Calc. Phos. 6x.

Uses: rheumatic pain.

Combination N
(New Era)

Combination of Calc. Phos. 6x, Kali. Mur. 6x, Kali. Phos. 6x, Mag. Phos. 6x.

Uses: menstrual pain.

Combination P
(New Era)

Combination of Calc. Fluor. 6x, Calc. Phos. 6x, Kali. Phos. 6x, Mag. Phos. 6x.

Uses: aching legs and feet.

Combination Q
(New Era)

Combination of Ferr. Phos. 6x, Kali. Mur. 6x, Kali. Sulph. 6x, Nat. Mur. 6x.

Uses: catarrh, sinus disorders.

Combination R
(New Era)

Combination of Calc. Fluor. 6x, Calc. Phos. 6x, Ferr. Phos. 6x, Mag. Phos. 6x, Silica 6x.

Uses: infants' teething pains.

Combination S
(New Era)

Combination of Kali. Mur. 6x, Nat. Phos. 6x, Nat. Sulph. 6x.

Uses: stomach upsets, sick headaches, biliousness.

Combuduron Lotion
(Weleda)

Dose: 1 teaspoonful in a cup of boiled water. Soak a piece of lint in the solution and apply as a compress. Keep moist. Apply the lotion undiluted to insect bites.
Constituents: small nettle (*Urtica urens*) ethanolic extract (1=2) 95 %, arnica (*Arnica montana*) ethanolic extract (1=2) 5 %. Nominal ethanol content 36 % v/v.
Uses: sunburn, insect bites, minor burns, minor rashes, nettle rash.
Caution: shake bottle before use.

Combuduron Ointment
(Weleda)

Dose: apply directly to the affected part or on a dry dressing.

Product licence: No. PL0298/5490.
Constituents: per 100 g: small nettle (*Urtica urens*) tincture (1=2) 9.5 ml, arnica (*Arnica montana*) tincture (1=2) 0.5 ml, lanolin, beeswax, vegetable oils.
Uses: to relieve minor burns and scalds.
Caution: some individuals may be sensitive to lanolin.

Comfrey Ointment
(Potters)

Dose: bathe the affected area in warm water and apply the ointment morning and night.
Product licence: No. PL0250/5121R.
Constituents: comfrey (*Symphytum officinale*) extract, base.
Uses: to relieve the discomfort and aid healing of bruises and sprains.
Caution: not to be used for long than 10 days at a time; not to be used on broken skin; not recommended during pregnancy or breastfeeding.

Complement Continus
(Napp)

A yellow tablet supplied at a strength of 100 mg and used as a source of vitamin B_6 to treat vitamin B_6 deficiency including that developed by the contraceptive pill.

Dose: 1 tablet a day.
Side effects:
Caution:
Not to be used for: children.
Not to be used with: levodopa.
Contains: pyridoxine hydrochloride.
Other preparations:

Concavit
(Wallace)

A capsule used as a multivitamin treatment for vitamin deficiencies.

Dose: 1 capsule a day.
Side effects:
Caution:
Not to be used for:
Not to be used with: levodopa.
Contains: vitamin A, thiamine, riboflavine, pyridoxine, calciferol, vitamin E, nicotinamide, calcium pantothenate, ascorbic acid, cyanocoblamin.
Other preparations: Concavit Drops, Concavit Syrup.

Conotrane
(Boehringer Ingelheim)

A cream used as an antiseptic for protecting the skin from water, nappy rash, bed sores.

Dose: apply to the affected area several times a day.
Side effects:
Caution:
Not to be used for:
Not to be used with:
Contains: benzalkonium chloride, dimethicone.
Other preparations:

Contac 400

Contac 400 contains phenylpropanolamine as a sympathomimetic and chlorpheniramine as an antihistamine.

Side effects: drowsiness, reduced reactions.

Caution: in patients suffering from liver or kidney disease.

Copholco
(Fisons)

A linctus used as an opiate, expectorant to treat laryngitis, inflammation of the windpipe.

Dose: adults 2 5 ml teaspoonsful 4-5 times a day; children over 5 years ½-1 teaspoonful 3 times a day.
Side effects: constipation.
Caution: in patients suffering from asthma.
Not to be used for: children under 5 years, or for patients suffering from liver disease.
Not to be used with: MAOIs.
Contains: pholcodine, menthol, cineole, terpin hydrate.
Other preparations:

Copholcoids
(Fisons)

A black pastille used as an opiate, expectorant to treat dry cough.

Dose: adults 1-2 pastilles sucked 3-4 times a day; children over 5 years 1 pastille sucked 3 times a day.
Side effects: constipation.
Caution: in patients suffering from asthma.
Not to be used for: children under 5 years or for patients suffering from liver disease
Not to be used with: MAOIs.
Contains: pholcodine, menthol, cineole, terpin hydrate.
Other preparations:

Copper Ointment
(Weleda)

Dose: apply thinly, and massage well into the affected area once or twice a day.
Product licence: No. PL0298/5211.
Constituents: per 100 g: Cuprum Metallicum Praep. 0.4 g in a base containing yellow soft paraffin.
Uses: the relief of muscular rheumatic pain.
Caution:

Corsodyl
(ICI)

A solution used as an antibacterial treatment for gingivitis, mouth ulcers, thrush, and for mouth hygiene.

Dose: rinse with 2 5 ml teaspoonsful for 1 minute twice a day.
Side effects: local irritation, stained tongue or teeth, may affect taste.
Caution:
Not to be used for:
Not to be used with:
Contains: chlorhexidine gluconate.
Other preparations: Corsodyl Gel.

Cough Drops
(Weleda)

Dose: 10-20 drops every 2 hours, to be taken in warm water.
Product licence: No. PL0298/5492.
Constituents: per 100 ml angelica (*Archangelica*) root 1.1 %, cinnamon (*Cinnamomum verum*) 1.5 %, clove (*Syzygium aromaticum*) 0.65 %, coriander (*Coriandrum sativum*) 0.75 %, lemon (*Citrus limon*) oil 0.06 %, lemon balm (*Melissa*) leaf 4.5 %, nutmeg (*Myristica fragrans*) 2.3 %, aqua cherry laurel

(*Laurocerasus*) 11 ml, nominal ethanol content 55 % v/v.
Uses: the relief of irritating coughs.
Special notes:
Caution: do not exceed the stated dose. Not recommended for children or during pregnancy or breastfeeding. May antidote any homoeopathic remedies you are taking.

Cradocap
(Napp Consumer)

A shampoo used as an antiseptic treatment for cradle cap, scurf cap.

Dose: shampoo twice a week.
Side effects: .
Caution:
Not to be used for:
Not to be used with:
Contains: cetrimide.
Other preparations:

Cranesbill
(Gerard House)

Dose: 1-2 tablets when necessary 3 times a day with water; children 12 years and over 1 tablet twice a day with water.
Product licence: No. 1661/5004R.
Constituents: wild cranesbill (*Geranium maculatum*) 270 mg, sugar 100 mg, talc 12 mg, magnesium stearate 3 mg, sodium starch glycollate 5 mg, lactose 50 mg, malto-dextrin 80 mg.
Uses: short-term relief of diarrhoea.
Special notes: vegetarian, yeast free.
Caution: not recommended for children under 12 years. Not to be used in pregnancy without practitioner supervision.

Cremalgin
(Rorer)

A balm used as an analgesic rub to treat rheumatism, fibrositis, lumbago, sciatica.

Dose: massage into the affected area 2-3 times a day.
Side effects: may be irritant.
Caution:
Not to be used for: areas near the eyes, broken or inflamed skin, or on membranes (such as the mouth).
Not to be used with:
Contains: methyl nicotinate, glycol salicylate, capsicum oleoresin.
Other preparations:

Cuplex
(SNP)

A gel used as a skin softener to treat warts, corns, and calluses.

Dose: at night apply 1-2 drops of gel to the wart after soaking in water and drying, remove the film in the morning and repeat the process, rubbing the area with a pumice stone between treatments.
Side effects:
Caution: do not apply to healthy skin.
Not to be used for: warts on the anal or genital areas
Not to be used with:
Contains: salicylic acid, lactic acid, copper acetate.
Other preparations:

Cuprum metallicum (Cuprum met.)
(Weleda 6c, 30c; Nelsons 6c)

Prepared from copper.

Uses: cramps and spasms, cramp in fingers, legs, or toes, nausea and vomiting with abdominal cramps, diarrhoea, metallic taste in mouth, spasmodic cough with shortness of breath and vomiting, cold hands and feet, bluish face and lips.
Symptoms better for: cold drinks.
Symptoms worse for: cold air, touch, before menstruation, coughing, after vomiting.
Low time: evening, night.

CX Powder
(Bio-Medical)

A powder used as a disinfectant to clean and disinfect the skin and prevent infection.

Dose: apply to the affected area 3 times a day.
Side effects:
Caution:
Not to be used for:
Not to be used with:
Contains: chlorhexidine acetate.
Other preparations:

Cyclospasmol
(SNP)

Drops used as an anticholinergic agent in ophthalmic procedures.

Dose: 1 or more drops into the eye as needed.
Side effects:
Caution:
Not to be used for: patients suffering from narrow angle glaucoma.

Not to be used with:
Contains: cyclopentolate hydrochloride.
Other preparations:

Cystemme see **Effercitrate**

Cystoleve see **Effercitrate**

Cystopurin see **Effercitrate**

Cytacon
(Duncan, Flockhart)

A white tablet supplied at a strength of 50 micrograms and used as a source of vitamin B_{12} to treat undernourishment, vitamin deficiencies, some types of anaemia, vitamin B_{12} deficiency after stomach surgery.

Dose: adults 1-3 tablet a day up to a maximum of 6 tablets a day for pernicious anaemia; children use liquid.
Side effects: rarely allergy
Caution:
Not to be used for:
Not to be used with: para-aminosalicylic acid, methyldopa, colchicine, cholestyramine, neomycin, biguanides, potassium chloride, cimetidine.
Contains: cyanocoblamin.
Other preparations: Cytacon Liquid.

Daktarin Cream
(Janssen)

A cream used as an antifungal treatment for infections of the skin and nails.

Dose: apply 1-2 times a day until 10 days.after the wounds have healed.
Side effects:
Caution:
Not to be used for:
Not to be used with:
Contains: miconazole nitrate.
Other preparations: Daktarin Twin Pack, Daktarin Spray Powder, Daktarin Powder.

Daktarin Oral Gel
(Janssen)

A gel supplied at a strength of 25 mg and used as an antifungal treatment for fungal infections of the mouth and pharynx.

Dose: adults hold 5-10 ml of gel in the mouth 4 times a day; children under 2 years use 2.5 ml twice a day, 2-6 years 5 ml gel twice a day, over 6 years 5 ml gel 4 times a day.
Side effects: mild stomach upset.
Caution:
Not to be used for:
Not to be used with: warfarin
Contains: miconazole.
Other preparations:

Dalivit Drops
(Paines & Byrne)

Drops used as a multivitamin preparation in the prevention and treatment of vitamin deficiency in children.

Dose: 0-1 year 7 drops a day, over 1 year 14 drops a day.
Side effects:

Caution:
Not to be used for:
Not to be used with: levodopa.
Contains: vitamin A, ergocalciferol, thiamine, riboflavine, pyridoxine, nicotinamide, ascorbic acid
Other preparations:

Daneral SA
(Hoechst)

An orange tablet supplied at a strength of 75 mg and used as an antihistamine to treat allergies.

Dose: adults 1-2 tablets at night.
Side effects: drowsiness, reduced reactions.
Caution: in nursing mothers.
Not to be used for:
Not to be used with: sedatives, MAOIs, alcohol.
Contains: pheniramine maleate.
Other preparations:

Daraprim
(Wellcome)

A white, scored tablet supplied at a strength of 25 mg and used as an antimalarial drug for the prevention of malaria.

Dose: adults and children over 10 years 1 tablet a week; children 5-10 years half adult dose.
Side effects: rash, anaemia.
Caution: in pregnant women, nursing mothers, and in patients suffering from liver or kidney disease.
Not to be used for: children under 5 years.
Not to be used with: co-trimoxazole, lorazepam.
Contains: pyrimethamine.
Other preparations:

Davenol
(Wyeth)

A linctus used as an antihistamine, sympathomimetic, and opiate preparation to treat cough.

Dose: adults 1-2 5 ml teaspoonsful 3-4 times a day; children no more than 1 teaspoonful 3-4 times a day.
Side effects: constipation, drowsiness, reduced reactions, anxiety, hands shaking, irregular or rapid heart rate, dry mouth, excitement, rarely skin eruptions.
Caution: in patients suffering from asthma, kidney disease, diabetes.
Not to be used for: children under 5 years or for patients suffering from liver disease, heart or thyroid disorders.
Not to be used with: MAOIs, alcohol, sedatives, tricyclics.
Contains: carbinoxamine maleate, ephedrine hydrochloride, pholcodine.
Other preparations:

Day Nurse

Day Nurse contains paracetamol, ascorbic acid, phenylpropanolamine, dextromethorphan, and alcohol. It is available in tablet and liquid form. Night Nurse omits the stimulant sympathomimetic. Side effects are similar to those of Actifed.

Debrisan
(Pharmacia)

A powder used as an absorbant to treat weeping wounds including ulcers.

Dose: wash the wound with a saline solution and, without drying first, coat with 3 mm of powder, and cover with a

perforated plastic sheet; repeat before the sheet is saturated.
Side effects:
Caution:
Not to be used for:
Not to be used with:
Contains: dextranomer.
Other preparations: Debrisan Paste.

De-Nol
(Brocades)

A white liquid used as a cell-surface protector to treat gastric and duodenal ulcer.

Dose: 10 ml diluted with 15 ml water twice a day 30 minutes before meals.
Side effects: black colour to tongue and stools.
Caution:
Not to be used for: children of for patients suffering from kidney failure.
Not to be used with:
Contains: tri-potassium dicitrato bismuthate.
Other preparations: De-Noltab

Derbac-M
(International)

A liquid used as a pediculicide and scabicide to treat scabies, lice in the head and pubic areas.

Dose: apply liberally and then shampoo after 24 hours.
Side effects:
Caution: keep out of the eyes.
Not to be used for:
Not to be used with:
Contains: malathion.

Other preparations:

Derbac Shampoo
(International)

A shampoo used as a pediculicide to treat head lice.

Dose: use as a shampoo, applying twice and then leaving the second treatment for 5 minutes before rinsing and drying.
Side effects:
Caution: keep out of the eyes.
Not to be used for:
Not to be used with:
Contains: carbaryl.
Other preparations:

Dermacort

Dermacort contains 0.1% hydrocortisone. It can be used sparingly to treat mild itchy skin conditions such as eczema and dermatitis. Overuse of steroids on the face can cause skin thinning, and skin infections of all sorts are made worse by steroids such as hydrocortisone.

Dermatodoron Ointment
(Weleda)

Dose: apply to the affected area 3-4 times a day.
Product licence: No. PL0298/5497.
Constituents: per 100 g: woody nightshade (*Solanum dulcamara*) ethanolic decoction (1=3) 15 ml, loosestrife (*Lysimachia nummularia*) ethanolic decoction (1=3) 15 ml, in a base containing lanolin, beeswax, and vegetable oils.
Uses: eczema.
Caution: some individuals may be sensitive to the lanolin

content.
Availability: pharmacies only.

Derminostat
(Cilag)

A cream used as an antifungal treatment for fungal infections of the skin and nails.

Dose: apply to the affected area twice a day until 10 days after the wounds have healed.
Side effects:
Caution:
Not to be used for:
Not to be used with:
Contains: miconazole nitrate.
Other preparations:

Dialamine
(S.H.S.)

Low-electrolyte, gluten-, galactose-, and lactose-free, orange-flavoured powder used as a source of essential amino acids, carbohydrate, ascorbic acid, certain minerals and trace elements for patients suffering from kidney failure, hypoproteinaemia, wound fistula leakage where there is loss of protein, and those patients who are on a diet where the nitrogen intake must be controlled.

Difflam
(3M Riker)

A cream used as an anti-inflammatory and analgesic rub to relieve muscular and skeletal pain.

Dose: massage gently into the affected area 3-6 times a day.
Side effects: may be irritant.
Caution:
Not to be used for: areas near the eyes, broken or inflamed skin, or on membranes (such as the mouth).
Not to be used with:
Contains: benzydamine hydrochloride.
Other preparations:

Difflam Oral Rinse
(3M Riker)

A solution used as an analgesic and anti-inflammatory treatment for painful inflammations of the throat and mouth.

Dose: rinse or gargle with 3 5 ml teaspoonsful every 90 minutes-3 hours..
Side effects: numb mouth.
Caution:
Not to be used for: children.
Not to be used with:
Contains: benzydamine hydrochloride.
Other preparations: Difflam Spray.

Digest
(Modern Health)

Dose: 2 tablets to be taken 3 times a day before meals.
Product licence: No. PL1146/5009R.
Constituents: parsley (*Petroselinum crispum*) 80 mg, centaury (*Centaurium erythraea*) 70 mg, marshmallow root (*Althaea officinalis*) 70 mg, excipients.
Uses: stimulates appetite, reduces flatulence, soothes the stomach, relieves spasm, aids digestion, tonic, relieves inflammation of mouth and stomach.
Special notes: not tested on animals.

Caution: not recommended for children under 12 years nor during pregnancy or breastfeeding unless prescribed.

Dimotane Expectorant
(Robins)

A liquid used as an antihistamine, expectorant, and sympathomimetic treatment for cough.

Dose: adults 1-2 5 ml teaspoonsful 3 times a day; children 2-6 years ½ teaspoonful 3 times a day, 7-12 years 1 teaspoonful 3 times a day.
Side effects: anxiety, hands shaking, rapid or abnormal heart rate, dry mouth, brain stimulation.
Caution: in patients suffering from diabetes.
Not to be used for: children under 2 years or for patients suffering from cardiovascular problems, overactive thyroid gland.
Not to be used with: MAOIs, tricyclics, alcohol, sedatives, anticholinergics.
Contains: brompheniramine maleate, guaiphenesin, pseudoephedrine hydrochloride.
Other preparations: Dimotane Co, Dimotane Co Paediatric.

Dimotane Plus
(Robins)

A liquid used as an antihistamine and sympathomimetic treatment for allergic rhinitis.

Dose: adults 2 5 ml teaspoonsful 3 times a day; children use Paediatric.
Side effects: drowsiness, reduced reactions, rarely stimulant effects.
Caution: in nursing mothers and in patients suffering from bronchial asthma.
Not to be used for: patients suffering from glaucoma, coma-

tose states, brain damage, epilepsy, retention of urine, cardio-vascular problems, overactive thyroid gland.
Not to be used with: MAOIs, tricyclics, alcohol, sedatives, anticholinergics.
Contains: brompheniramine maleate, pseudoephedrine hydrochloride.
Other preparations: Dimotane Plus Paediatric, Dimotane Plus LA, Dimotane LA, Dimotane Tablets, Dimotane Elixir.

Dimotapp LA
(Robins)

A brown tablet used as an antihistamine and sympathomimetic treatment for catarrh, allergic rhinitis, sinusitis.

Dose: adults 1-2 tablets night and morning; children use elixir.
Side effects: drowsiness, reduced reactions, rarely stimulant effects.
Caution: in nursing mothers and in patients suffering from bronchial asthma.
Not to be used for: patients suffering from glaucoma, coma-tose states, brain damage, epilepsy, retention of urine, cardio-vascular problems, overactive thyroid gland.
Not to be used with: MAOIs, tricyclics, alcohol, sedatives, anticholinergics.
Contains: brompheniramine maleate, phenylephrine hydrochloride, phenylpropanolamine hydrochloride.
Other preparations: Dimotapp Elixir, Dimotapp Elixir Paediatric.

Dioctyl Ear Drops
(Medo)

Drops used as a wax softener to remove wax from the ears.

Dose: 4 drops into the ear twice a day and plug with cotton wool.

Side effects:
Caution:
Not to be used for: patients suffering from perforated eardrum.
Not to be used with:
Contains: sodium docusate, polyethylene glycol.
Other preparations:

Dioralyte
(Rorer)

Cherry- or pineapple-flavoured powder supplied as sachets and used as a fluid and electrolyte replacement to treat acute watery diarrhoea including gastro-enteritis.

Dose: 1-2 sachets in 200-400 ml water after each occasion of diarrhoea; infants substitute equivalent volume of reconstituted powder to feeds.
Side effects:
Caution:
Not to be used for:
Not to be used with:
Contains: sodium chloride, potassium chloride, sodium bicarbonate, glucose.
Other preparations: Dioralyte Effervescent, Electrolade (Nicholas); Gluco-Lyte (Cupal); Rehidrat (Searle).

Diovol
(Pharmax)

A white suspension used as an antacid and anti-wind preparation to treat ulcers, hiatus hernias, wind, and acidity.

Dose: adults 10-20 ml as required; children over 6 years half adult dose.
Side effects: few; occasionally constipation.
Caution:

466

Not to be used for: infants.
Not to be used with: tetracycline antibiotics.
Contains: aluminium hydroxide, magnesium hydroxide, dimethicone.
Other preparations:

Disadine DP
(Stuart)

A powder spray used as an antiseptic for the prevention and treatment of infection in wounds such as burns, bed sores, varicose ulcers.

Dose: spray on to the affected area as needed.
Side effects:
Caution: care in treating severe burns.
Not to be used for: patients suffering from non-toxic colloid goitre.
Not to be used with:
Contains: povidone iodine.
Other preparations:

Disprol Paed
(Reckitt & Colman)

A suspensions supplied at a strength of 120 mg/5 ml teaspoonful and used as an analgesic to relieve pain and fever in children.

Dose: 3 months-1 year ½ 5 ml teaspoonful 4 times a day if needed, 1-6 years 1-2 teaspoonsful 4 times a day if needed, 6-12 years 2-4 teaspoonsful 4 times a day if needed.
Side effects:
Caution: in children suffering from liver or kidney disease.
Not to be used for:
Not to be used with:

Contains: paracetamol.
Other preparations:

Dithrocream
(Dermal)

A cream used as an antipsoriatic treatment for psoriasis.

Dose: apply to the affected area once a day and wash off after 30-60 minutes or apply at night and wash off in the morning.
Side effects: irritation, allergy.
Caution:
Not to be used for: patients suffering from acute psoriasis.
Not to be used with:
Contains: dithranol.
Other preparations: Dithrocream Forte, Dithrocream HP, Dithrocream 2%.

Dithrolan
(Dermal)

An ointment used as an antipsoriatic and skin softener to treat psoriasis.

Dose: before going to bed, bath and then apply the ointment to the affected area.
Side effects: irritation, allergy.
Caution:
Not to be used for: patients suffering from acute psoriasis.
Not to be used with:
Contains: dithranol, salicyclic acid.
Other preparations:

Diuretabs
(Potters)

Dose: 2 tablets 3 times a day.
Product licence: No. 0250/5167R.
Constituents: buchu leaf (*Agathosma betulina*), juniper (*Juniperus communis*) berry oil, parsley piert (*Aphanes arvensis*), uva ursi (*Arctostaphylos uva-ursi*), excipients.
Uses: diuretic, astringent, soothing, to aid water retention and premenstrual tension.
Special notes:
Caution: not intended for use in more serious conditions caused by poor heart function. The elderly should not use this product for more than a month at a time.

Dome-Acne
(Lagap)

A cream used as a skin softener to treat acne.

Dose: apply to the affected area night and morning.
Side effects: irritation, underactive thyroid gland.
Caution: keep out of the eyes, nose, and mouth.
Not to be used for: dark-skinned patients.
Not to be used with:
Contains: sulphur, resorcinol monoacetate.
Other preparations:

Dramamine
(Searle)

A white, scored tablet supplied at a strength of 50 mg and used as an antihistamine treatment for vertigo, nausea, vomiting, travel sickness.

Dose: adults 1-2 tablets 2-3 times a day; children 1-6 years ¼-½ tablet. 7-12 years ½-1 tablet 2-3 times a day.
Side effects: drowsiness, reduced reactions, rarely skin eruptions.

Caution: in patients suffering from liver or kidney disease.
Not to be used for:
Not to be used with: alcohol, sedatives, some antidepressants (MAOIs).
Contains: dimenhydrenate.
Other preparations:

Drapolene
(Wellcome)

A cream used as an antiseptic to treat nappy rash.

Dose: apply twice a day or each time the nappy is changed.
Side effects:
Caution:
Not to be used for:
Not to be used with:
Contains: benzalkonium chloride, cetrimide.
Other preparations:

Drosera
(Weleda 6c, 30c; Nelsons 6c)

Prepared from *Drosera rotundifolia* (round-leaved sundew) plant.

Uses: constant tickling cough, violent attacks of coughing which may end in vomiting, deep, hoarse, barking cough with retching, sore throat which is worse for swallowing, laryngitis with a dry throat making speech difficult.
Symptoms better for: open air.
Symptoms worse for: talking, laughing, drinking, lying down, warmth.
Low time: after midnight.

Droxalin
(Sterling Health)

A white tablet used as an antacid to treat acidity, dyspepsia, and hiatus hernia.

Dose: 1-3 tablets chewed as required, usually every 4 hours.
Side effects: few; occasionally constipation.
Caution:
Not to be used for: infants.
Not to be used with: tetracycline antibiotics.
Contains: alexitol sodium, magnesium trisilicate.
Other preparations:

Dual-Lax Extra Strong

As below, but contains 10 mg of aloin powder instead of aloes. This is a crystalline extract of aloes which is more readily absorbed and thus has a stronger action.

Dual-Lax Normal
(Lanes)

Dose: adults 1-3 tablets at night; children (7-14 years) 1 tablet at night.
Product licence: No. 1074/5014R.
Constituents: senna leaf powder B.P. 32 mg, aloes 33 mg, cascara sagrada (*Rhamnus purshiana*) extract 130 mg, calcium phosphate, corn starch, stearic acid, colloidal anhydrous silica, magnesium stearate, sodium starch glycollate, IMS, opaseal, sugar, calcium carbonate, talc, acacia, titanium dioxide, white dispersion, wax polish.
Uses: relief of temporary constipation.
Special notes: vegetarian, yeast free.
Caution: not recommended during pregnancy or breastfeeding nor for children under 7 years. May cause alkaline urine to turn red.

Dubam
(Norma)

An aerosol used as a topical analgesic to relieve muscular pain.

Dose: spray on to the affected area for 2 seconds up to 4 times a day.
Side effects: may be irritant.
Caution:
Not to be used for: areas near the eyes, broken or inflamed skin, or on membranes (such as the mouth).
Not to be used with:
Contains: glycol salicylate, methyl salicylate, ethyl salicylate, methyl nicotinate.
Other preparations:

Dulcolax
(Boehringer Ingelheim)
A yellow tablet supplied at a strength of 5 mg and used as a stimulant to treat constipation and for evacuation of the bowels before surgery.

Dose: adults 2 tablets at night; children under 10 years half adult dose.
Side effects:
Caution:
Not to be used for:
Not to be used with:
Contains: Bisacodyl.
Other preparations: Dulcolax suppositories.

Duocal Super Soluble
(S.H.S.)

Low-electrolyte, gluten-, protein-, and lactose-free powder used as a source of carbohydrate and fat for patients suffering from kidney failure, cirrhosis of the liver, intolerance to disaccharides, amino acid metabolic disorders, intolerance to whole protein, poor absorption states, and other conditions where a high-energy, low-fluid diet is needed.

Other preparations: Duocal Liquid

Duofilm
(Stiefel)

A liquid used as a skin softener to treat warts.

Dose: apply the liquid to the wart once a day, allow to dry, and cover, rubbing down between applications.
Side effects:
Caution: do not apply to healthy skin.
Not to be used for: warts on the face or anal and genital areas.
Not to be used with:
Contains: salicylic acid, lactic acid.
Other preparations:

Duphalac
(Duphar)

A syrup used as a laxative to treat constipation, brain disease due to liver problems.

Dose: children 0-1 year 2.5 ml twice a day; 1-4 years 5 ml twice a day; 5-10 years 10 ml twice a day; adults 15-50 ml 2-3 times a day until 2-3 soft stools are produced each day.
Side effects:
Caution:
Not to be used for: patients suffering from galactosaemia (an inherited disorder).

Not to be used with:
Contains: lactulose.
Other preparations: lactulose solution.

E45

E45 cream contains lanolin, white soft paraffin, and light liquid paraffin. It is a good cream for use in children as both a skin softener or protector, for example, in nappy rash.

Echinacea
(Gerard House)

Dose: 1-2 tablets 3 times a day after meals.
Product licence: No. 1661/5006R.
Constituents: coneflower (*Echinacea angustifolia*) 150 mg, purple coneflower (*Echinacea purpurea*) 52.5 mg, malto-dextrin 117.5 mg, sodium starch glycollate 2.5 mg, magnesium stearate 2.5 mg, talc 5 mg, iron oxide as coating.
Uses: antiseptic, useful for acne, spots, poor skin texture, mild eczema, boils, abscesses, sore throats, tonsillitis.
Special notes: vegan, yeast free.
Caution: not recommended for children under 12 years. Not to be used in pregnancy without practitioner supervision.

Ecostatin
(Squibb)

A cream used as an antifungal treatment for fungal infections of the skin.

Dose: apply to the affected area night and morning.
Side effects:
Caution:
Not to be used for:

Not to be used with:
Contains: econazole nitrate.
Other preparations: Ecostatin Lotion, Ecostatin Powder, Ecostatin Spray.

Eczema Ointment
(Potters)

Dose: apply twice a day to affected areas.
Product licence: No. PL0250/5123R.
Constituents: chickweed (*Stellaria media*) extract, lanolin, zinc oxide, salicylic acid, benzoic acid, base.
Uses: to relieve the symptoms of eczema.
Caution: remove jewellery. Not to be used on children under 5 years. Some individuals may be sensitive to lanolin.

Efcortelan

Efcortelan cream or ointment contains 1% hydrocortisone and is therefore ten times stronger than Dermacort . Consequently, it should be treated with even more respect. It should not be used for children.

Effercitrate
(Typharm)

A white effervescent tablet used as an alkalizing agent to treat cystitis.

Dose: adults and children over 6 years 2 tablets dissolved in water up to 3 times a day with meals; children 1-6 years half adult dose.
Side effects: raised potassium levels, stomach irritation, mild diuresis.
Caution: in patients suffering from kidney disease.

Not to be used for: infants under 1 year or for patients suffering from ulcerated or blocked small bowel.
Not to be used with: potassium-sparing diuretics.
Contains: citric acid, potassium bicarbonate.
Other preparations:

Effico
(Pharmax)

Effico is a good general tonic which contains nicotinamide, thiamine, caffeine, and gentian. Caffeine excess can lead to palpitations — the preparation Proplus is concentrated caffeine which is a stimulant but may also cause insomnia and palpitations.

Elantan
(Schwarz)

A white, scored tablet supplied at strengths of 10 mg, 20 mg, 40 mg and used as a nitrate treatment for the prevention of angina, and in addition to other treatments for congestive heart failure.

Dose: 10 mg twice a day at first increasing to 40-80 mg a day in 2 or 3 divided doses after meals to a maximum of 120 mg a day.
Side effects: headache, flushes, dizziness.
Caution:
Not to be used for: children.
Not to be used with:
Contains: isosorbide mononitrate.
Other preparations: Elantan LA, Imdur (Astra).

Elasto
(New Era)

Combination of Calc. Fluor. 6x, Calc. Phos. 6x, Ferr. Phos. 6x, Mag. Phos. 6x.

Uses: promotes the formation of elastin which is responsible for the repair and maintenance of the elastic tissues in the body; for varicose veins, aching legs.

Elderflower and Peppermint with Composition Essence
(Potters)

Dose: adults: 2 5 ml teaspoonsful 3 times a day in a third of a cupful of warm water; children over 5 years half the adult dose.
Product licence: P/L0250/5094R.
Constituents: bayberry bark (*Myrica cerifera*), hemlock spruce (*Tsuga canadensis*), elderflowers (*Sambucus*), peppermint (*Mentha piperita*) oil, syrup.
Uses: stimulant, diaphoretic (encourages perspiration). Elderflowers and peppermint have antiviral and antibacterial properties. Elderflower is anticatarrhal and expectorant, to relieve the symptoms of colds, chills, and sore throats.
Special notes:
Caution: shake the bottle before use. Not recommended for children under 5 years. Peppermint may antidote any homoeopathic remedies you are taking. Do not exceed the stated dose. Bayberry may cause nausea and flatulence in high doses.

Elemental 028
(S.H.S.)

An orange or flavour-free powder used as a source of amino acids, carbohydrate, fat, electrolytes, vitamins, and minerals for patients suffering from short bowel syndrome, intractable poor absorption, inflammatory bowel disease, bowel fistulas.

Caution: unsuitable as the only source of nutrition for children under 5 years.

Not to be used for: infants under 1 year.
Other preparations:

Elixir of Damiana and Saw Palmetto
(Potters)

Dose: 2 5 ml teaspoonsful 3 times a day for 1 week, then 1 5 ml teaspoonful 3 times a day.
Product licence: P/L0250/5071R.
Constituents: cornsilk (*Zea mays*), damiana (*Turnera diffusa*), saw palmetto (*Serenoa repens*), excipients.
Uses: tonic and restorative, nutritive, mild stimulant, laxative.
Special notes:
Caution: shake the bottle before use. Not recommended for children. Damiana has a slightly irritant effect on the genito-urinary mucosa. Not recommended in pregnancy or breastfeeding without practitioner supervision.

Eludril
(Pierre Fabre)

A solution used as an antibacterial treatment for throat and mouth infections, gingivitis, ulcers.

Dose: dilute 2 5 ml teaspoonsful with half a glass of warm water and gargle or rinse the mouth 3-4 times a day.
Side effects:
Caution:
Not to be used for: children under 6 years.
Not to be used with:
Contains: chlorhexidine digluconate, chlorbutol, chloroform.
Other preparations: Eludril Spray.

Ener-G
(General Designs)

Gluten-free preparation supplied as brown rice bread or tapioca bread used for patients suffering from disorders of the digestive system in which there is sensitivity to gluten, including herpetiformis, steatorrhoea, coeliac disease, dermatitis.

ENO
(Smith Kline Beecham)

ENO contains sodium bicarbonate, tartaric acid, and citric acid and is useful as an effervescent antacid. Care should be taken to avoid sodium overload. In contrast, Andrew's (Sterling Health) contains magnesium sulphate and acts as both an antacid and laxative. Andrew's Answer is another hangover remedy which contains paracetamol, caffeine, sodium bicarbonate, and citric acid.

Enrich
(Abbott)

Gluten- and lactose-free, vanilla-flavoured liquid feed used as a source of protein, carbohydrate, dietary fibre, fat, vitamins, and minerals for patients suffering from short bowel syndrome, intractable poor absorption, dysphagia, bowel fistulas, cachexia, anorexia nervosa, or for undernourished patients before surgery or after complete gastrectomy.

Caution: unsuitable as the only source of nutrition for children under 5 years.
Not to be used for: infants under 1 year.
Other preparations:

Ensure
(Abbott)

Low-electrolyte, gluten- and lactose-free, vanilla-flavoured liquid feed used as a source of protein, carbohydrate, fat, vitamins, and minerals for patients suffering from short bowel syndrome, intractable poor absorption, dysphagia, bowel fistulas, cachexia, anorexia nervosa, or for undernourished patients before surgery or after complete gastrectomy.

Caution: unsuitable as the only source of nutrition for children under 5 years.
Not to be used for: infants under 1 year.
Other preparations: Ensure Savoury; Ensure Plus.

Ephynal
(Roche)

A white tablet or a white, scored tablet according to strengths of 10 mg, 50 mg, 200 mg, and used as a source of vitamin E to treat vitamin E deficiency, tropical vitamin E deficiency.

Dose: adults 10-15 mg a day; children 1-10 mg per kg body weight a day.
Side effects:
Caution:
Not to be used for:
Not to be used with:
Contains: tocopheryl acetate.
Other preparations:

Epogam
(Scotia)

Dose: 4-6 capsules twice a day; children over 1 year 2-4 capsules twice a day.
Product licence: No. PL4382/0005
Constituents: oil from the pressed seeds of the evening primrose (*Oenothera biennis*) plant supplying GLA 40 mg, gelatin capsule.

Uses: Epogam is licensed as a medicine for the symptomatic relief of atopic eczema.

Possible uses under practitioner prescription/supervision only: a rich source of the essential fatty acid GLA (gamma linolenic acid) which belongs to the Omega-6 group. Therapeutic effect will depend on there being an existing deficiency of GLA. Studies suggest that evening primrose oil may reduce high cholesterol levels, reduce high blood pressure, may help prevent high blood pressure during pregnancy, help with auto-immune diseases, inhibit tumour growth, reduce itching and severity of eczema, reduce allergic response, reduce premenstrual tension including breast tenderness and swelling, help mastalgia, reduce inflammatory response, may help patients with lupus, help multiple sclerosis, may aid weight loss in those who are more than 10 per cent above ideal body weight, reduce Parkinsonian tremor, help Raynaud's syndrome, help rheumatoid arthritis, help scleroderma, in alcoholism may help prevent damage to liver and neurological system and aid withdrawal.

Special notes:

Caution: some patients may experience nausea, diarrhoea or headaches on high doses. Not to be taken by epileptic patients without medical supervision. Not recommended for children under 1 year. GLA can prolong bleeding time in high doses so should be avoided by haemophiliacs and people taking anticoagulants.

Eppy
(SNP)

Drops used as a sympathomimetic to treat glaucoma.

Dose: 1 drop into the eye 1-2 times a day.

Side effects: pain in the eye, headache, skin reactions, melanosis, red eye, rarely systemic effects.

Caution:

Not to be used for: patients suffering from absence of the lens, narrow angle glaucoma.

Not to be used with:

Contains: adrenaline.

Other preparations:

Eskamel
(S K B)

A cream used as a skin softener to treat acne.

Dose: apply a little to the affected area once a day.
Side effects: irritation.
Caution: in patients suffering from acute local infection; keep out of the eyes, nose, and mouth.
Not to be used for:
Not to be used with:
Contains: resorcinol, sulphur.
Other preparations:

Eskornade Spansule
(S K B)

A grey/clear capsule used as an antihistamine and sympathomimetic to treat congestion, running nose, and phlegm brought on by common cold, rhinitis, flu, sinusitis.

Dose: adults 1 capsule every 12 hours; children use syrup.
Side effects: drowsiness.
Caution: in patients suffering from diabetes.
Not to be used for: patients suffering from cardiovascular problems, overactive thyroid gland.
Not to be used with: MAOIs, tricyclics, alcohol.
Contains: phenylpropanolamine hydrochloride, diphenylpyraline hydrochloride.
Other preparations: Eskornade Syrup.

Euphrasia
(Weleda 6c, 30c; Nelsons 6c)

Prepared from entire plant *Euphrasia officinalis* (eyebright).

Uses: colds with watering eyes and streaming nose, hayfever, conjunctivitis with burning tears, photophobia, cough which comes only during the day and has copious mucus.
Symptoms better for: dim light, cold applications.
Symptoms worse for: sunlight, warmth, being indoors.
Low time: evening.

Eurax
(Geigy)

A lotion used as a scabicide to treat scabies.

Dose: apply to the body apart from the head and face after a hot bath.
Side effects:
Caution: keep out of the eyes.
Not to be used for: patients suffering from acute exudative dermatitis.
Not to be used with:
Contains: crotamiton.
Other preparations: Eurax Cream.

Exelderm
(ICI)

A cream used as an antifungal treatment for fungal infections of the skin.

Dose: rub into the affected area twice a day for 2-3 weeks after the wounds have healed.
Side effects:
Caution: keep out of the eyes; if the area becomes irritated, the treatment should be stopped.
Not to be used for:

Not to be used with:
Contains: sulconazole nitrate.
Other preparations:

Exlax
(Intercare)

Exlax contains phenolphthalein which is a powerful laxative only to be used when other simple remedies have failed.

Exolan
(Dermal)

A cream used as an antipsoriatic treatment for psoriasis.

Dose: apply to the affected area 1-2 times a day.
Side effects: irritation, allergy.
Caution:
Not to be used for: patients suffering from acute psoriasis.
Not to be used with:
Contains: dithranol triacetate.
Other preparations:

Expulin
(Galen)

A linctus used as an antihistamine, opiate, and sympathomimetic treatment for cough and congestion.

Dose: adults 2 5 ml teaspoonsful 4 times a day; children 2-6 years ½-1 teaspoonful 4 times a day, 7-12 years 1-2 teaspoonsful 4 times a day.
Side effects: constipation, drowsiness, reduced reactions, anxiety, hands shaking, irregular or rapid heart rate, dry mouth, excitement, rarely skin eruptions.

Caution: in patients suffering from asthma, kidney disease, diabetes.
Not to be used for: children under 5 years, or for patients suffering from liver disease, heart or thyroid disorders.
Not to be used with: MAOIs, alcohol, sedatives, tricyclics
Contains: pholcodine, pseudoephedrine hydrochloride, chlorpheniramine hydrochloride, chlorpheniramine maleate.
Other preparations: Expulin Paediatric.

Expurhin
(Galen)

A linctus used as an antihistamine and sympathomimetic treatment for congestion, phlegm, and running nose in children.

Dose: 3 months-1 year ½-1 5 ml teaspoonful twice a day, 1-5 years 1-2 teaspoonsful 3 times a day, 6-12 years 2-3 teaspoonsful 3 times a day.
Side effects: drowsiness, reduced reactions, anxiety, hands shaking, irregular or rapid heart rate, dry mouth, excitement, rarely skin eruptions.
Caution: in patients suffering from liver or kidney disease, diabetes.
Not to be used for: infants under 3 months, or for patients suffering from heart or thyroid disorders.
Not to be used with: alcohol, sedatives, some antidepressants (MAOIs), tricyclics
Contains: ephedrine hydrochloride, chlorpheniramine hydrochloride, chlorpheniramine maleate, menthol.
Other preparations:

Exterol
(Dermal)

Drops used as a wax softener to remove wax from the ears.

Dose: hold 5-1 drops in the ear 1-2 times a day for 3-4 days.
Side effects: slight fizzing.
Caution:
Not to be used for: patients suffering from perforated eardrum.
Not to be used with:
Contains: urea hydrogen peroxide, glycerin.
Other preparations:

Eye dew see **Brolene Eye Drops** and **Optrex**

Fefol Spansule
(S K & F)

A clear/green capsule used for the prevention of iron and folic acid deficiency in pregnancy.

Dose: 1 capsule a day.
Side effects: mild stomach upset.
Caution:
Not to be used for: children.
Not to be used with: tetracyclines.
Contains: ferrous sulphate, folic acid.
Other preparations:

Fefol-Vit Spansule
(S K & F)

A clear/white capsule used for the prevention of iron, folic acid, and vitamin deficiency in pregnancy.

Dose: 1 capsule a day.
Side effects: mild stomach upset.
Caution:
Not to be used for: children.
Not to be used with: tetracyclines.

Contains: ferrous sulphate, folic acid, thiamine mononitrate, riboflavine, pyridoxine hydrochloride, nicotinamide, ascorbic acid.
Other preparations:

Fefol Z Spansule
(S K & F)

A clear/blue capsule used for the prevention of iron and folic acid deficiency in pregnancy where zinc supplement is also needed.
Dose: 1 capsule a day.
Side effects: mild stomach upset.
Caution: in patients suffering from kidney disease
Not to be used for: children.
Not to be used with: tetracyclines.
Contains: ferrous sulphate, folic acid, zinc sulphate monohydrate.
Other preparations:

Femerital
(MCP)

A white, scored tablet used as an antispasmodic and analgesic for the relief of period pain.

Dose: 1-2 tablets 2-3 times a day beginning 2 days before the start of the period.
Side effects:
Caution: in patients suffering from liver or kidney disease.
Not to be used for: children.
Not to be used with:
Contains: ambucetamide, paracetamol.
Other preparations:

Fenostil Retard
(Zyma)

A white tablet supplied at a strength of 2.5 mg and used as an antihistamine treatment for rhinitis, urticaria, hay fever, other allergies.

Dose: adults 1 tablet night and morning.
Side effects: drowsiness, reduced reactions.
Caution: in nursing mothers.
Not to be used for: children.
Not to be used with: alcohol, sedatives, MAOIs.
Contains: dimethindene maleate.
Other preparations:

Fenulin
(Gerard House)

Dose: 2 tablets after meals 3 times a day.
Product licence: No. 1661/5008R
Constituents: fenugreek (*Trigonella foenum-graecum*) 275 mg, slippery elm (*Ulmus rubra*) 30 mg, golden seal (*Hydrastis*) 5 mg, malto-dextrin 139 mg, talc 16 mg, magnesium stearate 4 mg, sugar 50mg.
Uses: digestive upsets, dyspepsia, soothes irritated tissue.
Special notes: vegan, yeast free.
Caution: *Hydrastis* is not to be used in pregnancy or breastfeeding. Not recommended for children.

Feospan Spansule
(S K B)

A clear/red capsule supplied at a strength of 150 mg and used as an iron supplement to treat iron deficiency, anaemia.

Dose: adults 1-2 capsules a day; children 1-12 years 1 capsule

a day.
Side effects: mild stomach upset.
Caution:
Not to be used for: infants under 1 year.
Not to be used with: tetracyclines.
Contains: ferrous sulphate.
Other preparations:

Fergon
(Winthrop)

A red tablet supplied at a strength of 300 mg and used as an iron supplement to treat iron deficiency, anaemia.

Dose: adults treatment 4-8 tablets a day in divided doses 1 hour before food, prevention 2 tablets a day; children 6-12 years 1-3 tablets a day.
Side effects: nausea, constipation.
Caution:
Not to be used for: children under 6 years.
Not to be used with: tetracyclines.
Contains: ferrous gluconate.
Other preparations:

Ferrocontin Continus
(Degussa)

A red tablet supplied at a strength of 100 mg and used as an iron supplement to treat iron deficiency, anaemia.

Dose: 1 tablet a day.
Side effects:
Caution:
Not to be used for: children.
Not to be used with: tetracyclines.
Contains: ferrous glycine sulphate.

Other preparations: Ferrocontin Folic Continus.

Ferrograd
(Abbott)

A red tablet supplied at a strength of 325 mg and used as an iron supplement to treat iron deficiency, anaemia.

Dose: 1 tablet a day before food.
Side effects:
Caution: in patients suffering from slow bowel actions.
Not to be used for: children, or for patients suffering from diverticular disease, blocked intestine.
Not to be used with: tetracyclines.
Contains: ferrous sulphate.
Other preparations:

Ferrograd C
(Abbott)

A red, oblong tablet used as an iron supplement to treat iron deficiency, anaemia where absorption is difficult.

Dose: 1 tablet a day before food.
Side effects:
Caution: in patients suffering from slow bowel action.
Not to be used for: children, or for patients suffering from diverticular disease, blocked intestine.
Not to be used with: tetracyclines, Clinistix urine test.
Contains: ferrous sulphate, ascorbic acid.
Other preparations:

Ferrograd Folic
(Abbott)

A red yellow/tablet used as an iron supplement to treat anaemia in pregnancy.

Dose: 1 tablet a day before food.
Side effects:
Caution: in patients suffering from slow bowel movments.
Not to be used for: children, or for patients suffering from diverticular disease, intestinal blockage, vitamin B12 deficiency.
Not to be used with: tetracyclines.
Contains: ferrous sulphate, folic acid.
Other preparations:

Ferromyn
(Calmic)

An elixir used as an iron supplement to treat iron deficiency anaemia.

Dose: adults and children over 10 years 1 5 ml teaspoonful 3 times a day; children up to 2 years 1 ml twice a day, 2-5 years ½ teaspoonful 3 times a day, 5-10 years 1 teaspoonful twice a day.
Side effects: stomach upset.
Caution:
Not to be used for:
Not to be used with: tetracyclines, antacids.
Contains: ferrous succinate.
Other preparations:

Ferrum Phosphoricum (Ferr. Phos.)
(Weleda 6c, 30c; New Era 6x; Nelsons 6c)

Prepared from white phosphate of iron.

Uses: early stages of colds (after Aconite), early stages of fever and inflammation before exudation begins, anaemia, sluggish

venous circulation, hammering congestive headaches, nose-bleeds, rheumatism.
Suited to: pale, delicate people who flush easily on exertion.
Symptoms better for: cold applications, summer.
Symptoms worse for: touch, noise, cold.
Low time: night.

Fersaday
(Duncan, Flockhart)

A brown tablet supplied at a strength of 100 mg and used as an iron supplement to treat iron deficiency.

Dose: 1 tablet 1-2 times a day.
Side effects: stomach upset.
Caution: in patients with a history of peptic ulcer
Not to be used for: children.
Not to be used with: tetracyclines, antacids.
Contains: ferrous fumarate.
Other preparations:

Fersamal
(Duncan, Flockhart)

A brown tablet supplied at a strength of 65 mg and used as an iron supplement to treat iron deficiency, anaemia.

Dose: adults 1 tablet 3 times a day; children use Fersamal Syrup.
Side effects: stomach upset.
Caution: in patients with a history of peptic ulcer.
Not to be used for:
Not to be used with: tetracyclines, antacids.
Contains: ferrous fumarate.
Other preparations: Fersamal Syrup, Ferrocap (Consolidated).

Fesovit Spansule
(S K B)

A yellow/clear capsule used as an iron and vitamin supplement to treat iron deficiency anaemia needing vitamins B and C.

Dose: adults 1 capsule 1-2 times a day; children 1-12 years 1 capsule a day.
Side effects: mild stomach upset.
Caution:
Not to be used for: infants under 1 year.
Not to be used with: tetracyclines.
Contains: ferrous sulphate, ascorbic acid, thiamine mononitrate, riboflavine, pyridoxine hydrochloride, nicotinamide.
Other preparations:

Fesovit Z Spansule
(S K B)

An orange/clear capsule used as an iron, zinc, and vitamin supplement to treat iron deficiency anaemia where vitamins B and C and zinc are needed.

Dose: adults 1-2 capsules a day; children 1-12 years 1 capsule a day.
Side effects: mild stomach upset.
Caution: in patients suffering from kidney disease.
Not to be used for: infants under 1 year.
Not to be used with: tetracyclines.
Contains: ferrous sulphate, zinc sulphate monohydrate, ascorbic acid, thiamine mononitrate, riboflavine, pyridoxine hydrochloride, nicotinamide.
Other preparations:

Feverfew
(Weleda 6x)

Prepared from feverfew plant (*Chrysanthemum parthenium*).

Uses: to reduce frequency and severity of migraine attacks. The indications for homoeopathic feverfew are the same as for taking it as a herbal remedy. The potentized form has been prepared because some patients were complaining of mouth ulcers after taking the herbal form (which is not licensed as a medicine).

Finalgon
(Boehringer Ingelheim)

An ointment supplied with an applicator and used as an analgesic rub to relieve muscular and skeletal pain.

Dose: massage gently into the affected area as needed.
Side effects: may be irritant.
Caution:
Not to be used for: areas near the eyes, broken or inflamed skin, or on membranes (such as the mouth).
Not to be used with:
Contains: nonivamide, butoxyethyl nicotinate.
Other preparations:

Flexical
(Mead Johnson)

Gluten- and lactose-free powder used as a source of protein, carbohydrate, fat, vitamins, and minerals for patients suffering from short bowel syndrome, intractable poor absorption, bowel fistulas, cachexia, anorexia nervosa, or for undernourished patients before surgery or after complete gastrectomy.

Caution: unsuitable as the only source of nutrition for children under 5 years.
Not to be used for: infants under 1 year.
Other preparations:

Fluorescein
(SNP)

Drops used as a dye for staining purposes to enable abrasions or foreign bodies in the eye to be found.

Dose: 1 or more drops into the eye as needed.
Side effects:
Caution:
Not to be used for:
Not to be used with:
Contains: sodium fluorescein.
Other preparations:

Folex-350
(Rybar)

A pink tablet used as an iron supplement for the prevention of iron and folic acid deficiency in pregnancy.

Dose: 1 tablet a day.
Side effects: nausea, constipation.
Caution:
Not to be used for: children, or for patients suffering from megaloblastic anaemia.
Not to be used with: tetracyclines.
Contains: ferrous fumarate, folic acid.
Other preparations:

Forceval
(Unigreg)

A brown/red capsule used as a source of multivitamins and minerals to treat vitamin and mineral deficiencies.

Dose: adults 1 capsule a day; children over 5 years use Forceval Junior.
Side effects:
Caution:
Not to be used for: children under 5 years.
Not to be used with: levodopa.
Contains: multivitamins and minerals.
Other preparations: Forceval Junior.

Forceval Protein
(Unigreg)

Low-sodium, low-fat, galactose-, gluten- and lactose-free, natural-, vanilla-, orange-, or strawberry-flavoured powder used as a source of protein, carbohydrate, fat, vitamins, and minerals for patients suffering from short bowel syndrome, intractable poor absorption, dysphagia, inflammatory bowel disease, bowel fistulas, or for undernourished patients before surgery or after complete gastrectomy, where a low salt intake is needed.

Caution: unsuitable as the only source of nutrition for children under 5 years.
Not to be used for: infants under 1 year.
Other preparations:

Formula MCT (1)
(Cow & Gate)

Lactose-low powder used as a source of fatty acids, protein, carbohydrate, minerals, and electrolytes for patients suffering from liver failure, steatorrhoea with cystic fibrosis of the pancreas, intestinal lymphangiectasis, or in intestinal surgery.

Formula S
(Cow & Gate)

Gluten-, fructose-, sucrose- and lactose-free powder used as a source of protein, carbohydrate, fat, vitamins, and minerals for patients suffering from milk intolerance, lactose intolerance, galactosaemia, and low galactokinase.

Fortical
(Cow & Gate)

Low-electrolyte, gluten-, galactose-, sucrose-, lactose-, and protein-free liquid used as a source of high-energy carbohydrate for patients suffering from kidney failure, cirrhosis of the liver, or any conditions where a low-fluid, low-electrolyte, high-energy diet is needed.

Fortisip
(Cow & Gate)

Gluten-free and lactose-low, neutral-, banana-, orange-, tropical fruits-, mushroom-, or vanilla-flavoured liquid feed used as a source of protein, carbohydrate, vitamins, and minerals for patients suffering from short bowel syndrome, intractable poor absorption, dysphagia, bowel fistulas, cachexia, anorexia nervosa, inflammatory bowel disease, or for undernourished patients before surgery or after complete gastrectomy.

Caution: unsuitable as the only source of nutrition for children under 5 years.
Not to be used for: infants under 1 year.
Other preparations:

Fortison
(Cow & Gate)

Lactose-low and gluten-free liquid feed used as a source of protein, carbohydrate, fat, vitamins, and minerals for patients suffering from short bowel syndrome, intractable poor absorption, dysphagia, bowel fistulas, cachexia, anorexia nervosa, inflammatory bowel disease, cystic fibrosis, or for undernourished patients before surgery or after complete gastrectomy.

Caution: unsuitable as the only source of nutrition for children under 5 years (except Fortison Paediatric).
Not to be used for: infants under 1 year.
Other preparations: Fortison Energy Plus; Fortison Fibre; Fortison Paediatric; Fortison Soya.

Fosfor
(Chancellor)

A syrup used as a food supplement.

Dose: adults 4 5 ml teaspoonsful 3 times a day; children half adult dose.
Side effects:
Caution:
Not to be used for:
Not to be used with:
Contains: phosphorylcolamine.
Other preparations:

Fragador Tablets
(Weleda)

Dose: 2 tablets 3 times a day.
Product licence: No. PL0298/5512.
Constituents: scurvy grass (*Cochlearia officinalis*) 0.2 mg,

conchae 4 mg, wild strawberry (*Fragaria vesca*) fruit 2 mg, glycogen 10x 2 mg, lovage (*Levisticum*) root 5 mg, mel 1x 1 mg, natrum carbonicum 1x 2 mg, aniseed (*Pimpinella anisum*) fruit 3 mg, sage (*Salvia officinalis*) 2 mg, wheat germ 50 mg, stinging nettle (*Urtica dioica*) 10 mg, ferrum phosphoricum 4x 2 mg, excipients.
Uses: to relieve occasional nerviness and edginess brought on by everyday stress and strain.
Special notes:
Caution: not recommended during pregnancy or breastfeeding.

Fresubin
(Fresenius)

Low-electrolyte, low-lactose, gluten-free, vanilla-, peach-, nut-, mocha-, and chocolate-flavoured liquid feed used as a source of protein, carbohydrate, fat, vitamins, and minerals for patients suffering from short bowel syndrome, intractable poor absorption, dysphagia, bowel fistulas, cachexia, anorexia nervosa, or for undernourished patients before surgery or after complete gastrectomy.
Caution: unsuitable as the only source of nutrition for children under 5 years.
Not to be used for: infants under 1 year.
Other preparations: Fresubin Plus F.

Frost Cream
(Weleda)

Dose: apply directly to the affected part or on a dry dressing several times a day.
Product licence: No. PL0298/5513.
Constituents: per 100 g: Abrotanum ethanolic extract from 1 g of herb, balsam of Peru B.P.C. 0.4 g, petroleum 5 g, rosemary oil 1 g, Stibium Metallicum Praep. 0.1 g, base containing lanolin and yellow soft paraffin.

Uses: to relieve the symptoms of chilblains.
Caution: some individuals may be sensitive to lanolin.
Availability: pharmacies only.

Furadantin
(Norwich Eaton)

A yellow, pentagonal, scored tablet supplied at strengths of 50 mg, 100 mg, and used as an antiseptic to treat infection of the urinary tract.

Dose: adults treatment 100 mg 4 times a day with food or milk, prevention 100-200 mg a day; children 3 months-2½ years one-eighth adult dose, 2½-6 years quarter adult dose, 6-11 years half adult dose, 11-14 years three-quarters adult dose.
Side effects: stomach upset, allergy, jaundice, nerve inflammation, blood changes, possible liver damage.
Caution:
Not to be used for: infants under 1 month or for patients suffering from kidney problems resulting in reduced urine output.
Not to be used with:
Contains: nitrofurantoin.
Other preparations: Furadantin Suspension.

Fybranta
(Norgine)

A mottled, pale-brown, chewable 2 g tablet used as a bulking agent in the treatment of diverticular disease, irritable colon syndrome, constipation through a diet lacking in fibre.

Dose: adults 1-3 tablets with liquid 3-4 times a day; children in proportion.
Side effects:
Caution:

Not to be used for:
Not to be used with:
Contains: bran.
Other preparations:

Galactomin 17
(Cow & Gate)

Lactose-low, gluten-free powder used as a source of glucose, caseinates, vegetable oils, vitamins, minerals, and trace elements for patients suffering from galactosaemia and low galactokinase where there is also lactose intolerance.

Other preparations: Galactomin 19.

Galcodine
(Galen)

A linctus supplied at a strength of 15 mg and used as an opiate to treat dry cough.

Dose: adults 1 5 ml teaspoonful 4 times a day; children 1-5 years ½-1 teaspoonful 3-4 times a day, 6-12 years 1 teaspoonful 3-4 times a day..
Side effects: constipation.
Caution: in patients suffering from asthma.
Not to be used for: infants under 1 year, or for patients suffering from liver disease.
Not to be used with: MAOIs.
Contains: codeine phosphate.
Other preparations: Galcodine Paediatric.

Galenphol
(Galen)

A liquid supplied at a strength of 5 mg and used as an opiate to treat dry cough.

Dose: adults 1-2 5 ml teaspoonsful 3-4 times a day; children 1-5 years ½-1 teaspoonful 3-4 times a day, 6-12 years 1 teaspoonful 3-4 times a day.
Side effects: constipation.
Caution: in patients suffering from asthma.
Not to be used for: infants under 1 year, or for patients suffering from liver disease.
Not to be used with: MAOIs.
Contains: pholcodine.
Other preparations: Galenphol Linctus Strong, Galenphol Linctus Paediatric.

Galfer
(Galen)

A green/red capsule supplied at a strength of 290 mg and used as an iron supplement to treat iron deficiency anaemia.

Dose: adults 1 capsule a day before food; children as advised by a physician.
Side effects: nausea, constipation.
Caution:
Not to be used for:
Not to be used with: tetracyclines.
Contains: ferrous fumarate.
Other preparations:

Galfervit
(Galen)

An orange/maroon capsule used as an iron and vitamin supplement to treat iron deficiency anaemia where a vitamin supplement is also needed.

Dose: adults 1 capsule 1-2 times a day; children as advised by a physician.
Side effects: nausea, constipation.
Caution:
Not to be used for:
Not to be used with: tetracyclines, levodopa.
Contains: ferrous fumarate, ascorbic acid, thiamine mononitrate, riboflavine, pyridoxine hydrochloride, nicotinamide.
Other preparations:

Galpseud
(Galen)

A white tablet supplied at a strength of 60 mg and used as an sympathomimetic to treat congestion of the nose, sinuses, and upper respiratory tract.

Dose: adults 1 tablet 3 times a day; children use linctus.
Side effects: anxiety, hands shaking, irregular or rapid heart rate, dry mouth, excitement.
Caution: in patients suffering from diabetes.
Not to be used for: children under 2 years, or for patients suffering from heart or thyroid disorders.
Not to be used with: MAOIs, tricyclics.
Contains: pseudoephedrine hydrochloride.
Other preparations: Galpseud Linctus.

Gardolex
(Modern Health)

Dose: 1 tablet 3 times a day; children 5-12 years 1 tablet before going to bed.

Product licence: No. 1146/5001R.

Constituents: garlic oil 22 mg, marshmallow (*Althaea officinalis*) root 125 mg, parsley (*Petroselinum crispum*) 25 mg, excipients.

Uses: antibacterial, anti-inflammatory, expectorant, for colds, catarrh, and chest infections. See also notes under Garlic Preparations.

Caution: not be used in pregnancy or breastfeeding unless prescribed by a practitioner.

GARLIC PREPARATIONS

Opinions differ regarding the value of fresh garlic compared with that of supplements. It is commonly held that fresh garlic is the finest and most therapeutic form to take and that the supplements make it convenient to take daily and to reduce odour. There is also some evidence to suggest that too much fresh garlic may irritate or damage the lining of the digestive tract or cause anaemia.

Constituents: oil or powder from garlic (*Allium sativum*) plant.

Uses: garlic is licensed as an over-the-counter medicine to treat the symptoms of colds and catarrh.

Possible uses under practitioner prescription/supervision only: may lower blood pressure; studies suggest significant reduction of cholesterol and triglyceride levels during supplementation. Studies also suggest decreased tendency to thrombosis (formation of blood clots) and increased ability for the body to dissolve existing clots; may help protect against arteriosclerosis, expectorant, helps protect against colds, cleanser, antispasmodic, antibacterial. Studies demonstrate activity against 17 strains of fungus, and high efficacy against pathogenic yeasts, intestinal antiseptic; may help protect against amoebic dysentery and typhoid. Studies suggest possibility of inhibiting tumour growth.

Caution: Gerard House recommends that garlic supplements are not given to young children owing to a possible toxic hazard.

Gardolex
(Modern Health)

See separate entry.

Garlic Perles
(Gerard House)

Capsules of garlic oil 0.972 mg, soya bean oil 411 mg, gelatin
103 mg, glycerin 48mg.
Product licence: No. 1661/5030R.

Garlic Tablets
(Gerard House)

Pulverized garlic 198 mg, garlic oil 60 mg, sugar 55 mg, lactose
50 mg, tricalcium phosphate 10 mg, starch 9 mg, talc 4.5 mg,
povidone 3 mg, coating: titanium dioxide 1.5 mg, iron oxide,
kaolin, gum Arabic, syrup.
Product licence: No. 1661/5009R.

Garlic Tablets
(Potters)

Garlic powder and garlic oil
Product licence: No. 0250/5228R.

Lusty's Garlic Perles
(Lanes)

Essential oil of garlic 0.66 mg, soya bean oil, gelatin, glycerin.
Product licence: No. 1074/5041R.

Gastrocote
(MCP)

A white tablet used as an antacid and reflux suppressant to treat dyspepsia, hiatus hernia, oesophagitis.

Dose: adults 1-2 tablets 4 times a day; children over 6 years as adult.
Side effects: few; occasionally constipation.
Caution:
Not to be used for: infants.
Not to be used with: tetracycline antibiotics.
Contains: alginic acid, aluminium hydroxide, magnesium trisilicate, sodium bicarbonate.
Other preparations: Gastrocote Liquid.

Gastron
(Sterling Research Laboratories)

A white tablet used as an antacid and reflux suppressant to treat reflux symptom.

Dose: 1-2 tablets 3 times a day and 2 at bedtime.
Side effects: few; occasionally constipation.
Caution: in pregnant women and in patients suffering from high blood pressure, heart or kidney failure.
Not to be used for: infants.
Not to be used with: tetracycline antibiotics.
Contains: alginic acid, aluminium hydroxide, magnesium trisilicate, sodium bicarbonate.
Other preparations:

Gaviscon
(Reckitt & Colman)

A white tablet used as an antacid and reflux suppressant to treat reflux.

Dose: adults 1-2 tablets or 10-20 ml after meals and at night; children ½ infant sachet after meals.
Side effects: few; occasionally constipation.
Caution: in pregnant women, and in patients suffering from high blood pressure, heart or kidney failure.
Not to be used for: infants.
Not to be used with: tetracycline antibiotics.
Contains: sodium alginate, sodium bicarbonate, calcium carbonate.
Other preparations: Gaviscon Liquid, Gaviscon Infant.

Gelcosal
(Quinoderm)

A gel used as an antipsoriatic and skin softener to treat psoriasis, dermatitis, when the condition is scaling.

Dose: massage into the affected area twice a day.
Side effects:
Caution:
Not to be used for:
Not to be used with:
Contains: coal tar solution, tar, salicyclic acid.
Other preparations:

Gelcotar
(Quinoderm)

A gel used as an antipsoriatic treatment for psoriasis, dermatitis.

Dose: massage into the affected area twice a day.
Side effects: irritation, sensitivity to light

Caution:
Not to be used for: patients suffering from acute psoriasis.
Not to be used with:
Contains: coal tar solution, tar.
Other preparations: Gelcotar Liquid.

Gelsemium
(Weleda 6c, 30c; Nelsons 6c)

Prepared from bark of the root of *Gelsemium sempervirens* (yellow jasmine).

Uses: Influenza and its after-effects, fatigue, aching, trembling, weakness, heaviness, sneezing, sore throat, difficulty swallowing, headache, chills up and down the spine, vertigo, drooping eyelids, anticipatory fear.
Suited to: excitable, sensitive people who suffer from anticipatory fear.
Symptoms better for: urination, sweating.
Symptoms worse for: humidity, heat of sun, receiving bad news, shocks, anticipation, tobacco.
Low time: mid-morning.

Gelusil
(Warner-Lambert)

A white tablet used as an antacid to treat dyspepsia, heartburn.

Dose: adults 1-2 tablets after meals; children over 6 years half adult dose.
Side effects: few; occasionally constipation.
Caution:
Not to be used for: infants.
Not to be used with: tetracycline antibiotics.
Contains: magnesium trisilicate, aluminium hydroxide.
Other preparations:

Gencydo Ointment
(Weleda)

Dose: a small quantity to be inserted into each nostril twice daily, especially before retiring, or more often if required.
Product licence: No. PL0298/5516.
Constituents: per 100 g: concentrated lemon juice 20g, Quince seeds (Cydonia oblongata), Glycerine extract (1:10) 10g, Boric acid 2g, base.
Uses: to relieve hayfever symptoms.
Caution:
Availability: pharmacies only.

Gencydo Paint
(Weleda)

Dose: apply to the nasal mucosa several times a day. May also be diluted 1:5 in water as a nasal spray. Use in conjunction with Gencydo Ointment.
Product licence: No. PL0298/5517.
Constituents: per 100 g: concentrated lemon juice 20 g, quince seeds (*Cydonia oblonga*), glycerin extract (1:10) 10 g, boric acid 3 g.
Uses: to relieve the symptoms of hayfever.
Caution:
Availability: pharmacies only.

Generaid
(S.H.S.)

A powder used as source of protein, carbohydrate, and minerals for patients suffering from chronic liver disease, portohepatic encephalopathy.

Genisol
(Fisons)

A liquid used as an antipsioratic and anti-dandruff treatment for psoriasis, dandruff, seborrhoeic inflammation of the scalp.

Dose: shampoo once a week or as needed.
Side effects: irritation, sensitivity to light.
Caution:
Not to be used for: patients suffering from acute psoriasis.
Not to be used with:
Contains: coal tar, sodium sulphosuccinated undecylenic monoalkylomide.
Other preparations:

---

gentian mixture, acid

A tonic used to improve appetite.

Dose: 2-4 5 ml teaspoonsful ½ hour before a meal.
Side effects:
Caution:
Not to be used for: children.
Not to be used with:
Contains:
Other preparations: gentian mixture, alkaline.

Gerard 99
(Gerard House)

Dose: 2 tablets after meals 3 times a day.
Product licence: No. PL1661/5010R.
Constituents: hops (*Humulus lupulus*) 45 mg, passionflower (*Passiflora*) 100 mg, valerian (*Valeriana officinalis*) extract 20 mg, gentian extract 30 mg, malto-dextrin 87.50 mg, sugar 40 mg, talc 4 mg, magnesium stearate 1 mg, sodium starch

glycollate 2.5 mg. iron oxide and syrup as coating.
Uses: mild sedative, antispasmodic, to help with restlessness, irritability, nervousness, anxiety, tenseness.
Special notes: vegan, yeast free.
Caution: not to be used in pregnancy. Not recommended for children under 12 years. May cause drowsiness.

Germolene
(Smith Kline Beecham)

Germolene contains chlorhexidine, lanolin, paraffin, and salicylate and is available as a cream, ointment, or spray. It is a good general-purpose skin antiseptic useful for cleaning cuts and abrasions. Suitable for children.

Gevral
(Lederle)

A brown capsule used as a source of multivitamins and minerals to treat vitamin and mineral deficiencies.

Dose: 1 capsule a day.
Side effects:
Caution:
Not to be used for:
Not to be used with: levodopa.
Contains: multivitamins and minerals.
Other preparations:

Givitol
(Galen)

A maroon/red capsule used as an iron, folic acid, and vitamin supplement to treat iron and folic acid deficiences in pregnancy where vitamin supplements are also needed.

Dose: 1 capsule a day before food.
Side effects: nausea, constipation.
Caution:
Not to be used for: children.
Not to be used with: tatracyclines, levodopa.
Contains: ferrous fumarate, ascorbic acid, riboflavine, pyridoxine hydrochloride, nicotinamide, folic acid.
Other preparations:

Gladlax
(Gerard House)

Dose: 1-2 tablets as required, to be taken at bedtime.
Product licence: 1661/5011R
Constituents: Cape aloes 50 mg, fennel (*Foeniculum vulgare*) 15 mg, valerian 30 mg, holy thistle (*Cnicus benedictus*) 60 mg, myrrh (*Commiphora molmol*) 15 mg, malto-dextrin 90 mg, sodium starch glycollate 12.5 mg, talc 3 mg, sugar 40 mg, lactose 20 mg, magnesium stearate 1.5 mg, starch 3mg.
Uses: occasional or non-persistent constipation. Aloes acts as a laxative and stool softener, valerian is to reduce and to prevent griping, fennel is anti-inflammatory, holy thistle is to stimulate and aid digestion.
Special notes: vegetarian, yeast free.
Caution: not to be taken with other laxatives, during pregnancy or breastfeeding, or by children under 12 years.

Glandosane
(Fresenius)

An aerosol used to provide artificial saliva for dry mouth and throat.

Dose: spray into the mouth and throat for 1-2 seconds as needed.
Side effects:

Caution:
Not to be used for:
Not to be used with:
Contains: carboxymethylcellulose sodium, sorbitol, potassium chloride, sodium chloride, magnesium chloride, calcium chloride, dipotassium hydrogen phosphate.
Other preparations:

Glucotard
(MCP)

Mini-tablets in 5 g sachets used as a bulking agent to treat diabetes.

Dose: 1 sachet taken with water 1-3 times a day before main meals.
Side effects: wind swollen abdomen.
Caution: glucose levels should be checked initially.
Not to be used for: children or for patients suffering from blocked intestine, oesophageal disease.
Not to be used with:
Contains: guar gum.
Other preparations:

Glutafin
(Nutricia)

Gluten-free preparation supplied as biscuits, macaroni, spaghetti, pasta spirals for patients with digestive conditions that are sensitive to gluten.

Glutarol
(Dermal)

A solution used as a virucidal, skin-drying agent to treat warts.

Dose: apply the solution to the wart twice a day and rub down hard skin.
Side effects: staining of the skin.
Caution: do not apply to healthy skin.
Not to be used for: warts on the face or anal and genital areas.
Not to be used with:
Contains: glutaraldehyde.
Other preparations:

Glutenex
(Cow & Gate)

Gluten- and milk-free biscuit used as a source of protein and sucrose for patients with digestive conditions sensitive to gluten.

Glykola
(Sinclair)

A liquid used as a tonic.

Dose: 1-2 5 ml teaspoonsful 3 times a day.
Side effects:
Caution: in patients with a history of peptic ulcer.
Not to be used for: children.
Not to be used with:
Contains: caffeine, calcium glycerophosphate, kola liquid extract, chloroform suspension, alcohol, ferrous perchloride liquid.
Other preparations:

Golden Seal Compound
(Gerard House)

Dose: 2 tablets 3 times a day between meals.

Product licence: No. 1661/5005R.

Constituents: marshmallow (*Althaea officinalis*) root 100 mg, golden seal (*Hydrastis*) 10 mg, cranesbill (*Geranium maculatum*) 30 mg, dandelion root (*Taraxacum officinale*) 60 mg, maltodextrin 130 mg, talc 5 mg, magnesium stearate 2.50 mg, sodium starch glycollate 2.5 mg, sugar 60 mg, ethyl cellulose as coating.

Uses: indigestion, heartburn, flatulence, nausea, gastric irritation.

Special notes: vegan, yeast free.

Caution: not to be used in pregnancy or breastfeeding. Not recommended for children under 12 years.

Graphites
(Weleda 6c, 30c; Nelsons 6c)

Prepared from amorphous carbon.

Uses: eczema which cracks and weeps, thickening and hardening of skin, cracks and fissures, wounds which tend to suppurate, styes, overweight, constipation, anal fissures, tinnitus, hot flushes, dandruff.

Suited to: cautious, indecisive people who tend to put on weight.

Symptoms better for: touch, more clothing, eating.

Symptoms worse for: during and after menstruation, cold, light.

Low time: night.

Guanor
(R P Drugs)

A liquid used as an expectorant, antihistamine, mucus softener to treat cough, bronchial congestion.

Dose: adults 1-2 5 ml teaspoonsful every 2-3 hours; children 1-

5 years ½ teaspoonful every 3-4 hours, 6-12 years 1 teaspoonful every 3-4 hours.
Side effects: drowsiness, reduced reactions, rarely skin eruptions.
Caution: in patients suffering from liver or kidney disease.
Not to be used for: infants under 1 year.
Not to be used with: alcohol, sedatives, some antidepressants (MAOIs).
Contains: ammonium chloride, diphenhydramine hydrochloride, sodium citrate, menthol.
Other preparations:

Guarem
(Rybar)

Dispersible granules in a 5 g sachet used as a bulking agent to treat diabetes.

Dose: 1 sachet taken with water 1-3 times a day before main meals.
Side effects: wind swollen abdomen.
Caution: glucose levels should be checked.
Not to be used for: children or for patients suffering from blocked intestine, oesophageal disease.
Not to be used with:
Contains: guar gum.
Other preparations: Guarina (Norgine).

Halycitrol
(LAB)

An emulsion used as a multivitamin preparation to treat vitamin A and vitamin D deficiencies.

Dose: adults and children over 6 months 1 5 ml teaspoonful a day; infants under 6 months ½ teaspoonful a day.

Side effects: vitamin poisoning
Caution: in patients suffering from kidney disease, sarcoidosis (a chest disease that affects calcium levels).
Not to be used for:
Not to be used with:
Contains: vitamin A, vitamin D.
Other preparations:

Hamamelis
(Weleda 6c, 30c; Nelsons 6c)

Prepared from fresh bark of twigs and roots of *Hamamelis virginica* (witch hazel).

Uses: varicose veins, haemorrhoids, bruised soreness, chilblains with bluish colour, nosebleeds, venous congestion.
Symptoms better for:
Symptoms worse for: injuries, bruises, day, touch, pressure, humidity.
Low time: night.

Hayfever
(Nelsons)

Combination of 6c *Allium cepa*, 6c *Euphrasia officinalis*, 6c *Sabadilla officinarum*.

Uses: relief of hayfever.

Haymine
(Pharmax)

A yellow tablet used as an antihistamine and sympathomimetic treatment for allergies.

Dose: 1 tablet in the morning and 1 tablet at night if needed.
Side effects: drowsiness, reduced reactions, dizziness.
Caution:
Not to be used for: children, or for patients suffering from overactive thyroid gland, high blood pressure, coronary thrombosis.
Not to be used with: alcohol, sedatives, MAOIs.
Contains: chlorpheniramine maleate, ephedrine hydrochloride.
Other preparations:

Hayphryn
(Winthrop)

A spray used as a sympathomimetic, antihistamine treatment for blocked nose resulting from allergy.

Dose: adults 2 sprays into the nostrils every 3-4 hours; children over 7 years half adult dose.
Side effects:
Caution: in patients suffering from overactive thyroid gland, cardiovascular disease; do not use for periods longer than 7 days.
Not to be used for: children under 7 years
Not to be used with: MAOIs.
Contains: phenylephrine hydrochloride, thenyldiamine hydrochloride.
Other preparations:

Heemex
(Lanes)

Dose: apply freely to haemorrhoids night and morning, and after each bowel movement.
Product licence: No. PL1074/5023.
Constituents: witch hazel (*Hamamelis*) water 25 %, tinct.

benzoin 8.3 %, zinc oxide 5.1 %, emulsified base 61.6 %.
Uses: relieves pain and itching of haemorrhoids, and heals broken bleeding tissues.
Caution:

Helonias Compound
(Gerard House)

Dose: 1 tablet 3 times a day after meals.
Product licence: No. 1661/5017R.
Constituents: unicorn root (*Helonias*) 120 mg, parsley 60 mg, black cohosh (*Cimicifuga racemosa*) 30 mg, raspberry leaf extract 16.7 mg, chlorophyllin 0.10 mg, malto-dextrin 100 mg, sugar 63.20 mg, talc 6 mg, magnesium stearate 1.5 mg, sodium starch glycollate 2.5 mg, ethyl cellulose as coating.
Uses: diuretic, uterine tonic, to help premenstrual tension with fluid retention, abdominal bloating and tenderness.
Special notes: vegan, yeast free.
Caution: not to be used during pregnancy or breastfeeding. Not to be used for children or for the elderly.

Hepar Sulphuris (Hepar Sulph.)
(Weleda 6c, 30c; Nelsons 6c)

Prepared from a sulphide of calcium made by burning the white interior of oyster shells and sulphur together.

Uses: hypersensitivity, irritability, intolerance of pain, skin highly sensitive to touch, eczema, acne, intense chilliness, croup, cough brought on by exposure to cold air, wheezing, sensation of splinter at back of throat, tonsillitis, earache; all wounds tend to suppurate; will hasten abcesses; establishes suppuration around and removes foreign body.
Symptoms better for: warmth, humidity.
Symptoms worse for: cold dry air, winter, drafts, touch, noise, exertion.

Low time: night.

Hepatic Aid II
(Kendall)

Chocolate-, chocolate mint-, custard-, or egg nog-flavoured powder used as a source of amino acids, fat, oil, and lecithin for patients suffering from chronic liver disease where the diet must be controlled.

Caution: blood ammonia, BUN levels, serum electrolytes, glucose, and liver should be monitored regularly.
Not to be used for: children or for patients suffering from severe encephalopathy, coma caused by liver failure, phenylketonuria, or other malfunctions of amino acid metabolism.
Other preparations:

Herbal Powder No. 8
(Gerard House)

Dose: half-a-teaspoon 3 times a day after meals.
Product licence: 1661/5018R.
Constituents: half-a-teaspoonful will deliver approximately dandelion (*Taraxacum officinale*) 528 mg, uva ursi 132 mg, couch grass (*Agopyron repens*) 132 mg, buchu (*Agathosma betulina*) 88 mg.
Uses: diuretic, antiseptic, to relieve fluid retention, cystitis.
Special notes: vegan, yeast free.
Caution: not recommended for children under 12 years. Not to be used in pregnancy without practitioner supervision.

Herbheal Ointment
(Potters)

Dose: apply to affected parts night and morning.
Product licence: No. PL0250/5118R.
Constituents: colophony (from *Pinus palustris*), marshmallow (*Althaea officinalis*) root, chickweed (*Stellaria media*), lanolin, starch, sublimed sulphur, zinc oxide, base.
Uses: for skin conditions where irritation and itching is present.
Caution: not for children under 5 years. Some individuals may be sensitive to lanolin.

Hexopal
(Winthrop)

A white, scored tablet supplied at a strength of 500 mg and used as a vasodilator to treat Raynaud's phenomenon (a condition caused by spasm of the blood vessels), intermittent claudication (difficulty walking caused by circulation disorders).

Dose: 2 tablets 3-4 times a day.
Side effects:
Caution: in pregnant women.
Not to be used for: children.
Not to be used with:
Contains: inositol nicotinate.
Other preparations: Hexopal Forte, Hexopal Suspension.

Hibiscrub
(ICI)

A solution used as a disinfectant for cleansing and disinfecting skin and hands.

Dose: use as a liquid soap.
Side effects:
Caution:
Not to be used for:
Not to be used with:

Contains: chlorhexidine gluconate.
Other preparations:

Hibisol
(ICI)

A solution used as a disinfectant for cleansing and disinfecting skin and hands.

Dose: rub vigorously on to the skin until dry.
Side effects:
Caution:
Not to be used for:
Not to be used with:
Contains: chlorhexidine gluconate, isopropyl alcohol.
Other preparations:

Hibitane
(ICI)

A cream used as a disinfectant for cleansing and disinfecting hands and skin before surgery, and for prevention of infections in wounds, and after surgery.

Dose: apply freely to the affected area as needed.
Side effects:
Caution:
Not to be used for:
Not to be used with:
Contains: chlorhexidine gluconate.
Other preparations: Hibitane Obstetric Cream, Hibitane Concentrate, Hibitane 20% Gluconate.

Hioxyl
(Quinoderm)

A cream used as a disinfectant to treat minor wounds, infections, bed sores, leg ulcers.

Dose: apply freely as needed and cover with a dressing.
Side effects:
Caution:
Not to be used for:
Not to be used with:
Contains: hydrogen peroxide.
Other preparations:

Hiprex
(3M Riker)

A white, oblong, scored tablet supplied at a strength of 1 g and used as an antibacterial treatment for infections of the urinary tract.

Dose: adults 1 g twice a day; children 6-12 years half adult dose.
Side effects: stomach upset, rash, bladder irritation.
Caution:
Not to be used for: patients suffering from severe dehydration, severe kidney failure, or electrolyte changes.
Not to be used with: sulphonamides, alkalizing agents.
Contains: hexamine hippurate.
Other preparations:

Hirudoid

Hirudoid contains heparin (blood-thinning) components and is useful in dissolving skin bruises and local clots of blood. It may also reduce the tenderness in varicose veins.

Histalix
(Wallace)

A syrup used as qan antihistamine, expectorant, and sputum softener to treat bronchial and nasal congestion.

Dose: adults 1-2 5 ml teaspoonsful every 3 hours; children hald adult dose.
Side effects: drowsiness, reduced reactions, rarely skin eruptions.
Caution: in patients suffering from liver or kidney disease.
Not to be used for:
Not to be used with: alcohol, sedatives, MAOIs.
Contains: diphenhydramine hydrochloride, ammonium chloride, sodium citrate, menthol.
Other preparations:

Histryl Spansule
(S K & F)

A pink/clear capsule supplied at a strength of 5 mg and used as an antihistamine to treat rhinitis, severe allergic conditions, insect bites and stings, allergies to food or other drugs.

Dose: 1-2 capsules night and morning.
Side effects: drowsiness, reduced reactions, dry mouth, blurred vision, dizziness.
Caution: in nursing mothers.
Not to be used for: children.
Not to be used with: alcohol, sedatives, MAOIs.
Contains: diphenyl pyraline hydrochloride.
Other preparations: Histryl Paediatric.

Horehound and Aniseed Cough Mixture
(Potters)

Dose: adults 2 5 ml teaspoonsful 3 times a day; children over 5 years 1 5 ml teaspoonful 3 times a day.
Product licence: P/L0250/5096R.
Constituents: pleurisy root (*Asclepias tuberosa*), elecampane (*Inula helenium*), horehound (*Marrubium vulgare*), skunk cabbage (*Symplocarpus foetidus*), lobelia (*Lobelia inflata*), syrup.
Uses: to relieve coughs.
Special notes:
Caution: not recommended during pregnancy or breastfeeding nor for children under 5 years. Do not exceed the stated dose.

Hycal
(Beecham Products)

Low-electrolyte, lactose-, sucrose-, fructose-, and protein-free, flavoured liquid feed used as a source of carbohydrate for patients suffering from kidney failure, cirrhosis of the liver, or any conditions where a high-energy, low-electrolyte, low-fluid diet is needed.

Hypericum
(Weleda 6c, 30c; Nelsons 6c)

Prepared from entire plant *Hypericum perforatum* (perforate St John's wort).

Uses: painful injuries to parts rich in nerve endings especially fingers and toes, lacerated wounds involving nerve endings, violent shooting pains, falls injuring spine especially coccyx, blows or crush injuries to fingers or toes, headache after blow to the occiput.
Symptoms better for: bending backwards, rubbing.
Symptoms worse for: shock, touch, movement, cold damp.
Low time:

Hypericum/Calendula Ointment
(Weleda)

Dose: apply directly to the affected part or on a dry dressing.
Constituents: per 100 g: perforate St John's wort (*Hypericum perforatum*) tincture (1=3) 15 ml, marigold (*Calendula officinalis*) tincture (1=2) 10 ml, in a base containing lanolin, beeswax, vegetable oils.
Uses: to aid healing of minor cuts and sores.
Caution: some individuals may be sensitive to lanolin.
Not to be used for: patients where a deep infection is present because *Calendula* promotes surface healing and may seal in sepsis.

Hypotears
(Iolab)

Drops used to moisten dry eyes.

Dose: 1-2 drops every 3-4 hours or as needed.
Side effects:
Caution:
Not to be used for: patients who wear soft contact lenses.
Not to be used with:
Contains: polyethylene glycol, polyvinyl alcohol.
Other preparations:

Iceland Moss Compound
(Gerard House)

Dose: 1-2 tablets as necessary every 4 hours; children (5-12 years) 1 tablet each morning and night.
Product licence: No. 1661/5013R.
Constituents: Iceland moss (*Cetraria islandica*) 250 mg, liquorice (*Glycyrrhiza glabra*) 30 mg, lobelia (*Lobelia inflata*) 20 mg, malto-dextrin 100 mg, lactose 100 mg, talc 16 mg, magnesium

stearate 4 mg.
Uses: relief of congestion in the respiratory tract, chesty coughs, colds.
Special notes: vegetarian, yeast free.
Caution: not recommended for children under 5 years. Not to be used during pregnancy without practitioner supervision. Do not exceed the stated dose.

Ignatia
(Weleda 6c, 30c; Nelson 6c)

Prepared from the seeds of the *Ignatia amara* tree.

Uses: grief, fright, bereavement, exhaustion from prolonged grief, sighing, spasms, sensation of lump in throat, sore throat which is better for swallowing, piercing headache, haemorrhoids which are better when walking, croup, irritating cough which worsens with coughing, constipation.
Suited to: sensitive, emotional people who prefer to be alone.
Symptoms better for: being alone, eating.
Symptoms worse for: emotion, worry, coffee, tobacco smoke.
Low time: morning.

Indian Brandee
(Potters)

Dose: 1 5 ml teaspoonful in or with a little water. Repeat once or twice if necessary.
Product licence: P/L0250/5098R.
Constituents: capsicum tincture, strong ginger (*Zingiber officinale*) tincture, compound rhubarb tincture.
Uses: a warming remedy which helps relieve nausea and digestive discomfort.
Special notes:
Caution: not recommended for children or during pregnancy.

Indigestion and Flatulence Naturtabs
(Larkhall)
'Cantassium'

Dose: 1-2 tablets to be taken after meals.
Product licence: No. PL/0912/5997R.
Constituents: capsicin B.P. 30 mg, valerian (*Valerian officinalis*) extract 14 mg, fennel (*Foeniculum vulgare*) 14 mg, myrrh (*Commiphora molmol*) 19 mg, papain B.P.C. 1 mg, excipients.
Uses: to aid digestive discomfort.
Special notes: vegan, yeast free, hypoallergenic.
Caution: not recommended for children or during pregnancy or breastfeeding.

Indigestion and Flatulence Tablets
(Booker)
'Heath & Heather'

Dose: 2 tablets to be taken with water 3 times a day after meals.
Product licence: No. PL1713/5064R.
Constituents: peppermint (*Mentha piperita*) oil 0.01 ml, fennel (*Foeniculum vulgare*) oil 0.005 ml, capsicum oleoresin 0.1 mg, dicalcium phosphate, microcrystalline cellulose, silica, magnesium stearate, stearic acid.
Uses: to relieve the symptoms of indigestion and flatulence.
Special notes: vegan, yeast free.
Caution: not to be taken during early pregnancy without practitioner supervision. Not recommended for children. May antidote any homoeopathic remedies you are taking. Susceptible individuals may be sensitive to the menthol content of peppermint oil.

Indigestion Mixture
(Potters)

Dose: 1 5 ml teaspoonful after meals 3-4 times a day.

Product licence: No. PL0250/5065R.
Constituents: meadowsweet (*Filipendula ulmaria*) extract, concentrated compound gentian infusion, spindle tree (*Euonymus*) tincture.
Uses: to relieve the symptoms of indigestion, heartburn, and flatulence. Meadowsweet is the herbalist's antacid, gentian and *Euonymus* tone the liver and improve digestive function.
Special notes:
Caution: not recommended for children or during pregnancy or breastfeeding.

Indigestion Naturtabs
(Larkhall)
'Cantassium'.

Dose: 1-2 tablets to be taken after meals.
Product licence: No. PL0912/7313R.
Constituents: myrrh (*Commiphora molmol*) 20 mg, fennel (*Foeniculum vulgare*) 15 mg, valerian (*Valeriana officinalis*) extract 4 mg, papain 1.5 mg, capsicin 0.3 mg, calcium carbonate, calcium sulphate dihydrate, sago flour, calcium phosphate tribasic, vegetable fatty acid, magnesium trisilicate.
Uses: to relieve indigestion.
Special notes: vegan, yeast free, hypoallergenic.
Caution: not recommended for children or during pregnancy or breastfeeding.

Inner Fresh Tablets
(Booker)
'Heath & Heather'

Dose: 1-2 tablets to be taken before going to bed.
Product licence: No. P/L1713/5031R.
Constituents: alder buckthorn bark (*Rhamnus frangula*) extract equivalent to total glucofrangulins 20 mg, dicalcium phosphate, microcrystalline cellulose, stearic acid, magnesium

stearate, coating: hypromellose, polyethylene glycol, vegetable carbon, titanium dioxide.

Uses: a stimulant laxative for the relief of occasional constipation.

Special notes: vegan, yeast free.

Caution: may cause griping pain in susceptible individuals. Not recommended for children or during pregnancy. Discoloration of the urine, which may occur, is harmless.

Intralgin
(3M Riker)

A gel used as an analgesic rub to treat muscle strains, sprains.

Dose: massage gently into the affected area as needed.
Side effects: may be irritant.
Caution:
Not to be used for: areas near the eyes, broken or inflamed skin, or on membranes (such as the mouth).
Not to be used with:
Contains: salicylamide, benzocaine.
Other preparations:

Ionax
(Alcon)

A gel used as an abrasive, antibacterial preparation to clean the skin in the treatment of acne.

Dose: wet the face, then rub in once a day, and rinse.
Side effects:
Caution:
Not to be used for: children under 12 years.
Not to be used with:
Contains: polyethylene granules, benzalkonium chloride.
Other preparations:

Ionil T
(Alcon)

A shampoo used as an antipsoriatic treatment for seborrhoeic inflammation of the scalp.

Dose: shampoo once a day if needed.
Side effects: irritation, sensitivity to light.
Caution:
Not to be used for: patients suffering from acute psoriasis.
Not to be used with:
Contains: coal tar solution, salicyclic acid, benzalkonium chloride.
Other preparations:

Ipecacuanha (Ipecac.)
(Weleda 6c, 30c: Nelsons 6c)

Prepared from dried root of *Cephaelis ipecacuanha* plant.

Uses: nausea, vomiting, morning sickness, travel sickness, gastric upset with clean tongue, bronchitis, loose coarse rattle in chest without expectoration, nausea and shortness of breath accompany most complaints.
Symptoms better for: open air, rest, closing eyes, cold drinks, pressure.
Symptoms worse for: warmth, overeating, change of weather, vomiting, motion.
Low time:

Irofol C
(Abbott)

A red, oblong tablet used as an iron, folic acid, and vitamin supplement for the prevention and treatment of iron and folic acid deficiency in pregnancy where vitamin supplement is also needed.

Dose: 1 tablet a day before food.
Side effects:
Caution: in patients suffering from slow bowel action.
Not to be used for: children or for patients suffering from megaloblastic anaemia, diverticular disease, intestinal blockage.
Not to be used with: tetracyclines, Clinistix urine test.
Contains: ferrous sulphate, folic acid, ascorbic acid.
Other preparations:

Isocal
(Mead Johnson)

Lactose- and gluten-free liquid feed used as a source of protein, carbohydrate, fat, vitamins, and minerals for patients suffering from short bowel syndrome, intractable poor absorption, dysphagia, bowel fistulas, cachexia, anorexia nervosa, or for undernourished patients before surgery or after complete gastrectomy.

Caution: unsuitable as the only source of nutrition for children under 5 years.
Not to be used for: infants under 1 year.
Other preparations:

Isomil
(Abbott)

Milk protein-, gluten- and lactose-free powder used as a source of protein, carbohydrate, fat, vitamins, and minerals for patients suffering from galactosaemia, intolerance to lactose and milk, low galactokinase.

Isopto Alkaline
(Alcon)

Drops used to lubricate the eyes.

Dose: 1-2 drops into the eye 3 times a day.
Side effects:
Caution:
Not to be used for: patients who wear soft contact lenses.
Not to be used with:
Contains: hypromellose.
Other preparations:

Isopto Frin
(Alcon)

Drops used to lubricate the eyes when no infection is present.

Dose: 1-2 drops into the eye 3 times a day.
Side effects:
Caution: in infants and in patients suffering from narrow angle glaucoma.
Not to be used for: patients who wear soft contact lenses.
Not to be used with:
Contains: phenylephrine hydrochloride.
Other preparations:

Isopto Plain
(Alcon)

Drops used to moisten dry eyes.

Dose: 1-2 drops into the eye 3 times a day.
Side effects:
Caution:
Not to be used for: patients who wear soft contact lenses.

Not to be used with:
Contains: hypromellose.
Other preparations:

Isordil
(Wyeth)

A white, scored tablet supplied at strengths of 10 mg, 30 mg and used as a nitrate for the prevention of angina, acute congestive heart failure.

Dose: 5-15 mg under the tongue every 2-3 hours at first, then 10-60 mg swallowed 4 times a day. 40-120 mg for the prevention of angina.
Side effects: headache, flushes, dizziness, may make chest pain worse.
Caution: heart function should be checked in the case of heart failure.
Not to be used for: children.
Not to be used with:
Contains: isosorbide dinitrate.
Other preparations: Isordil Sublingual, Isordil Tembids.

Jamaican Sarsaparilla
(Potters)

Dose: 2 5 ml teaspoonsful in water 3 times a day.
Product licence: No. P/L0250/5093R.
Constituents: sarsaparilla (*Smilax reqelii*) root extract, syrup.
Uses: to relieve minor skin complaints, blemishes, and rashes.
Special notes:
Caution: not to be used for children or during pregnancy or breastfeeding without practitioner supervision.

Juvela
(Nutricia)

Gluten-free preparation supplied as loaf, fibre loaf, and mixes for patients with digestive conditions sensitive to gluten.

Other preparations: Juvela Low Protein.

Kalium Bichromicum (Kali. Bich.)
(Weleda 6c, 30c: Nelsons 6c)

Prepared from potassium bichromate.

Uses: catarrh which is stringy and tenacious, hard cough with plugs of mucus, pain in small spots (can be covered with point of finger), sore throat, migraine with blurred vision preceding the attack.
Suited to: reserved, conscientious people with a tendency to put on weight.
Symptoms better for: movement, pressure.
Symptoms worse for: alcohol, hot weather.
Low time: morning, 2-3 am.

Kalium Muriaticum (Kali. Mur.)
(New Era 6x)

Prepared from potassium chloride.

Uses: a blood purifier and cleanser, may help prevent blood from clotting too easily; white or greyish-white coated tongue and throat, sore throat, swollen glands, tonsillitis, thick white sticky catarrh, deafness from catarrh and blocked eustachian tubes, indigestion from fatty food, rheumatic swellings.
Symptoms better for: cold drinks, rubbing.
Symptoms worse for: open air, menstruation, movement, dampness, rich food.

Low time:

Kalium Phosphoricum (Kali. Phos.)
(Weleda 6c, 30c; New Era 6x; Nelsons 6c)

Prepared from potassium phosphate.

Uses: nervous exhaustion, nervousness, insomnia, depression, anxiety, vertigo, headache with humming in the ears, shingles, nervous asthma, hoarseness, dry tongue; night fears in children.
Symptoms better for: sleep, eating, gentle movement.
Symptoms worse for: worry, excitement, touch, pain, overwork.
Low time:

Kalium Sulphuricum (Kali. Sulph.)
(New Era 6x)

Prepared from potassium sulphate.

Uses: skin problems with scaling, psoriasis, athlete's foot, brittle nails, yellow slimy coating on the tongue, yellow catarrh, rheumatism which moves from joint to joint.
Symptoms better for: cool open air, walking.
Symptoms worse for: warmth of room, noise.
Low time: evening.

Kalms
(Lanes)

Dose: 2 tablets twice a day after meals and 2 more at bedtime.
Product licence: No. 1074/5045R.
Constituents: valerian (*Valeriana officinalis*)extract 33.75 mg (equivalent to valerian 135 mg), hops (*Humulus lupulus*) 45 mg, gentian (*Gentiana lutea*) extract 22.5 mg (equivalent to gentian

90 mg), corn starch, gum acacia, sugar, sodium starch glycollate, magnesium stearate, vegetable stearic acid, silica, shellac, industrial methylated spirit, calcium carbonate, talc, titanium dioxide, white dispersion, wax polish.

Uses: anxiety, irritability, insomnia, flushing and cold sweats of menopause.

Special notes: vegetarian, yeast free.

Caution: not to be taken during pregnancy or breastfeeding. Not recommended for children. Not recommended for those suffering from clinical depression. Valerian should not be taken in large doses for extended periods of time. Seek medical advice if you are taking other medications.

Kamillosan Ointment
(Norgine)

Dose: adults apply twice a day or after breastfeeding; infants apply at each nappy change.

Constituents: volatile camomile oil 0.5 %, camomile extract 10 %, base.

Uses: chapped skin, sore and cracked nipples, nappy rash.

Caution:

Availability: pharmacies.

---

kaolin

Kaolin preparations are useful for mild diarrhoea; they are not absorbed into the body and so have limited side effects. Products containing kaolin include Kaopectate, Kaodene, Enterosan (with belladonna and morphine), and Collis Browne's (with morphine, peppermint oil, and calcium carbonate).

Kas-Bah Herb
(Potters)

Dose: 3 level 5 ml teaspoonsful (about 6 g) infused in 1 pint of boiling water and taken daily in portions when cool enough.
Product licence: No. PL0250/5150R
Constituents: buchu (*Agathosma betulina*), clivers (*Galium aparine*), couchgrass (*Agropyron repens*), horsetail (*Equisetum*), uva ursi (*Arctostaphylos uva-ursi*), senna leaf Alexandrian (*Cassia senna*), excipients.
Uses: diuretic, soothing, astringent, antihaemorrhagic, urinary antiseptic, to relieve urinary and bladder discomfort and associated backache.
Special notes:
Caution: senna is not to be used in colitis or spastic colon. Not to be used for children or during pregnancy or breastfeeding without practitioner supervision. Senna may cause harmless discoloration of urine or stools.

KELP PREPARATIONS

Dose: see product pack.
Constituents: dried kelp (*Fucus vesiculosus*), excipients.
Uses: nutritional supplement, obesity associated with low thyroid function, relief of rheumatic pain, mild diuretic.
Special notes: (Gerard House) vegan, yeast free.
Caution: not recommended for children under 5 years. Not to be taken during pregnancy or by patients taking thyroxin or thyroid drugs without practitioner supervision.

Kelp Tablets
(Gerard House)

kelp 300 mg plus 12 mg kelp extract, sugar 118 mg, starch 16 mg, talc 2 mg, magnesium stearate 2mg.
Product licence: No. PL1661/5014R.

Malted Kelp Tablets
(Potters)

kelp, malt extract, anise oil.
Product licence: No. PL0250/5205R.

Keralyt
(Westwood)

A gel used as a skin softener to treat thickened skin.

Dose: wet the skin for 5 minutes and then apply once a day at night.
Side effects:
Caution: keep out of the eyes, nose, and mouth.
Not to be used for:
Not to be used with:
Contains: salicyclic acid.
Other preparations:

Kleer
(Modern Health)

Dose: 2 tablets 3 times a day before meals; children 5-12 years 1 tablet 3 times a day before meals.
Product licence: No. 1146/5006R.
Constituents: purple coneflower (*Echinacea*) 75 mg, stinging nettle (*Urtica dioica*) 75 mg, burdock root (*Arctium lappa*) 50 mg, excipients.
Uses: skin disorders, eczema, boils, acne, urticaria, psoriasis, purifies system and increases resistance to infection.
Special notes: not tested on animals.
Caution: not recommended for children under 5 years or during pregnancy and breastfeeding unless prescribed.

Kloref
(Cox)

A white effervescent tablet used as a potassium supplement to treat potassium deficiency.

Dose: adults 1-2 tablets in water 3 times a day; children as advised by a physician.
Side effects:
Caution: in patients suffering from kidney disease.
Not to be used for: patients suffering from increased chloride levels or other rare metabolic disorders.
Not to be used with:
Contains: betaine hydrochloride, potassium bezoate, potassium bicarbonate, potassium chloride.
Other preparations: Kloref-S.

Kolanticon
(Merrell Dow)

A gel used as an antacid, anti-spasm, and anticholinergic preparation to treat bowel/stomach spasm, acidity, wind, ulcers.

Dose: 10-20 ml every 4 hours.
Side effects: occasionally constipation, blurred vision, confusion, dry mouth.
Caution:
Not to be used for: infants or for patients suffering from glaucoma, inflammatory bowel disease, intestinal obstruction, or enlarged prostate.
Not to be used with: tetracycline antibiotics.
Contains: aluminium hydroxide, magnesium oxide, dicyclamine hydrochloride, dimethicone.
Other preparations:

Labiton
(LAB)

A liquid used as a tonic.

Dose: 2-4 5 ml teaspoonsful twice a day.
Side effects:
Caution:
Not to be used for: children, or for patients suffering from hepatitis or who are taking sedatives.
Not to be used with:
Contains: thiamine hydrochloride, p-aminobenzoic acid, kola nut dried extract, alcohol, caffeine.
Other preparations:

Labosept
(LAB)

A red hexagonal-shaped pastille supplied at a strength of 0.25 mg and used as an antiseptic treatment for mouth and throat infections.

Dose: 1 pastille every 4 hours.
Side effects:
Caution:
Not to be used for:
Not to be used with:
Contains: dequalinium chloride.
Other preparations:

Lachesis
(Weleda 6c)

Prepared from venom of *Trigonocephalus lachesis* snake (surukuku).

Uses: throbbing headache with head feeling hot and heavy, hot flushes, hot perspiration, menopause, intolerance of touch, pressure of clothing aggravates, symptoms occur more on left side of body or travel from left to right, poor circulation with bluish mottled appearance, sore throat extending to ear — better for swallowing solids but worse for liquids, tonsillitis.
Suited to: talkative excitable people.
Symptoms better for: open air, cold drinks, menstruation.
Symptoms worse for: sleep, heat, spring, summer, sun, touch, pressure, alcohol, hot drinks.
Low time: morning.

Lacri-Lube
(Allergan)

An ointment used for lubricating the eyes and protecting the cornea.

Dose: apply into the eye as needed.
Side effects:
Caution:
Not to be used for:
Not to be used with:
Contains: liquid paraffin, wool fat.
Other preparations:

Larch Resin Comp. Lotion
(Weleda)

Dose: apply sparingly around the eyes on the lids and temples as required.
Product licence: No. PL0298/5524.
Constituents: ananassa fruit extract 2.5 %, lavender oil 1 %, larch resin 5 %.
Uses: to relieve tired strained eyes.
Caution: keep out of the eyes. Shake bottle before use. Do not

use to treat inflamed conditions of the eyes. If you experience any irritation, discontinue using this product.

Laxative Tablets
(Seven Seas)

Dose: 1-2 tablets as required, preferably on going to bed. Initially the lowest recommended dose should be taken and, if required, increased by half each day, until a satisfactory bowel movement is obtained. Maximum dose 8 tablets in 24 hours. Children 6-12 years half the adult dose: 1 tablet to be taken in 24 hours, preferably in the morning. For children under 6 years, consult the doctor.
Product licence: No. PL2210/5046
Constituents: dandelion root extract (*Taraxacum officinale*) 60 mg, peppermint oil (*Mentha piperita*) 0.6 mg, senna extract to give 7.5 mg total sennosides A and B, dicalcium phosphate, maize starch, hydroxypropylmethylcellulose, magnesium stearate, talc, silica, ethylcellulose, glycerol, titanium dioxide, iron oxides.
Uses: the relief of occasional constipation.
Special notes:
Caution: laxative preparations should not be given when any undiagnosed acute or persistent abdominal symptoms such as pain, nausea, or vomiting are present. Should not be taken for long periods of time without consulting your doctor. Senna may colour the urine or stools. Not recommended during pregnancy or breastfeeding. May antidote any homoeopathic remedies you are taking.

Ledum
(Weleda 6c)

Prepared from entire plant *Ledum palustre*.

Uses: puncture wounds, insect bites, bee stings, bruised or bloodshot eyes, cold blue swellings, chilliness, rheumatic or arthritic conditions which start in the lower limbs and ascend, gout.

Symptoms better for: cold applications, resting.
Symptoms worse for: warmth, movement, alcohol.
Low time: night.

Lemsip

Lemsip contains paracetamol, caffeine, and phenylephrine. Mildly stimulant and pain relieving — caffeine may cause tremors. Coldrex is similar and has additional ascorbic acid.

Lenium
(Winthrop)

An anti-dandruff preparation.

Dose: twice a week for the first two weeks, once a week for two further weeks, then once every 3-6 weeks.
Side effects:
Caution: keep out of the eyes and any areas of broken skin; do not use within 48 hours of waving or colouring substances.
Not to be used for:
Not to be used with:
Contains: selenium sulphide.
Other preparations:

Leo K
(Leo)

A white, oval tablet used as a potassium supplement to treat potassium deficiency.

Dose: adults 3-5 tablets a day in divided doses; children as advised by a physician.
Side effects: ulcers or blockage in the small bowel.
Caution: in patients suffering from kidney disease.

Not to be used for:
Not to be used with:
Contains: potassium chloride.
Other preparations:

Lergoban
(3M Riker)

An off-white tablet supplied at a strength of 5 mg and used as an antihistamine to treat allergies.

Dose: 1-2 tablets every 12 hours.
Side effects: drowsiness, reduced reactions, dizziness, headache, flushing, anorexia, dry mouth.
Caution: in nursing mothers.
Not to be used for: children.
Not to be used with: alcohol, sedatives, MAOIs.
Contains: diphenylpyraline hydrochloride.
Other preparations:

Life Drops
(Potters)

Dose: 11 drops (O.2 ml) in 1-2 tablespoonsful of warm water every hour when required; children over 7 years adult dose every 2 hours when required.
Product licence: No. P/L0250/5100R.
Constituents: capsicum, elderflower (*Sambucus*), peppermint (*Mentha piperita*) oil.
Uses: to relieve the discomfort of colds, flu, fever, chills, and sore throat. Peppermint oil has potent antimicrobial activity.
Special notes:
Caution: may antidote any homoeopathic remedies you are taking.

Liga
(Cow & Gate)

Gluten-free rusks used for patients with digestive conditions sensitive to gluten.

Lightning Cough Remedy
(Potters)

Dose: adults 2 5 ml teaspoonfuls 3-4 times a day; children over 5 years 1 5 ml teaspoonful every 5-6 hours.
Product licence: P/L0250/5099R
Constituents: liquorice (*Glycyrrhiza glabra*) extract, anise (*Pimpinella anisum*) oil, excipients.
Uses: to relieve cough symptoms.
Special notes:
Caution: not to be used in pregnancy or breastfeeding nor for children under 5 years.

Ligvites
(Gerard House)

Dose: 2 tablets after breakfast and after evening meal.
Product licence: No. 1661/5016R.
Constituents: guaiacum (*Guaiacum officinale*) resin 40 mg, black cohosh (*Cimicifuga racemosa*) 35 mg, white willow bark (*Salix alba*) 100 mg, sarsaparilla extract 25 mg, poplar bark extract 17 mg, malto-dextrin 6 mg, sodium starch glycollate 14 mg, talc 7.20 mg, titanium dioxide 1700 and syrup as coating.
Uses: analgesic, anti-inflammatory, for the relief of rheumatic and arthritic aches and pains, backache, joint stiffness, fibrositis.
Special notes: vegan, yeast free.
Caution: not to be used in pregnancy or breastfeeding. Not recommended for children under 12 years.

Liminate
(Modern Health)

Dose: 2 tablets to be taken before going to bed; children over 7 years 1 tablet to be taken before going to bed.
Product licence: No. PL1146/5010R.
Constituents: Turkey rhubarb 150 mg, senna leaf 60 mg, Irish moss (*Chondrus crispus*) 40 mg, excipients.
Uses: laxative, lubricates and softens stools. Irish moss soothes irritated mucous membrane.
Special notes: not tested on animals.
Caution: senna is not to be used in colitis or spastic colon. Large doses of senna cause nausea, griping pain, and red coloration of urine. Not to be used in pregnancy or breastfeeding. Not recommended for children under 7 years.

Lipoflavonoid
(Lipomed)

A black/pink capsule used as a multivitamin treatment for vitamin B deficiency.

Dose: 3 capsules 3 times a day for 2-3 months reducing to 2 capsules 3 times a day.
Side effects:
Caution:
Not to be used for: children.
Not to be used with:
Contains: choline bitartrate, inositol, methionine, ascorbic acid, lemon bioflavonoid complex, thiamine, riboflavine, nicotinamide, pyridoxine, panthenol, hydroxocobalamin.
Other preparations:

Lipotriad
(Lipomed)

A clear/pink capsule used as a multivitamin treatment for vitamin B deficiency.

Dose: 3 capsules 3 times a day for 2-3 months reducing to 2 capsules 3 times a day.
Side effects:
Caution:
Not to be used for: children.
Not to be used with: levodopa.
Contains: choline bitartrate, inositol, di-methionine, thiamine, riboflavine, nicotinamide, pyridoxine, panthenol, hydroxocobalamin.
Other preparations: Lipotriad Liquid.

Liquifilm Tears
(Allergan)

Drops used to lubricate dry eyes.

Dose: 1 drop into the eye as needed.
Side effects:
Caution:
Not to be used for: patients who wear soft contact lenses.
Not to be used with:
Contains: polyvinyl alcohol.
Other preparations:

Liquigen
(S.H.S.)

Low-electrolyte emulsion used as milk substitute to supply triglycerides for patients suffering from steatorrhoea with cystic fibrosis of the pancreas, intestinal lymphangiectasis, chronic liver disease, cirrhosis of the liver, poor absorption, and in intestinal surgery or where a ketogenic diet is needed for control of epilepsy and Type 1 hyperlipoproteinaemia.

Liquisorb
(Merck)

Gluten-free and lactose-low, plain, chocolate-, strawberry-, banana-, or vanilla-flavoured liquid feed used as a source of protein, carbohydrate, fat, vitamins, minerals, and trace elements for patients suffering from short bowel syndrome, intractable poor absorption, dysphagia, bowel fistulas, inflammatory bowel disease, cachexia, anorexia nervosa, or for undernourished patients before surgery or after complete gastrectomy.

Caution: unsuitable as the only source of nutrition for children under 5 years.
Not to be used for: infants under 1 year.
Other preparations:

Liquisorb MCT
(Merck)

Gluten- and fructose-free, low-lactose, plain, chocolate-, strawberry-, or vanilla-flavoured liquid feed used as a source of protein, carbohydrate, fat, vitamins, minerals, and trace elements for patients suffering from short bowel syndrome, intractable poor absorption, dysphagia, bowel fistulas, inflammatory bowel disease, cachexia, anorexia nervosa, or for undernourished patients before surgery or after complete gastrectomy.

Caution: unsuitable as the only source of nutrition for children under 5 years.
Not to be used for: infants under 1 year.
Other preparations:

Liquorice Formula
(Bio-Strath: imported by Cedar Health Ltd)

Dose: 20 drops (0.6 ml) in a lttle water 3 times a day before meals.
Product licence: No. PL04210/0006.
Constituents: liquorice root (*Glycyrrhiza glabra*) extract 22.5 %, German camomile flowers (*Matricaria chamomilla*) extract 22.5 %, gentian root (*Gentiana lutea*) extract 5 %, torula utilis yeast plasmolysate 50 %, (ethanol content 35.5 % v/v approx.).
Uses: to aid digestion.
Special notes:
Caution: do not exceed the recommended dose. Large doses of liquorice may cause sodium retention and potassium loss leading to water retention, high blood pressure, headache, and shortness of breath.

Loasid
(Calmic)

A white tablet used as an antacid and anti-wind preparation to treat ulcers, oesophagitis, gastritis, hiatus hernia, heartburn.

Dose: 1-2 tablets when required.
Side effects: few; occasionally constipation.
Caution: in patients suffereing from kidney failure.
Not to be used for: infants.
Not to be used with: tetracycline antibiotics.
Contains: aluminium hydroxide, dimethicone.
Other preparations:

Lobelia Compound
(Gerard House)

Dose: 1 tablet every 4 hours as necessary.
Product licence: No. 0904/5001R.

Constituents: lobelia (*Lobelia inflata*) 60 mg, gum ammoniacum 30 mg, squill extract 30 mg, cayenne 10 mg, sugar 100 mg, lactose 70 mg, sodium starch glycollate 8.75 mg, talc 3.75 mg, magnesium stearate 2.50 mg; coating iron oxide, titanium dioxide, and syrup.

Uses: expectorant, respiratory stimulant, anti-spasmodic, helpful for coughs, catarrh, sinusitis.

Special notes: vegetarian, yeast free.

Caution: not recommended for children under 12 years. Not to be used in pregnancy without practitioner supervision. Do not exceed the stated dose. Large doses of *Lobelia* may cause nausea and vomiting.

Locasol
(Cow & Gate)

Low-calcium food product used for patients needing calcium-controlled diets.

Lofenlac
(Mead Johnson)

A low-phenylalanine, gluten-, and lactose-free powder used as a source of protein, carbohydrate, fat, vitamins, and minerals for patients suffering from phenylketonuria.

Lorexane
(Care)

A cream used as a scabicide and pediculicide to treat scabies and lice.

Dose: apply to the affected areas as directed.
Side effects:
Caution: keep out of the eyes.

Not to be used for:
Not to be used with:
Contains: lindane.
Other preparations: Lorexane Medicated Shampoo.

Lotussin
(Searle)

A linctus used as an antihistamine, antussive treatment for cough.

Dose: adults 2 5 ml teaspoonsful 3 times a day; children 1-5 years ½-1 teaspoonful 3 times a day, 5-12 years 1-2 teaspoonsful 3 times a day.
Side effects: drowsiness, reduced reactions, constipation, rarely skin eruptions.
Caution: in patients suffering from kidney disease, asthma.
Not to be used for: infants under 1 year, or for patients suffering from liver disease.
Not to be used with: alcohol, sedatives, some antidepressants (MAOIs).
Contains: diphenhydramine hydrochloride, dextromethorphan hydrobromide.
Other preparations:

Lusty's Herbalene
(Lanes)

Dose: ½-1 5 ml teaspoonful placed on the tongue and washed down with a little warm water first thing in the morning and last thing at night; children (7-14 years) half the adult dose.
Product licence: No.1074/5043/R.
Constituents: senna (*Cassia senna* B.P.) 64 %, buckthorn (*Rhamnus frangula* B.P.)4 %, elder leaves (*Folia sambuci*) 8 %, fennel (*Foeniculum vulgare*) mate (*Ilex paraguariensis*) 8 %.
Uses: relief of temporary or occasional constipation.

Special notes: vegan, yeast free.
Caution: not recommended for children under 7 years. Not to be used during pregnancy without practioner supervision.

Lycopodium
(Weleda 6c, 30c; Nelsons 6c)

Prepared from *Lycopodium clavatum* plant (common club moss).

Uses: abdominal bloating and flatulence, excessive hunger but a few mouthfuls satiate, loud rumbling especially in lower abdomen, craving sweets although they aggravate, symptoms are mainly on the right side of body or moving from right to left, ailments from anticipation, fear of failure, cystitis, gout.
Suited to: people who may appear proud or argumentative but are lacking in self-confidence.
Symptoms better for: warm drinks, movement, eructations.
Symptoms worse for: pressure of clothes, eating, sleep, bread, onions, cabbage, wine, coffee, smoking.
Low time: late afternoon to mid-evening.

Maalox
(Rorer)

A white tablet used as an antacid to treat gastric and duodenal ulcer, hiatus hernias, wind, and acidity.

Dose: 1-2 tablets after meals and at bedtime.
Side effects: few; occasionally constipation.
Caution:
Not to be used for: infants.
Not to be used with: tetracycline antibiotics.
Contains: aluminium hydroxide, magnesium hydroxide.
Other preparations: Maalox Suspension, Maalox Plus Suspension and Tablets (with dimethicone), Maalox TC (higher-dose aluminium suspension and tablets); Mucogel (Pharmax).

Magnesia Phosphorica (Mag. Phos.)
(New Era 6x)

Prepared from magnesium phosphate.

Uses: colic, cramps, spasms, neuralgic pains, right-sided complaints, sharp lightning-like pains, writer's cramp, menstrual cramp, facial neuralgia, headache relieved by warmth, sciatica.
Suited to: dark-haired, thin, nervous people.
Symptoms better for: warmth, hot bathing, pressure, rubbing, doubling up.
Symptoms worse for: cold, being uncovered.
Low time: night.

Malatex
(Norton)

A solution used as an anti-inflammatory preparation to treat varicose and indolent ulcers, bed sores, burns.

Dose: cleanse the affected area with the solution and then apply the cream twice a day.
Side effects:
Caution:
Not to be used for:
Not to be used with:
Contains: propylene glycol, malic acid, benzoic acid, salicylic acid.
Other preparations: Malatex Solution

Malinal
(Robins)

A scored, white chewable tablet supplied at a strength of 500 mg and used as an antacid to treat indigestion, ulcers, hyperacidity.

Dose: 2 tablets at mealtimes and at bedtime.
Side effects:
Caution:
Not to be used for: children.
Not to be used with: tetracycline antibiotics.
Contains: almasilate.
Other preparations:

Manusept
(Hough, Hoseason)

A solution used as a disinfectant for cleansing and disinfecting skin and hands before surgery.

Dose: rub into the skin until dry.
Side effects:
Caution: keep out of the eyes.
Not to be used for:
Not to be used with:
Contains: triclosan, isopropyl alcohol.
Other preparations:

Maxamaid
(S.H.S.)

Leucine, isoleucine, and valine-free powder used as a source of amino acids, carbohydrate, vitamins, minerals, and trace elements for patients suffering from maple syrup urine disease.

Not to be used for: children under 2 years.
Other preparations: Maxamaid RVHB; Maxamaid XLYS TRY; Maxamaid XMET, THRE, VAL, ISOLEU; Maxamaid XPHEN, TYR: Maxamaid XP; Maxamaid XP BAR.

Maxamum XP
(S.H.S.)

Phenylalanine-free, orange- or unflavoured powder used as a source of amino acids, carbohydrate, minerals, vitamins, and trace elements for patients suffering from phenylketonuria.

Not to be used for: children under 8 years.

Maxijul Super Sol
(S.H.S.)

Gluten-, sucrose-, galactose-, fructose-, and lactose-free powder used as a source of polyglucose polymer, sodium, and potassium for patients suffering from kidney failure, cirrhosis of the liver, intolerance of disaccharide, amino acid metabolic disorders, poor absorption, and hypoglycaemia where a high-energy, low-fluid diet is needed.

Other preparations: Maxijul Liquid; Maxijul LE.

Maxipro HBV Super Soluble
(S.H.S.)

A protein powder used for patients suffering from hypoproteinaemia, short bowel syndrome, intractable poor absorption, inflammatory bowel disease, bowel fistulas, dysphagia, and for undernourished patients before surgery or in complete gastrectomy where salt intake must be reduced.

Caution: unsuitable as the only source of nutrition for children under 5 years.
Not to be used for: infants under 1 year.

MCT Pepdite
(S.H.S.)

Gluten-, sucrose-, and lactose-free powder used as a source of protein, carbohydrate, fat, vitamins, minerals, and trace elements for patients suffering from intolerance to whole protein, short bowel syndrome, intractable poor absorption, bowel fistulas, inflammatory bowel disease, where fat is difficult to absorb.

Caution: use correct formulation depending upon the patient's age.
Other preparations: MCT Pepdite 2+.

Medicated Extract of Rosemary
(Potters)

Dose: massage gently into scalp twice a day.
Product licence: No. PL0250/5105R.
Constituents: rosemary oil, rosegeranium oil, methyl salicylate, bay oil.
Uses: to improve hair condition.
Caution:

Medicoal
(Lundbeck)

Effervescent granules used as an adsorbent to treat acute poisoning, overdose of drugs.

Dose: 5-10 g in 100 ml of water, repeat up to a maximum of 50 g.
Side effects:
Caution:
Not to be used for: poisoning where there is a known antidote or for poisoning by acids, alkalis, iron salts, cyanides, malathion, DDT, sulphonylureas.

Not to be used with: drugs taken by mouth.
Contains: activated charcoal.
Other preparations:

Medilave
(Martindale)

A gel used as an antiseptic and local anaesthetic to treat abrasions or ulcers in the mouth, teething.

Dose: apply to the affected area without rubbing in 3-4 times a day.
Side effects:
Caution:
Not to be used for: infants under 6 months.
Not to be used with:
Contains: benzocaine, cetylpyridinium.
Other preparations:

Meditar
(Brocades)

A waxy stick used as an antipsoriatic treatment for psoriasis, eczema.

Dose: apply to the affected area 1-2 times a day.
Side effects: irritation, sensitivity to light.
Caution:
Not to be used for: patients suffering from acute psoriasis.
Not to be used with:
Contains: coal tar.
Other preparations:

Melissa Compound
(Weleda)

Dose: 10-20 drops to be taken in a little water every hour as required.
Product licence: No. PL0298/5529
Constituents: Archangelica root 1.1 %, cinnamon (*Cinnamomum verum*) 1.5 %, clove (*Syzygium aromaticum*) 0.65 %, coriander (*Coriandrum sativum*) 0.75 %, lemon (*Citrus limon*) oil 0.6 %, lemon balm (*Melissa officinalis*) 4.5 %, nutmeg 2.2 %, nominal ethanol content 62 % v/v.
Uses: to relieve nausea, stomach upsets, occasional diarrhoea, period pains.
Special notes:
Caution: not recommended during pregnancy. May antidote any homoeopathic remedies you are taking.

Mercurius Solubilis (Merc. Sol.)
Weleda 6c, 30c, Nelsons 6c.

Prepared from dimercurous ammonium nitrate.

Uses: suppuration, abcesses, mouth ulcers, sore throat, tonsillitis, excessive saliva, metallic taste in mouth, bad breath, tongue swollen and flabby showing imprint of teeth, profuse sweats, feverish head cold with offensive green/yellow catarrh, earache, diarrhoea with straining, tremor.
Suited to: those who are hurried and impulsive.
Symptoms better for: even temperature, rest.
Symptoms worse for: temperature changes.
Low time: night.

Merocaine
(Merrell Dow)

A green lozenge supplied at a strength of 1.4 mg and used as an antiseptic and local anaesthetic to treat painful infections of the throat and mouth, and as an additional treatment for tonsillitis and pharyngitis.

Dose: 1 lozenge allowed to dissolve in the mouth every 2 hours up to a maximum of 8 lozenges in 24 hours.
Side effects:
Caution:
Not to be used for: children.
Not to be used with:
Contains: cetylpyridinium chloride, benzocaine.
Other preparations:

Merocet
(Merrell Dow)

A solution used as an antiseptic to treat infections of the throat and mouth.

Dose: rinse the mouth or gargle with the solution diluted or undiluted every 3 hours or as needed.
Side effects:
Caution:
Not to be used for: children under 6 years.
Not to be used with:
Contains: cetylpyridinium chloride.
Other preparations:

Metatone
(Warner-Lambert)

A liquid used as a source of vitamin B1 and minerals and used as a tonic.

Dose: adults 1-2 5 ml teaspoonsful twice a day.
Side effects:
Caution:
Not to be used for: children under 6 years.
Not to be used with:
Contains: thiamine hydrochloride, calcium glycerophosphate,

manganese, potassium, sodium.
Other preparations:

Midrid
(Sinclair)

A red capsule used as an analgesic to treat migraine.

Dose: 2 capsules at the beginning of the migraine attack, then 1 capsule every hour to a maximum of 5 capsules in 12 hours.
Side effects: dizziness.
Caution: in pregnant women and nursing mothers.
Not to be used for: children, or for patients suffering from severe kidney, liver, or heart disease, gastritis, severe high blood pressure, or glaucoma.
Not to be used with: MAOIs.
Contains: isometheptene mucate, paracetamol.
Other preparations:

Migraleve
(International)

A pink tablet and a yellow tablet according to strength and contents and used as an analgesic, antihistamine treatment for migraine.

Dose: adults and children over 10 years 2 pink tablets at the beginning of the attack and then 2 yellow tablets every 4 hours if needed to a maximum of 2 pink tablets and 6 yellow tablets in 24 hours.
Side effects: drwsiness.
Caution: in patients suffering from liver or kidney disease.
Not to be used for: children under 10 years.
Not to be used with: .
Contains: pink: buclizine hydrochloride, paracetamol, codeine phosphate; yellow: paracetamol, codeine phosphate.

Other preparations:

Milk of Magnesia

Milk of Magnesia contains magnesium hydroxide and is available in liquid and tablet form, as well as in combination with paraffin as Milpar.

Milupa lpd
(Milupa)

Low-protein, demineralized powder used as a source of vegetable oil, starch, sucrose, monoglycerides, potassium citrate, and calcium phosphate for children suffering from amino acid disorders.

Not to be used for: infants under 1 year.

Minafen
(Cow & Gate)

Low-phenylalanine powder used as a source of protein, carbohydrate, fat, vitamins, and minerals for infants and young children suffering from phenylketonuria.

Minamino
(Chancellor)

A syrup used as a source of amino acids, B vitamins, and minerals to treat vitamin and mineral deficiences.

Dose: adults 4 5 ml teaspoonsful 3 times a day; children half adult dose.
Side effects:

Caution:
Not to be used for:
Not to be used with: levodopa.
Contains: multivitamins and minerals.
Other preparations:

Minims Saline
(SNP)

Drops used to irrigate the eyes.

Dose: use as needed.
Side effects:
Caution:
Not to be used for: patients who wear soft contact lenses.
Not to be used with:
Contains: sodium chloride.
Other preparations:

Mintec
(Bridge)

A green/ivory capsule used as an anti-spasm treatment for irritable bowel syndrome, spastic colon.

Dose: adults 1-2 capsules 3 times a day before meals.
Side effects:
Caution:
Not to be used for:
Not to be used with:
Contains: peppermint oil.
Other preparations:

Mintezol
(MSD)

A pink, scored, chewable tablet supplied at a strength of 500 mg and used to treat worms and other associated conditions and infections.

Dose: under 60 kg body weight 25 mg per kg twice a day with food; over 60 kg body weight 1.5 g twice a day with food.
Side effects: reduced alertness, stomach and brain disturbances, allergy, liver damage, changes to sight and hearing, low blood pressure, bed wetting.
Caution: in patients suffering from liver or kidney disease.
Not to be used for:
Not to be used with: xanthine derivatives (such as theophylline).
Contains: thiabendazole.
Other preparations:

Mixed Pollen
(Weleda 30c)

Prepared from the following pollens: grasses — bent, brome, cocksfoot, crested dogtail, false oat, fescue, meadowgrass, rye grass, timothy grass, vernal, Yorkshire fog; trees — alder, ash, beech, silver birch, elm, hazel, oak, plane, poplar, willow; flowering plants — heather, nettle, plantain, fat hen, mugwort, borage, rape.

Uses: the relief of hayfever resulting from the above pollens.

Modjul Flavour
(S.H.S.)

A blackcurrant-, pineapple-, orange-, or tomato-flavoured carbohydrate, saccharin, citric and malic acid powder used to flavour unflavoured preparations for patients where metabolic disorders need dietary control.

Molcer
(Wallace)

Drops used as a wax softener to soften ear wax.

Dose: fill the ear with the drops and plug with cotton wool; leave for 2 nights and then clean out.
Side effects:
Caution:
Not to be used for: patients suffering from perforated eardrum.
Not to be used with:
Contains: sodium docusate.
Other preparations:

Monphytol
(LAB)

A paint used as an antifungal treatment for athlete's foot.

Dose: paint on to the affected area twice a day at first, then once a week.
Side effects:
Caution:
Not to be used for: children or pregnant women.
Not to be used with:
Contains: chlorbutol, methyl undecoanate, salicylic acid, methyl salicylate, propyl salicylate, propyl undecoanate.
Other preparations:

Motherwort Compound
(Gerard House)

Dose: 2 tablets 3 times a day after meals.

Product licence: No. PL1661/5012R.

Constituents: passionflower (*Passiflora*) 90 mg, motherwort extract (*Leonurus cardiaca*) 50 mg, lime flower (*Tilia cordata*) extract 670 mg, sugar 75 mg, talc 2.75 mg, magnesium stearate 2.75 mg, sodium starch glycollate 5.5 mg, lactose 35 mg, starch 1500 2mg.

Uses: sedative, anti-spasmodic, lowers blood pressure, mild diuretic, to calm and soothe those who are hyperactive, overexcitable, anxious or nervous.

Special notes: vegetarian, yeast free.

Caution: not recommended for children. Not to be used in pregnancy without practitioner supervision.

M.S.U.D. Aid
(S.H.S.)

A leucine-, isoleucine-, and valine-free powder used as a source of amino acids, vitamins, minerals, and trace elements for patients suffering from maple syrup urine disease.

Multivite
(Duncan, Flockhart)

A brown pellet used as a multivitamin treatment for vitamin deficiencies.

Dose: adults 2 pellets a day; children 1 pellet a day.
Side effects:
Caution:
Not to be used for:
Not to be used with:
Contains: vitamin A, thiamine, calciferol, ascorbic acid.
Other preparations:

Murine see **Brolene** and **Optrex**

Natracalm
(English Grains Healthcare)

Dose: 1 tablet 3 times a day, with a further tablet at bedtime if required. Tablet should be swallowed without chewing.
Product licence: No. PL0418/5104R.
Constituents: passionflower (*Passiflora incarnata*) aqueous alcoholic extractive from 500 mg of herb, lactose base.
Uses: to relieve the symptoms of nervous tension and the stresses and strains of everyday life.
Special notes:
Caution: not recommended for children or during pregnancy or breastfeeding.

Natrum Muriaticum (Nat. Mur.)
(Weleda 6c, 30c; New Era 6x; Nelsons 6c)

Prepared from sodium chloride.

Uses: excessive moisture or dryness in any part of the system, profuse watery colds, hayfever, severe headache, migraine, vertigo, pain in eyes from reading, effects of longstanding grief, depression, dry skin, eczema, cold sores, warts, menstrual pain, constipation, incontinence.
Suited to: thin, pale, reserved people who, though emotionally sensitive, dislike consolation.
Symptoms better for: open air, cool bathing.
Symptoms worse for: sun, emotion, consolation, touch, noise, music, salt, seaside.
Low time: mid- to late morning

Natrum Phosphoricum (Nat. Phos.)
(New Era 6x)

Prepared from sodium phosphate.

Uses: an acid neutralizer; helps remove excesses of lactic and uric acid from the body and thus aids digestive and rheumatic disorders, sour vomiting, yellow creamy coating at base of tongue, dyspepsia, tightness of muscles and tendons, gout.
Symptoms better for: cold.
Symptoms worse for: sugar, milk, fatty food.
Low time: evening.

Natrum Sulphuricum (Nat. Sulph.)
(New Era 6x)

Prepared from sodium sulphate.

Uses: regulates density of intercellular fluids by eliminating excess water; aids the healthy functioning of the liver, biliousness, bitter taste in mouth, brown tongue, yellow diarrhoea, painful flatulence, rumbling abdomen, photophobia, inflammation of nailbed.
Symptoms better for: open air, changing position.
Symptoms worse for: all forms of damp, night air, music.
Low time: morning.

Naturest
(Lanes)

Dose: 2 tablets 3 times a day and up to 3 more at bedtime.
Product licence: No. 1074/5049R.
Constituents: passionflower (*Passiflora*) extract 22 mg (equivalent to passionflower 66 mg), sugar, glucose, magnesium stearate.
Uses: temporary or occasional insomnia.
Special notes: vegan, yeast free.
Caution: not to be taken during pregnancy or breastfeeding. Not recommended for children under 12 years.

Naxogin 500
(Farmitalia CE)

A white scored tablet supplied at a strength of 500 mg and used as an antiprotozoal treatment for acute ulcerative gingivitis.

Dose: 1 tablet twice a day for 2 days.
Side effects: stomach upset.
Caution: in pregnant women.
Not to be used for: children, nursing mothers, or for patients siffereing from kidney weakness or brain disease.
Not to be used with: alcohol.
Contains: nimorazole.
Other preparations:

Neocate
(S.H.S.)

Gluten-, sucrose-, and lactose-free preparation used as a source of protein, carbohydrate, fat, vitamins, minerals, and trace elements for patients suffering from intolerance to whole protein, inflammatory bowel disease, bowel fistulas.

Neophryn
(Winthrop)

A spray or nasal drops used as a sympathomimetic treatment for blocked nose.

Dose: adults 2-3 drops or 2 sprays in each nostril every 3-4 hours; children over 7 years 1-2 drops into each nostril every 3-4 hours.
Side effects:
Caution: in patients suffering from cardiovascular disease or overactive thyroid. Do not use for longer than 7 days.
Not to be used for: children under 7 years

Not to be used with: MAOIs.
Contains: phenylephrine hydrochloride.
Other preparations:

Nericur
(Schering)

A gel used as an antibacterial skin softener to treat acne.

Dose: wash and dry the affected area, then apply the gel once a day.
Side effects: irritation, peeling.
Caution: keep out of the eyes, nose, mouth.
Not to be used for: children.
Not to be used with:
Contains: benzoyl peroxide.
Other preparations:

Nervone
(New Era)

Combination of Calc. Phos. 6x, Kali. Mur. 6x, Kali. Phos. 6x, Mag. Phos. 6x.

Uses: nervous debility, nerve pains and allied conditions.

Nestargel
(Nestle)

A carob seed flour, calcium lactate preparation used for patients suffering from vomiting and regurgitation.

Newrelax (formerly Neurelax)
(Potters)

Dose: 2 tablets 3 times a day.
Product licence: No. 0250/5199R.
Constituents: hops (*Humulus lupulus*), scullcap (*Scutellaria lateriflora*), valerian (*Valeriana officinalis*), vervain (*Verbena officinalis*), excipients.
Uses: sedative, antispasmodic, mild analgesic, to relieve tension, irritability, agitation, and restlessness. May help modify withdrawal symptoms in patients coming off conventional sedatives (this is best done under practitioner supervision). Gives best results when taken as a continuous course for a few weeks.
Special notes:
Caution: not to be used in pregnancy or breastfeeding. Not recommended for children.

Nicorette
(Lundbeck)

Chewing gum supplied at strengths of 2 mg and 4 mg, and used as an alkaloid to end smoking addiction.

Dose: 1 when required.
Side effects: addiction, hiccoughs, indigestion, irritated throat.
Caution: in patients suffering from coronary disease, angina, gastritis, peptic ulcer.
Not to be used for: children or pregnant women.
Not to be used with:
Contains: nicotine.
Other preparations:

Niferex
(Tillotts)

An elixir used as an iron supplement to treat iron deficiency anaemia.

Dose: adults treatment 1 5 ml teaspoonful 1-2 times a day,

prevention ½ teaspoonful a day; children 0-2 years 1 drop per 0.45 kg body weight a day, 2-6 years ½ 5 ml teaspoonful a day, 6-12 years 1 teaspoonful a day.
Side effects:
Caution: in patients with a history of peptic ulcer.
Not to be used for:
Not to be used with: tetracyclines.
Contains: polysaccharide-iron complex.
Other preparations: Niferex Tablets, Niferex-150.

Nilstim
(De Witt)

A green tablet used as a bulking agent to treat obesity.

Dose: 2 tablets to be broken into pieces and taken with liquid 15 minutes before meals.
Side effects:
Caution:
Not to be used for: children or for patients suffering from blocked intestine.
Not to be used with:
Contains: cellulose, methyl cellulose.
Other preparations:

Nine Rubbing Oils
(Potters)

Dose: rub into the affected part as required.
Product licence: No. PL0250/5102R.
Constituents: amber oil, clove oil, eucalyptus oil, linseed oil, methyl salicylate, volatile mustard oil, rectified turpentine oil, thyme oil, peppermint oil, arachis oil.
Uses: to relieve symptoms of muscular pain and stiffness including backache, sciatica, lumbago, fibrositis, rheumatic pain, and strains.

Caution: may antidote any homoeopathic remedies you are taking. Clove and thyme oil are not recommended during pregnancy.

Nivaquine
(M & B)

A yellow tablet supplied at a strength of 200 mg and used as an antimalarial drug for the prevention and treatment of malaria.

Dose: adults prevention 2 tablets on the same day once a week; treatment as advised by the physician; children use Nivaquine Syrup.
Side effects: headache, stomach upset, skin eruptions, hair loss, eye disorders, blood disorders, loss of pigment.
Caution: in pregnant women, nursing mothers, and in patients suffering from porphyria (a rare blood disorder), liver or kidney disease, psoriasis. The eyes should be tested before and during prolonged treatment
Not to be used for:
Not to be used with:
Contains: chloroquine sulphate.
Other preparations: Nivaquine Syrup, Nivaquine Injection.

Noctura
(Nelsons)

Combination of Kali. Brom. 6c, *Coffea* 6c, *Passiflora* 6c, *Avena sativa* 6c, valerian 6c.

Uses: to encourage restful sleep.

Noradran
(Norma)

A syrup used as an antussive to treat bronchitis, bronchial asthma.

Dose: adults 2 5 ml teaspoonsful every 4 hours; children over 5 years 1 5 ml teaspoonful every 4 hours.
Side effects: sedation, dry mouth, nervousness, restlessness, hands shaking, abnormal heart rhythm, stomach upset.
Caution: in patients suffering from heart or liver disease, diabetes.
Not to be used for: children under 5 years, or for patients suffering from high blood pressure, overactive thyroid, coronary disease, cardiac asthma
Not to be used with: MAOIs, sympathomimetics, tricyclics, alcohol, cimetidine, erythomycin, interferon, ciprofloxaxin.
Contains: guaiphenesin.
Other preparations:

Normasol
(Seton-Prebbles)

A solution in a sachet used for washing out eyes, burns, wounds.

Dose: use as needed.
Side effects:
Caution:
Not to be used for:
Not to be used with:
Contains: sodium chloride.
Other preparations:

Nu-K
(Consolidated)

A blue capsule supplied at a strength of 600 mg and used as a potassium supplement to treat potassium deficiency.

Dose: 1-6 capsules a day in divided doses after food..
Side effects: ulcers or blockage in the small bowel.
Caution:
Not to be used for: children or for patients suffering from advanced kidney disease.
Not to be used with:
Contains: potassium chloride.
Other preparations:

Nulacin
(Bencard)

A beige tablet used as an antacid to treat dyspepsia, acidity, oesophagitis, hiatus hernia.

Dose: 1 or more tablets as required.
Side effects: diarrhoea.
Caution: in patients suffering from kidney impairment.
Not to be used for: children, or for patients suffering from coeliac disease.
Not to be used with: tetracycline antibiotics.
Contains: milk solids with dextrins and maltose, magnesium oxide, magnesium carbonate, magnesium trisilicate.
Other preparations:

Nurofen
(Boots)

A magenta-coloured, oval tablet supplied at strengths of 200 mg, 400 mg, 600 mg, and used as a non-steroid anti-inflammatory drug to treat pain, rheumatoid arthritis, ankylosing spondylitis, osteoarthritis, seronegative arthritis, peri-articular disorders, soft tissue injuries.

Dose: adults 1200-1800 mg a day in divided doses, to a maximum of 2400 mg a day; children 20 mg per kg body weight a day.

Side effects: dyspepsia, stomach bleeding, rash, rarely low blood platelet levels.

Caution: in pregnant women, and in patients suffering from asthma or allergy to aspirin or anti-inflammatory drugs.

Not to be used for: patients suffering from peptic ulcer.

Not to be used with:

Contains: ibuprofen.

Other preparations: Apsifen (APS), Brufen (Boots), Ebufac (DDSA), Lidifen (Berk), Motrin (Upjohn), Paxofen (Steinhard).

Nutramigen
(Mead Johnson)

Gluten-, fructose-, and lactose-free powder used as a source of protein, carbohydrate, fat, vitamins, and minerals for patients suffering from sensitivity to milk, intolerance to lactose, galactosaemia, or low galactokinase.

Nux vomica (Nux vom.)
(Weleda 6c, 30c; Nelsons 6c)

Prepared from seeds of *Strychnos nux-vomica* (strychnine) tree.

Uses: hypersensitivity to external stimuli, irritability, effects of overwork, effects of overeating, hangover, headache with nausea or dizziness, dyspepsia, nausea, vomiting, travel sickness, hiccough, raw sore throat, colds, hayfever, violent cough, spasms, menstrual cramps, colic, constipation with ineffectual urging, itching haemorrhoids.

Suited to: solid, compact, muscular people who are inclined to be impatient, irritable, and fastidious.

Symptoms better for: warmth, evening, resting.

Symptoms worse for: cold, alcohol, coffee, noise, light, odours, music, mental exertion, vexation.
Low time: early morning.

Octovit
(S K B)

A maroon, oblong tablet used as a multivitamin treatment for vitamin and mineral deficiencies.

Dose: 1 tablet a day.
Side effects:
Caution:
Not to be used for: children
Not to be used with: tetracyclines, levodopa.
Contains: vitamin A, thiamine, riboflavine, nicotinamide, pyridoxine, cyanocoblamin, ascorbic acid, cholecalciferol, tocopheryl acetate, calcium hydrogen phosphate, ferrous sulphate, magnesium hydroxide, zinc.
Other preparations:

Oleum Rhinale
(Weleda)

Dose: 2-4 drops of the oil to be instilled into and around the opening of each nostril twice a day.
Product licence: No. PL0298/5540.
Constituents: per 100 ml: oil extract from marigold (*Calendula*) 1 g, *Mercurius sulphuratus ruber* 3x 0.1 g, peppermint oil 0.3 ml, eucalyptus oil 0.3 ml.
Uses: the relief of catarrh, sinus congestion, dry rhinitis.
Caution: shake bottle before use. May antidote any homoeopathic remedies which you are taking.

Optimine
(Kirby-Warrick)

A white, scored tablet supplied at a strength of 1 mg and used as an antihistamine and serotonin antagonist (hormone blocker) to treat bites and stings, itch, allergic rhinitis, urticaria.

Dose: adults 1-2 tablets twice a day; children over 1 year use syrup.
Side effects: drowsiness, reduced reactions, greater appetite, anorexia, nausea, headache, anticholinergic effects.
Caution:
Not to be used for: infants under 1 year or for patients suffering from prostate enlargement, retention of urine, glaucoma, peptic ulcer causing blockage.
Not to be used with: sedatives, MAOIs, alcohol.
Contains: azatadine maleate.
Other preparations: Optimine Syrup.

Optrex eye preparations
Optrex eye preparations contain dilute solutons of witch hazel. This reduces eye reddening, and the solution acts to irrigate the eye. Some people are particularly sensitive to witch hazel and the treatment should not be continued if symptoms persist or worsen. Local sensitivity will present as stinging in or around the eye.

Opulets Saline
(Alcon)

Drops used to irrigate the eyes.

Dose: use as needed.
Side effects:
Caution:
Not to be used for:

Not to be used with:
Contains: sodium chloride.
Other preparations:

Orabase
(Squibb)

An ointment used as a mucoprotectant to protect lesions in the mouth.

Dose: apply to the affected area without rubbing in.
Side effects:
Caution:
Not to be used for:
Not to be used with:
Contains: carmellose sodium, pectin, gelatin.
Other preparations:

Oralcer
(Vitabiotics)

A green pellet used as an antibacterial, antifungal treatment for mouth ulcers.

Dose: adults allow 6-8 pellets to dissolve slowly near the ulcer on the first day, reducing to 4-6 pellets on the second day; children 3-4 pellets a day.
Side effects: local irritation.
Caution: do not use for extended periods.
Not to be used for: patients suffering from kidney or liver disease, overactive thyroid, intolerance to iodine.
Not to be used with:
Contains: clioquinol, ascorbic acid.
Other preparations:

Oraldene
(Warner-Lambert)

A solution used as an antiseptic rinse to treat thrush, gingivitis, ulcers, bad breath, stomatitis.

Dose: rinse out the mouth or gargle with 3 5 ml teaspoonsful 2-3 times a day.
Side effects: local irritation.
Caution:
Not to be used for:
Not to be used with:
Contains: hexetidine.
Other preparations:

Orovite
(Bencard)

A maroon tablet used as a source of multivitamins to aid recovery from feverish illness, infection or surgery, and to treat confusion in the elderly, mild alcoholic disorders, or for treatment after intravenous vitamin therapy.

Dose: adults 1 tablet 3 times a day; children use syrup.
Side effects:
Caution:
Not to be used for:
Not to be used with: levodopa.
Contains: thiamine, riboflavine, pyridoxine, nicotinamide, ascorbic acid.
Other preparations: Orovite Syrup.

Orovite 7
(Bencard)

Granules in a sachet used as a multivitamin treatment for vitamin deficiencies.

Dose: 1 sachet in water once a day.
Side effects:
Caution:
Not to be used for: children under 5 years.
Not to be used with: levodopa.
Contains: vitamin A palmitate, calciferol, thiamine, riboflavine, pyridoxine, nicotinamide, ascorbic acid.
Other preparations:

Osmolite
(Abbott)

Gluten- and lactose-free liquid feed used as a source of protein, carbohydrate, fat, vitamins, and minerals for patients suffering from short bowel syndrome, intractable poor absorption, dysphagia, bowel fistulas, inflammatory bowel disease, cachexia, anorexia nervosa, or for undernourished patients before surgery or after complete gastrectomy.

Caution: unsuitable as the only source of nutrition for children under 5 years.
Not to be used for: infants under 1 year.
Other preparations:

Ossopan 800
(Sanofi)

A buff-coloured tablet supplied at a strength of 830 mg and used as a calcium-phosphorus supplement to treat osteoporosis, rickets, osteomalacia (bone disorders).

Dose: adults 4-8 tablets a day in divided doses before food; children as advised by a physician.

Side effects:
Caution: in patients suffering from kidney disease, severe loss of movement, or a history of kidney stones.
Not to be used for: patients suffering from raised blood or urine calcium.
Not to be used with:
Contains: hydroxyapatite compound.
Other preparations: Ossopan Powder.

Ostersoy
(Farley)

Milk protein-, gluten-, sucrose-, and lactose-free powder used as a source of protein, carbohydrate, fat, vitamins, and minerals for patients suffering from intolerance of cow's milk, lactose, or sucrose, or galactosaemia, or low galactokinase.

Otrivine-Antistin
(Ciba)

A spray or drops used as a sympathomimetic, antihistamine treatment for hay fever, allergic rhinitis.

Dose: 2-3 drops or 1 spray into each nostril 2-3 times a day.
Side effects: itching nose, headache, sleeplessness, rapid heart rate.
Caution: Do not use for extended periods.
Not to be used for: children.
Not to be used with: MAOIs.
Contains: xylometazoline hydrochloride, antazoline sulphate.
Other preparations:

Otrivine-Anistin
(Zyma)

Drops used as a sympathomimetic, antihistamine treatment for allergic conjunctivitis and other eye inflammations.

Dose: adults 1-2 drops into the eye 2-4 times a day; children over 2 years 1 drop 2-4 times a day.
Side effects: temporary smarting, headache, sleeplessness, drowsiness, rapid heart rate, congestion.
Caution: in patients suffering from high blood pressure, enlarged prostate, coronary disease, diabetes.
Not to be used for: patients suffering from glaucoma or who wear soft contact lenses.
Not to be used with: MAOIS.
Contains: xylometazoline hydrochloride.
Other preparations:

Out of Sorts Tablets
(Potters)

Dose: 1-2 tablets at bedtime when necessary.
Product licence: 0250/5188R.
Constituents: senna, Cape aloe (*Aloe ferox*), cascara sagrada (*Rhamnus purshiana*) bark, dandelion root (*Taraxacum officinale*), fennel seed (*Foeniculum vulgare*), excipients.
Uses: relief of occasional constipation and bloatedness.
Special notes:
Caution: not to be used in pregnancy or breastfeeding.

Paediasure
(Abbott)

A preparation used as a source of protein, carbohydrate, fat, vitamins, minerals, and trace elements for patients suffering from short bowel syndrome, intractable poor absorption, dysphagia, bowel fistulas, inflammatory bowel disease, cachexia, or for undernourished patients before surgery.

Not to be used for: adults or for infants under 1 year.

Paedilyte RS
(Abbott)

A solution used to supply electrolytes in the treatment of dehydration.

Dose: adults dose as required; children equivalent amount to estimated fluid loss in divided doses given over 6-8 hours.
Side effects:
Caution: in patients suffering from dehydration.
Not to be used for: patients suffering from kidney disease with kidney failure, blocked intestine, bowel paralysis, severe vomiting, severe dehydration where intravenous fluid treatment is needed.
Not to be used with:
Contains: glucose, sodium chloride, sodium citrate, potassium citrate.
Other preparations: Ossopan Powder.

Pain Relief Naturtabs
(Larkhall)
'Cantassium'

Dose: 1-2 tablets up to 4 times a day.
Product licence: No. PL0912/7226R.
Constituents: willow bark (*Salix alba*) extract 250 mg (7.5 % salicin), passionflower (*Passiflora*) extract 10 mg, valerian (*Valeriana officinalis*) extract 15 mg, calcium phosphate tribasic 40 mg, calcium sulphate dihydrate 30 mg, potato starch 20 mg, vegetable fatty acid 2mg.
Uses: for general relief of pain, willow contains salicin and salicylic acid and is considered the natural form and origin of aspirin.
Special notes: vegan, yeast free.

Caution: not recommended for children or during pregnancy or breastfeeding.

Palaprin Forte
(Nicholas)

An orange, oval, scored tablet supplied at a strength of 600 mg and used as a non-steroid anti-inflammatory drug to treat rheumatoid arthritis, osteoarthritis, spondylitis.

Dose: 1 tablet per 6.5 kg body weight a day in divided doses dispersed in water, sucked, chewed, or swallowed.
Side effects: stomach upsets, allergy, asthma.
Caution: in pregnant women, the elderly, and in patients with a history of allergy to aspirin, asthma, impaired kidney or liver function, indigestion.
Not to be used for: children, nursing mothers, or for patients suffering from haemophilia or ulcers.
Not to be used with: anticoagulants (blood-thinning drugs), some antidiabetic drugs, anti-inflammatory agents, methotrexate, spironolactone, steroids, some antacids, some uric-acid lowering drugs.
Contains: aloxiprin.
Other preparations:

Paludrine
(ICI)

A white, scored tablet supplied at a strength of 100 mg and used as an antimalarial drug for the prevention of malaria.

Dose: adults and children over 12 years 1-2 tablets a day after meals; children under 1 year ¼ tablet, 1-4 years ½ tablet, 5-8 years ¾ tablet, 9-12 years 1 tablet after meals.
Side effects: stomach upset.
Caution:

Not to be used for:
Not to be used with:
Contains: proguanil hydrochloride.
Other preparations:

Panoxyl
(Stiefel)

A gel used as an antibacterial skin softener to treat acne.

Dose: wash and dry the affected area, then apply once a day.
Side effects: irritation, peeling.
Caution: keep out of the eyes, nose, mouth.
Not to be used for:
Not to be used with:
Contains: benzoyl peroxide..
Other preparations: Panoxyl Aquagel, Panoxyl Wash.

Papaya Plus
(Gerard House)

Dose: 1 tablet before meals 3 times a day.
Product licence: 1661/5019R.
Constituents: charcoal 100 mg, papain 60 mg, slippery elm
(*Ulmus rubra*) 60 mg, golden seal (*Hydrastis*) 10 mg, sugar 135
mg, povidone 15 mg, talc 8 mg, magnesium stearate 2 mg, ethyl
cellulose as coating.
Uses: papaya contains the enzyme papain which acts as an aid
to digestion, charcoal acts to reduce/control gas in the stomach,
slippery elm and *Hydrastis* soothe gastro-intestinal inflammation. Helpful for indigestion, heartburn, hyperacidity, and flatulence.
Special notes: vegan, yeast free.
Caution: not recommended for children, not to be used in
pregnancy or breastfeeding.

---

paracetamol tablets

A tablet supplied at a strength of 500 mg and used as an analgesic to relieve pain and reduce fever.

Dose: adults 1-2 tablets 4 times a day; children 6-12 years ½-1 tablet 4 times a day.
Side effects:
Caution: in patients suffering from kidney or liver disease.
Not to be used for: children under 6 years.
Not to be used with:
Contains:
Other preparations: paracetamol soluble, paracetamol elixir, Panadol (Winthrop), Panasorb (Winthrop).

Paracodol
(Fisons)

A white, effervescent tablet used as an analgesic to relieve pain.

Dose: adults 1-2 tablets in water every 4-6 hours to a maximum of 8 tablets in 24 hours; children 6-12 years ½-1 tablet to a maximum of 4 doses in 24 hours.
Side effects:
Caution: in patients suffering from kidney or liver disease, or who are on a limited consumption of salt.
Not to be used for: children under 6 years.
Not to be used with:
Contains: paracetamol, codeine phosphate.
Other preparations:

Parahypon
(Calmic)

A pink, scored tablet used as an analgesic to relieve pain.

Dose: adults 1-2 tablets 4 times a day; children 6-12 years half adult dose.
Side effects:
Caution: in patients suffering from kidney or liver disease.
Not to be used for: children under 6 years.
Not to be used with:
Contains: paracetamol, caffeine, codeine phosphate.
Other preparations:

Parake
(Galen)

A white tablet used as an analgesic to relieve pain and reduce fever.

Dose: 2 tablets every 4 hours to a maximum of 8 tablets in 24 hours.
Side effects:
Caution: in patients suffering from kidney or liver disease.
Not to be used for: children.
Not to be used with:
Contains: paracetamol, codeine phosphate.
Other preparations:

Pardale
(Martindale)

A white, scored tablet used as an analgesic to relieve headache, rheumatism, period pain.

Dose: 1-2 tablets 3-4 times a day.
Side effects:
Caution: in patients suffering from kidney or liver disease.
Not to be used for: children.
Not to be used with:
Contains: paracetamol, caffeine hydrate, codeine phosphate.

Other preparations:

Paroven
(Zyma)

A yellow capsule supplied at a strength of 250 mg and used as a vein constrictor to treat ankle swelling, varicose veins.

Dose: 3-4 capsules a day with food at first, then reduce.
Side effects: stomach disturbances, flushes, headache.
Caution:
Not to be used for: children.
Not to be used with:
Contains: oxerutins.
Other preparations:

Passiflora
(Potters)

Dose: to aid sleep: 2 tablets at tea-time and 2 at bedtime; daytime use 1-2 tablets 4 times a day
Product licence: 0250/5210R.
Constituents: passionflower (*Passiflora incarnata*) extract, excipients.
Uses: sedative, antispasmodic, mild analgesic.
Special notes:
Caution: not to be used in pregnancy or breastfeeding. Not to be used for children without practitioner supervision. May cause drowsiness.

Pavacol-D
(Boehringer Ingelheim)

A mixture containing opiate and demulcents used to treat cough.

Dose: adults 1-2 5 ml teaspoonsful as needed; children 1-2 years ½ teaspoonful 3-4 times a day, 3-5 years 1 teaspoonful 3 times a day, 6-12 years 1 teaspoonful 4-5 times a day.
Side effects: constipation.
Caution: in patients suffering from asthma.
Not to be used for: infants under 1 year, or for patients suffering from liver disease.
Not to be used with: MAOIs.
Contains: pholcodine, aromatic oils.
Other preparations:

Paynocil
(S K B)

A white, scored tablet used as an analgesic to relieve pain, reduce fever, and to treat rheumatoid arthritis and other rheumatic conditions.

Dose: 1 tablet dissolved on the tongue every 4-6 hours. For rheumatic conditions 2-3 tablets 3 times a day for 2-3 weeks reducing to 1-2 tablets 3 times a day.
Side effects: stomach upsets, allergy, asthma.
Caution: in pregnant women, the elderly, or in patients with a history of allergy to aspirin, asthma, impaired kidney or liver function, indigestion.
Not to be used for: children, nursing mothers, or for patients suffering from haemophilia or ulcers.
Not to be used with: anticoagulants (blood-thinning drugs), some antidiabetic drugs, anti-inflammatory agents, methotrexate, spironolactone, steroids, some antacids, some uric-acid lowering drugs.
Contains: aspirin, glycine.
Other preparations:

Peerless Composition Essence
(Potters)

Dose: adults: 1-2 5 ml teaspoonsful every 3 hours when necessary; children over 8 years 1 5 ml teaspoonful every 3 hours when necessary.

Product licence: No. PL0250/5091R.

Constituents: oak bark (*Quercus robur*), hemlock spruce (*Tsuga canadensis*), poplar bark, prickly ash bark (*Zanthoxylum americanum*), bayberry bark (*Myrica cerifera*), capsicum, herbal oils, syrup base.

Uses: to alleviate colds and chills, astringent, drying to mucous membranes. Prickly ash is a circulatory stimulant, poplar is a mild analgesic because of its salicylic glycosides, capsicum and ginger give the mixture a pleasantly hot taste.

Special notes:

Caution: Not recommended in pregnancy or breastfeeding nor for children under 8 years.

Pepdite
(S.H.S.)

Gluten-, sucrose-, and lactose-free powder used as a source of protein, carbohydrate, fat, vitamins, minerals, and trace elements for patients suffering from intolerance to whole protein or lactose, short bowel syndrome, intractable poor absorption, bowel fistulas, inflammatory bowel disease.

Caution: use the formulation suitable for the age of the patient.

Other preparations: Pepdite 2+.

Peptamen
(Clintec)

A preparation used as a source of protein, carbohydrate, fat, vitamins, minerals, and trace elements for patients suffering from short bowel syndrome, intractable poor absorption, dysphagia, bowel fistulas, inflammatory bowel disease, cachexia, anorexia nervosa, or for undernourished patients before surgery or after complete gastrectomy.

Caution: unsuitable as the only source of nutrition for children under 5 years.
Not to be used for: infants under 1 year.

Pepti-2000 LF
(Cow & Gate)

Powder used as a source of protein, carbohydrate, fat, vitamins, and minerals for patients suffering from intractable poor absorption, bowel fistulas, cachexia, and after complete gastrectomy.

Caution: unsuitable as the only source of nutrition for children under 5 years.
Not to be used for: infants under 1 year.
Other preparations: Pepti-2000 LF Liquid.

Pepti-Junior
(Cow & Gate)

Low-lactose powder used as a source of protein, carbohydrate, fat, vitamins, and minerals for patients suffering from intolerance to lactose and sucrose with protein intolerance in steatorrhoea associated with cystic fibrosis and other poor absorption conditions.

Peptisorb
(Merck)

Gluten- and fructose-free, low-lactose liquid used as a source of protein, carbohydrate, fat, vitamins, minerals, and trace elements for patients suffering from intractable poor absorption, bowel fistulas, cachexia, or after complete gastrectomy.

Not to be used for: children.

Peptisorbon
(Merck)

Low-lactose, gluten-, sucrose, fructose, and galactose-free powder used as a source of protein, carbohydrate, fat, vitamins, minerals, and trace elements for patients suffering from intractable poor absorption, bowel fistulas, cachexia, or after complete gastrectomy.

Caution: unsuitable as the only source of nutrition for children under 5 years.
Not to be used for: infants under 1 year.

Peptobismol

Peptobismol contains bismuth salicylate (see also De-Nol). Bismuth may colour the stools black and should be used with caution in patients suffering from kidney disease.

Periactin
(MSD)

A white, scored tablet supplied at a strength of 4 mg and used as an antihistamine , serotonin antagonists (hormone blocker) to improve appetite and to treat allergies, itchy skin conditions.

Dose: adults and children over 7 years1 tablet 3-4 times a day; children 2-6 years 2 tablets a day or ½ tablet 3-4 times a day.
Side effects: anticholinergic effects, reduced reactions, drowsiness, excitement.
Caution: in pregnant women, and in patients suffering from bronchial asthma, raised eye pressure, overactive thyroid, cardiovascular disease, high blood pressure.

Not to be used for: newborn infants, nursing mothers, the elderly, or patients suffering from glaucoma, enlarged prostate, bladder obstruction, retention of urine, stomach blockage, peptic ulcer, or debilitation.
Not to be used with: alcohol, sedatives, MAOIs.
Contains: cyproheptadine hydrochloride.
Other preparations: Periactin Syrup.

Pevaryl
(Cilag)

A cream used as an antifungal treatment for inflammation of the penis, inflammation of the vulva, thrush-like nappy rash, other skin infections such as tinea or nail infections.

Dose: massage gently into the affected area 2-3 times a day.
Side effects: irritation.
Caution:
Not to be used for:
Not to be used with:
Contains: econazole nitrate.
Other preparations: Pevaryl Lotion, Pevaryl Spray, Pevaryl Powder.

Phenergan
(M & B)

A blue tablet supplied at a strength of 10 mg, 25 mg and used as an antihistamine to treat allergies.

Dose: adults 10-20 mg 2-3 times a day; children 1-5 years 5-15 mg a day, over 5 years 10-25 mg a day.
Side effects: drowsiness, reduced reactions, dizziness, disorientation, sensitivity to light, convulsions on high doses, extrapyramidal reactions (shaking and rigidity).
Caution:

Not to be used for: infants under 1 year
Not to be used with: alcohol, sedatives, MAOIs.
Contains: promethazine hydrochloride.
Other preparations: Phenergan Elixir, Phenergan Injection.

Phensedyl
(M & B)

A linctus used as an antihistamine, opiate, sympathomimetic treatment for cough.

Dose: adults 1-2 5 ml teaspoonsful 2-3 times a day; children 2-5 years ½ teaspoonful 2-3 times a day, 6-12 years ½-1 teaspoonful 2-3 times a day.
Side effects: constipation, drowsiness, reduced reactions, anxiety, hands shaking, irregular or rapid heart rate, dry mouth, excitement, rarely skin eruptions.
Caution: in patients suffering from asthma, kidney disease, diabetes.
Not to be used for: children under 2 years, or for patients suffering from liver disease, heart or thyroid disorders.
Not to be used with: MAOIs, alcohol, sedatives, tricyclics.
Contains: promethazine hydrochloride, codeine phosphate, ephedrine hydrochloride.
Other preparations: Galcodine Paediatric.

Phenylephrine
(SNP)

Drops used as a sympathomimetic pupil dilator.

Dose: 1 drop into the eye as needed.
Side effects:
Caution:
Not to be used for: patients suffering from narrow angle glaucoma, high blood pressure, coronary disease, overactive

thyroid.
Not to be used with: ß-blockers.
Contains: phenylephrine.
Other preparations:

---

pHiso-Med
(Winthrop)

A solution used as a disinfectant to treat acne, and for disinfecting infants' skin, cleansing and disinfecting skin before surgery.

Dose: use as a liquid soap.
Side effects:
Caution: in newborn infants dilute 10 times.
Not to be used for:
Not to be used with:
Contains: chlorhexidine gluconate.
Other preparations:

Pholcomed-D
(Galen)

A linctus used as an opiate and bronchial relaxant to treat dry, irritating cough.

Dose: adults 2-3 5 ml teaspoonsful 3-4 times a day; children under 2 years years ½ teaspoonful 3-4 times a day, 2-12 years 1 teaspoonful 3-4 times a day.
Side effects: constipation.
Caution: in patients suffering from asthma.
Not to be used for: children under 1 year, or for patients suffering from liver disease.
Not to be used with: MAOIs.
Contains: pholcodine, papaverine hydrochloride.
Other preparations: Pholcomed Capsules, Pholcomed, Pholcomed Forte, Pholcomed Forte Diabetic, Pholcomed Expectorant.

Pholtex
(3M Riker)

A liquid used as an opiate and antihistamine treatment for dry cough.

Dose: adults 1 5 ml teaspoonful 2-3 times a day; children ½-1 teaspoonful 2-3 times a day.
Side effects: constipation.
Caution: in patients suffering from asthma.
Not to be used for: children under 5 years, or for patients suffering from liver disease.
Not to be used with: MAOIs.
Contains: pholcodine, phenyltoloxamine.
Other preparations:

Phosphate
(Sandoz)

A white, effervescent tablet used as a phosphate supplement to treat elevated calcium levels.

Dose: adults and children over 5 years up to 6 tablets a day; children under 5 years half adult dose.
Side effects: diarrhoea.
Caution: in patients suffering from kidney disease, congestive heart disease, high blood pressure.
Not to be used for: patients on a low sodium diet.
Not to be used with: antacids.
Contains: sodium acid phosphate, sodium bicarbonate, potassium bicarbonate.
Other preparations:

Phosphorus
(Weleda 6c, 30c; Nelsons 6c)

Prepared from red amorphous phosphorus.

Uses: cough with difficult rapid breathing, bronchitis, painful hoarseness, laryngitis, vomiting, diarrhoea, heartburn, burning sensations in small areas, need to eat often, anxiety, oversensitivity, vertigo, exhaustion with weakness and trembling, tendency to bleed or bruise easily.
Suited to: tall, slender, fine-boned, sensitive people.
Symptoms better for: cold food, ices, sleep.
Symptoms worse for: cold, thunderstorms, emotional upset, warm food, mental fatigue, lying on left side.
Low time: evening.

Phytex
(Pharmax)

A paint used as an antifungal treatment for skin and nail infections.

Dose: paint on to the affected area morning and evening, and after bathing for 2-3 weeks after the symptoms have gone.
Side effects:
Caution:
Not to be used for: children under 5 years or pregnant women.
Not to be used with:
Contains: tannic acid, boric acid, salicylic acid, methyl salicylate, acetic acid.
Other preparations:

Phytocil
(Fisons)

A cream used as an antifungal treatment for tinea infections.

Dose: apply to the affected area 2-3 times a day.
Side effects:
Caution:
Not to be used for:
Not to be used with:
Contains: phenoxypropanol, chlorophenoxyethanol, salicylic acid, menthol.
Other preparations: Phytocil Powder.

Phytolacca
(Weleda 6c)

Prepared from roots, berries and leaves of *Phytolacca decandra* plant (Virginian pokeweed).

Uses: mastitis, breast abscess, sore throat with intense burning and dryness, tonsillitis, rheumatism, shooting pains like shocks through the body, teething pains which are better when infant bites on something.
Symptoms better for: lying on abdomen, rest.
Symptoms worse for: movement, menstruation, cold damp, swallowing hot drinks.
Low time:

Piletabs
(Potters)

Dose: 2 tablets 3 times a day; elderly 2 tablets morning and night.
Product licence: 0250/5202R.
Constituents: pilewort (*Ranunculus ficaria*), agrimony (*Agrimonia eupatoria*), cascara sagrada (*Rhamnus purshiana*), stone root (*Collinsonia*).
Uses: relief of haemorrhoids.
Special notes:
Caution: not recommended during pregnancy or breastfeeding.

Pilewort Compound
(Gerard House)

Dose: 1-2 tablets at night before going to bed.
Product licence: 1661/5020R.
Constituents: pilewort (*Ranunculus ficaria*) extract 12 mg, senna leaf 30 mg, cranesbill (*Geranium maculatum*) extract 80 mg, cascara sagrada (*Rhamnus purshiana*) extract 54 mg, lactose 48 mg, sodium starch glycollate 8 mg, talc 6 mg, magnesium stearate 2 mg, iron oxide and syrup as coating.
Uses: relief of haemorrhoids and constipation.
Special notes: vegetarian, yeast free.
Caution: not recommended for children under 12 years. Not to be used in pregnancy or breastfeeding.

Pilewort Ointment
(Potters)

Dose: apply to affected parts twice a day.
Product licence: No. PL0250/5130R.
Constituents: pilewort (*Ranunculus ficaria*) herb extract, base.
Uses: to relieve the discomfort of piles.
Caution:

Piriton
(A & H)

A cream-coloured tablet supplied at a strength of 4 mg and used as an antihistamine treatment for allergies.

Dose: adults 1 tablet 3-4 times a day; children 6-12 years ½-1 tablet 3-4 times a day, under 6 years use syrup.
Side effects: drowsiness, reduced reactions, dizziness, excitation.
Caution: in nursing mothers.
Not to be used for:

Not to be used with: MAOIs, sedatives, alcohol.
Contains: chlorpheniramine maleate.
Other preparations: Piriton Syrup, Piriton Spandets, Piriton Injection.

PK Aid III
(S.H.S.)

Phenylalanine-free preparation used as a source of amino acids for patients suffering from phenylketonuria.

PKU 2
(Milupa)

Phenylalanine-free, vanilla-flavoured granules used as a source of amino acids, carbohydrate, vitamins, minerals, and trace elements for patients suffering from phenylketonuria.

Not to be used for: infants under 1 year.

PKU Drink
(Nutricia)

Phenylalanine-low milk substitute used for patients suffering from phenylketonuria.

Plesmet
(Napp)

A syrup used as an iron supplement to treat iron-deficiency anaemia.

Dose: adults 1-2 5 ml teaspoonsful 3 times a day; children ½-1 teaspoonful 2-3 times a day.

Side effects:
Caution:
Not to be used for:
Not to be used with: tetracyclines.
Contains: ferrous glycine sulphate.
Other preparations:

Polial
(Ultrapharm)

Gluten-, wheat starch-, milk protein-, egg-, and lactose-free, biscuit used for patients suffering from gluten-sensitive digestive disorders.

Polleneze

Polleneze contains astemozole and is a useful antihistamine for hay fever.

Side effects: drowsiness, reduced reactions, dizziness, excitation.
Caution: in nursing mothers.

Polycal
(Cow & Gate)

A carbohydrate powder used for patients suffering from kidney failure, cirrhosis of the liver, intolerance of disaccharide and protein, hypoglycaemia, amino acid metabolic disorders, and poor absorption conditions where a high-energy, low-fluid diet is needed.

Caution: do not give to infants without diluting.

Polytar Liquid
(Stiefel)

A liquid used as an antipsoriatic treatment for psoriasis of the scalp, dandruff, seborrhoea, eczema..

Dose: shampoo once or twice a week.
Side effects:
Caution:
Not to be used for:
Not to be used with:
Contains: tar, cade oil, coal tar, arachis oil, coal tar extract, oleyl alcohol.
Other preparations:

Polyvite
(Medo)

A red, oval capsule used as a multivitamin treatment for vitamin deficiencies.

Dose: 1-2 capsules a day.
Side effects:
Caution:
Not to be used for:
Not to be used with: levodopa.
Contains: vitamin A, calciferol, thiamine, riboflavine, pyridoxine, ascorbic acid, calcium pantothenate, nicotinamide.
Other preparations:

Ponoxylan
(Rorer)

A gel used as an antibacterial treatment for infection and inflammation of the skin.

Dose: apply to the affected area as needed.
Side effects:
Caution:
Not to be used for:
Not to be used with:
Contains: polynoxylin.
Other preparations:

Portagen
(Mead Johnson)

Gluten-, fructose-, and lactose-free powder used as a source of protein, carbohydrate, fat, vitamins, and minerals for patients suffering from poor fat absorption with intolerance of lactose, cachexia..

Posalfilin
(Norgine)

An ointment used as a skin softener to treat warts.

Dose: protect healthy skin, apply the ointment to the wart, and cover; repeat 2-3 times a week.
Side effects: pain when the ointment is first applied.
Caution: do not use on healthy skin.
Not to be used for: pregnant women or on warts on the face or anal and genital areas.
Not to be used with:
Contains: salicyclic acid, podophyllum resin.
Other preparations:

Pragmatar
(Bioglan)

A cream used as an anti-itch, antiseptic, skin softener to treat scaly skin, scalp seborrhoea, and similar disorders.

Dose: apply weekly, or daily in severe cases, to wet hair.
Side effects: irritation.
Caution: dilute the cream first when using for infants.
Not to be used for:
Not to be used with:
Contains: cetyl alcohol/coal tar distillate, sulphur, salicyclic acid.
Other preparations:

Prefil
(Norgine)

Brown granules used as a bulking agent to treat obesity.

Dose: 2 5 ml teaspoonsful swallowed with water ½-1 hour before eating.
Side effects:
Caution:
Not to be used for: patients suffering from blocked intestine.
Not to be used with:
Contains: sterculia.
Other preparations:

Pregaday
(Duncan, Flockhart)

A brownish-red tablet used as an iron and folic acid supplement in the prevention of iron and folic acid deficiency in pregnancy.

Dose: 1 tablet a day.
Side effects: stomach upset, allergy.
Caution: in patients with a history of peptic ulcer or who are in the first three months of pregnancy..
Not to be used for: patients suffering from vitamin B_{12} defi-

ciency.

Not to be used with: tetracyclines, antacids, anticonvulsant drugs, co-trimoxazole.

Contains: ferrous fumarate, folic acid.

Other preparations:

Pregestimil
(Mead Johnson)

Gluten-, sucrose-, fructose-, and lactose-free powder used as a source of protein, carbohydrate, fat, vitamins, and minerals for patients suffering from galactosaemia, low galactokinase, intolerance of sucrose and lactose, poor fat absorption, intolerance of protein, cachexia.

Pregnavite Forte F
(Bencard)

A lilac-coloured tablet used as an iron, folic acid, and vitamin supplement to treat iron and vitamin deficiencies.

Dose: 1 tablet 3 times a day after meals starting at least 1 month before conception and continuing at least until the second missed period date.

Side effects: stomach upset.

Caution:

Not to be used for: children or for patients suffering from megaloblastic anaemia.

Not to be used with: tetracyclines, levodopa.

Contains: ferrous sulphate, folic acid, calciferol, thiamine hydrochloride, riboflavine, pyridoxine hydrochloride, nicotinamide, ascorbic acid, calcium phosphate.

Other preparations:

Prejomin
(Milupa)

Gluten-, sucrose-, galactose-, fructose-, lactose-, and casein residue-free powder used as a source of protein, carbohydrate, fat, vitamins, minerals, and trace elements for patients suffering from galactosaemia, low galactokinase, intolerance of sucrose, fructose, lactose, or protein.

Prementaid
(Potters)

Dose: 2 tablets 3 times a day on uncomfortable days. It is important to take these regularly for several days to gain proper benefit.
Product licence: 0250/5211R.
Constituents: vervain (*Verbena officinalis*), motherwort (*Leonurus cardiaca*) extract, wild anemone (*Pulsatilla*) extract, uva ursi (*Arctostaphylos uva-ursi*), valerian (*Valeriana officinalis*).
Uses: to relieve the bloating and abdominal discomfort associated with premenstrual tension.
Special notes:
Caution: not to be used in pregnancy or breastfeeding.

Prioderm
(Napp Consumer)

A lotion used as a pediculicide and scabicide to treat scabies, lice in the head and pubic areas.

Dose: rub in and shampoo after 2-12 hours; repeat after 7-9 days.
Side effects:
Caution: keep out of the eyes.
Not to be used for:
Not to be used with:

Contains: malathion.
Other preparations: Prioderm Cream Shampoo.

Priory Cleansing Herbs
(Gerard House)

Dose: ¼ teaspoonful, or more, to be taken on going to bed, washed down with warm water.
Product licence: No. 1661/5022R.
Constituents: ¼ teaspoon will deliver senna leaf 378 mg, buckthorn (*Frangula alnus*) 54 mg, fennel (*Foeniculum vulgare*) 54 mg, psyllium (*Plantago*) seeds 54 mg, all as powder.
Uses: relief of short-term, non-persistent constipation.
Special notes: vegan, yeast free.
Caution: not recommended for children under 12 years. Not to be taken in pregnancy without practitioner supervision. Senna is not to be used in colitis or spastic colon and it may cause harmless coloration of urine and stools.

Pripsen
(Reckitt & Colman)

A sachet used to treat worms.

Dose: adults and children over 6 years 1 sachet and then a second dose of 1 sachet after 14 days; infants 3 months-1 year ⅓ sachet then a second dose after 14 days; children 1-6 years ⅔ sachet then a second dose after 14 days.
Side effects: rarely sight disorders, vertigo.
Caution: in nursing mothers and in patients suffering from nervous disorders.
Not to be used for: patients suffering from epilepsy, liver or kidney disease.
Not to be used with:
Contains: piperazine phosphate, sennoside.
Other preparations:

Pro-Actidil
(Wellcome)

A white tablet supplied at a strength of 10 mg and used as an antihistamine treatment for allergies.

Dose: 1 tablet a day 5-6 hours before going to bed.
Side effects: drowsiness, reduced reactions, rarely skin eruptions.
Caution: in nursing mothers, and in patients suffering from liver or kidney disease.
Not to be used for: children.
Not to be used with: MAOIs, sedatives, alcohol.
Contains: triprolidine hydrochloride.
Other preparations:

Promod
(Abbott)

Powder used as a source of protein and carbohydrate for patients suffering from hypoproteinaemia.

Propain
(Panpharma)

A yellow, scored tablet used as an analgesic, antihistamine treatment for headache, migraine, muscle pain, period pain.

Dose: 1-2 tablets every 4 hours to a maximum of 10 tablets in 24 hours.
Side effects: drowsiness.
Caution: in patients suffering from liver or kidney disease.
Not to be used for: children.
Not to be used with: alcohol, sedatives.
Contains: codeine phosphate, diphenhydramine hydrochloride, paracetamol, caffeine.

Other preparations:

Prosobee Liquid
(Mead Johnson)

Gluten-, sucrose-, fructose-, and lactose-free, liquid used as a source of protein, carbohydrate, fat, vitamins, minerals, and trace elements for young children suffering from intolerance to lactose, sucrose, and cow's milk, and galactosaemia, and low galactokinase.

Caution: dilute the liquid.
Other preparations: Prosobee Powder.

Protat
(Potters)

Dose: 1 5 ml teaspoonful 3 times a day.
Product licence: No. PL0250/5079R.
Constituents: cornsilk (*Zea mays*), kava (*Piper methysticum*), excipients.
Uses: short-term symptomatic relief of bladder discomfort.
Special notes:
Caution:

Protifar
(Cow & Gate)

Protein powder used for patients suffering from hypoproteinaemia.

Psoradrate
(Norwich Eaton)

A gel used as an antipsoriatic, drying agent to treat psoriasis.

Dose: wash and dry the area, then apply the cream twice a day.
Side effects: irritation, hypersensitivity.
Caution:
Not to be used for: pustular psoriasis.
Not to be used with:
Contains: dithranol, urea.
Other preparations:

Psorasolv Ointment
(Potters)

Dose: apply up to 4 times a day, as often as practicable.
Product licence: No. PL0250/5131R.
Constituents: pokeweed root (*Phytolacca americana*), clivers (*Galium aparine*), starch, sublimed sulphur, zinc oxide.
Uses: antiseptic, anti-inflammatory, to relieve the symptoms of mild psoriasis.
Caution: remove jewellery. Do not apply on top of any other product.

Psoriderm
(Dermal)

An emulsion used as an antipsoriatic to treat psoriasis.

Dose: add 30 ml of the emulsion to the bath water, soak for 15 minutes, dry, then apply the cream to the affected area.
Side effects: irritation, sensitivity to light.
Caution:
Not to be used for: patients suffering from acute psoriasis.
Not to be used with:
Contains: coal tar.
Other preparations: Psoriderm Cream, Psoriderm Scalp Lotion.

Psorigel
(Alcon)

A gel used as an antipsoriatic treatment for psoriasis.

Dose: rub into the affected area and allow to dry 1-2 times a day.
Side effects: irritation, sensitivity to light.
Caution:
Not to be used for: patients suffering from acute psoriasis.
Not to be used with:
Contains: coal tar solution.
Other preparations:

Psorin
(Thames)

An ointment used as an antipsoriatic skin softener to treat psoriasis, eczema.

Dose: apply to the affected area twice a day.
Side effects:
Caution: keep out of the eyes, and avoid direct sunlight.
Not to be used for: patients suffering from unstable psoriasis.
Not to be used with:
Contains: coal tar, dithranol, salicyclic acid.
Other preparations:

Pulsatilla
(Weleda 6c, 30c; Nelsons 6c)

Prepared from entire flowering *Pulsatilla nigricans* plant (wind anemone).

Uses: changeability of symptoms and of mood, pains which move and change, menstrual irregularities, menstrual pain, colds with thick bland yellow catarrh, thick coated white tongue,

stomach upsets from rich fatty foods, thirstless even though mouth is dry, weepy, yielding, babies who are quiet only when carried, styes, arthritis, cystitis, poor circulation, varicose veins.
Suited to: affectionate, emotional people easily moved to laughter or tears, fair haired, tend to put on weight easily.
Symptoms better for: open air, slow movement, consolation.
Symptoms worse for: rich foods, stuffy rooms.
Low time: evening.

Pyralvex
(Norgine)

A liquid used as an anti-inflammatory treatment for mouth inflammations.

Dose: apply to the affected area 3-4 times a day.
Side effects: local irritation.
Caution:
Not to be used for: children under 6 years.
Not to be used with:
Contains: anthraquinone glycosides, salicylic acid.
Other preparations:

Quellada
(Stafford-Miller)

A lotion used as a scabicide to treat scabies.

Dose: apply as directed.
Side effects:
Caution: keep out of the eyes.
Not to be used for: infants under 1 month.
Not to be used with:
Contains: lindane.
Other preparations: Quellada Application PC.

Quiet Days
(Larkhall)
'Cantassium'.

Dose: 1-2 tablets 3 times a day.
Product licence: No. PLR0912/7222.
Constituents: scullcap (*Scutellaria*) 75 mg, hops (*Humulus lupulus*) 25 mg, valerian (*Valeriana officinalis*) extract 42.5 mg, tricalcium phosphate 10.8 mg, mannitol 10 mg, sago flour 11.5 mg, magnesium trisilicate 5 mg, acacia gum 1 mg, stearic acid 1 mg, 10 % gum solution 0.0320 ml.
Uses: for the relief of mild anxiety during the day.
Special notes: vegan, yeast free, hypoallergenic.
Caution: not recommended for children. Not to be taken during pregnancy or breastfeeding without practitioner supervision.

Quiet Life
(Lanes)

Dose: 2 tablets twice a day after meals and 2-3 at bedtime.
Product licence: No. 1074/5032R.
Constituents: hops (*Humulus lupulus*) 75 mg, wild lettuce (*Lactuca virosa*) extract 7.25 mg (equivalent to wild lettuce 29 mg), valerian (*Valeriana officinalis*) extract 12.5 mg (equivalent to valerian 50 mg), motherwort (*Leonorus cardiaca*) 34 mg, passionflower (*Passiflora incarnata*) 58 mg, vitamin B$_1$ 0.71 mg, vitamin B$_2$ 0.57 mg, nicotinamide 4.49 mg, gum acacia, sugar, sodium starch glycollate, magnesium stearate, vegetable stearic acid, silica, shellac, IMS, calcium carbonate, talc, titanium dioxide, opalux pink, wax polish.
Uses: irritability, nervousness, tension, insomnia, to aid relaxation.
Special notes: vegetarian, yeast free.
Caution: high doses may cause headaches or sickness in sensitive individuals. Not recommended during pregnancy or breastfeeding, nor for children, nor for those suffering from clinical depression. Seek medical advice if you are taking other medication.

Quiet Night Tablets
(Booker)
'Heath & Heather'

Dose: 2 tablets to be taken with water 1 hour before going to bed.
Product licence: P/L1713/5061R
Constituents: valerian (*Valeriana officinalis*) 160 mg, hops (*Humulus lupulus*)200 mg, passionflower (*Passiflora*) 130 mg, dicalcium phosphate, microcrystalline cellulose, stearic acid, magnesium stearate; coating hypromellose, titanium dioxide, iron oxide, polyethylene glycol.
Uses: to aid sleep.
Special notes: vegan, yeast free.
Caution: not recommended for children. Not to be used in pregnancy. Drowsiness may persist into next day — if affected do not drive or operate machinery, and avoid alcoholic drink.

Quiet Nite Sleep
(Larkhall)
'Cantassium'.

Dose: 2-3 tablets to be taken at night preferably with a little water.
Product licence: No. PLR0912/7323.
Constituents: valerian (*Valeriana officinalis*) extract 30 mg, hops (*Humulus lupulus*) extract 15 mg, wild lettuce (*Lactuca virosa*) extract 10 mg, passionflower (*Passiflora incarnata*) extract 10 mg, camomile extract 15 mg, dicalcium phosphate 84.8 mg, sago flour 30.7 mg, stearic acid 1mg.
Uses: for the relief of occasional insomnia.
Special notes: vegan, yeast free, hypoallergenic.
Caution: not to be used in pregnancy of breastfeeding. Not recommended for children.

Quiet Time
(Larkhall)
'Cantassium'

Dose: see product pack.
Product licence: No. PL0912/7227R.
Constituents: scullcap (*Scutellaria*) 10 mg, hops (*Humulus lupulus*) 10 mg, passionflower (*Passiflora*) 10 mg, valerian (*Valeriana officinalis*) extract 15 mg, starch, sodium starch glycollate, calcium phosphate tribasic, calcium sulphate dihydrate, vegetable fatty acid, gum acacia.
Uses: the relief of mild anxiety.
Special notes: vegan, hypoallergenic.
Caution: not recommended for children, not to be used in pregnancy or breastfeeding.

Quinoderm Cream
(Quinoderm)

A cream used as an antibacterial skin softener to treat acne, acne-like eruptions, inflammation of the follicles.

Dose: massage into the affected area 1-3 times a day.
Side effects: irritation, peeling.
Caution: keep out of the eyes, nose, mouth.
Not to be used for:
Not to be used with:
Contains: potassium hydroxyquinolone sulphate, benzoyl peroxide.
Other preparations: Quinoderm Cream 5, Quinoderm Lotio-Gel, Quinoderm Lotio-Gel 5%, Quinoderm with Hydrocortisone.

Quinoped
(Quinoderm)

A cream used as a steroid, antifungal, antibacterial treatment for skin disorders where there is also infection.

Dose: massage into the affected area 2-3 times a day.
Side effects: fluid retention, suppression of adrenal glands, thinning of the skin may occur.
Caution: use for short periods of time only.
Not to be used for: patients suffering from acne or any other skin infections caused by tuberculosis, ringworm, viruses, or funguses, or continuously especially in pregnant women.
Not to be used with:
Contains: potassium hydroxyquinolone sulphate, hydrocortisone.
Other preparations:

Raspberry Leaf
(Potters)

Dose: 2 tablets 3 times a day after meals.
Product licence: No. PL0250/5212R.
Constituents: raspberry leaf (*Rubus idaeus*), excipients.
Uses: to strengthen, tone, and relax the uterus, for painful menstruation.
Special notes:
Caution: not now recommended in pregnancy except where labour has begun.

Reabilan
(Roussel)

Gluten- and lactose-free liquid feed used as a source of oligopeptides, carbohydrate, fat, vitamins, minerals and trace elements used as a complete nutrition for patients suffering from short bowel syndrome, intractable poor absorption, dysphagia, bowel fistulas, Inflammatory bowel syndrome, cachexia, or for undernourished patients before surgery or after complete gastrectomy.

Caution: unsuitable as the only source of nutrition for children under 5 years.
Not to be used for: infants under 1 year.

Redoxon
(Roche)

A white tablet supplied at strengths of 25 mg, 50 mg, 200 mg, and used as a vitamin C treatment for scurvy, and as an additional treatment for wounds and infections.

Dose: adults 500 mg-1 g 2-3 times a day; children under 4 years quarter adult dose, 4-12 years half adult dose, 12-14 years three-quarters adult dose.
Side effects: diarrhoea.
Caution:
Not to be used for:
Not to be used with:
Contains: ascorbic acid.
Other preparations: Redoxon Effervescent.

Rehidrat
(Searle)

A lemon and lime, and orange-flavoured powder used to provide electrolytes in fluid and electrolyte loss.

Dose: adults and children until thirst is quenched: infants substitute for feeds or after breast feeding.
Side effects:
Caution:
Not to be used for: patients suffering from kidney disease, blocked intestine, bowel paralysis.
Not to be used with:
Contains: sodium chloride, potassium chloride, sodium bicarbonate, citric acid, glucose, sucrose, laevulose.

Other preparations:

Resonium-A
(Winthrop)

A powder used for ion-exchange to lower potassium levels.

Dose: 15 g 3-4 times a day.
Side effects:
Caution: potassium and sodium levels should be checked regularly.
Not to be used for:
Not to be used with:
Contains: sodium polystyrene sulphonate.
Other preparations:

Rheumadoron Ointment
(Weleda)

Dose: massage into the affected area morning and evening.
Product licence: No. PL0928/5554.
Constituents: per 100 g: wolfbane (*Aconitum napellus*) extract from 1 g of plant, arnica (*Arnica montana*) extract from 3.5 g of plant, birch (*Betula*) extract from 2 g of plant, mandrake (*Mandragora*) extract from 0.3 g of plant, rosemary oil 1 g, base containing lanolin, beeswax, and vegetable oils.
Uses: to relieve the symptoms of muscular rheumatic pain.
Caution: do not apply to broken skin. Some individuals may be sensitive to lanolin.
Availability: pharmacies only.

Rheumadron
(English Grains Healthcare)

Dose: 1 tablet 3 times a day with meals.

Product licence: No. PL0418/5053R.
Constituents: guaiacum (*Guaiacum officinale*) resin 90 mg, prickly ash bark (*Zanthoxylum americanum*) aqueous extractive from 115 mg bark, excipients.
Uses: antirheumatic, anti-inflammatory, for the relief of muscular pain and stiffness associated with backache, sciatica, lumbago, fibrositis, rheumatism and painful joints.
Special notes:
Caution: not recommended for children, nor in pregnancy and breastfeeding without practitioner supervision.

Rheumadron 102A Drops
(Weleda)

Dose: 5-10 drops 3-4 times a day.
Product licence: No. PL0298/5553.
Constituents: per 100 ml aconite 3x 10 ml, arnica (1:2) 37.5 ml, birch (*Betula*) (1:3) 3.6 ml, mandragora root 1x 3 ml.
Uses: relief of muscular rheumatic pain.
Special notes:
Caution: do not exceed the stated dose. Not to be used during pregnancy or breastfeeding.
Availability: pharmacies only.

Rheumatic Pain
(Larkhall)
'Cantassium'

Dose: 1-2 tablets to be taken after each meal.
Constituents: dandelion root (*Taraxacum officinale*)24 mg, celery (*Apium graveolens*) extract 7.5 mg, buckbean (*Menyanthes trifoliata*) extract 7.5 mg, guaiacum resin 50 mg, capsicum oleoresin, calcium phosphate tribasic, calcium sulphate dihydrate, sago starch, magnesium trisilicate, vegetable fatty acid.
Uses: the relief of rheumatic aches and pains.

Special notes: vegan, hypoallergenic.
Caution: not recommended for children, nor in pregnancy or childbirth without practitioner supervision.

Rheumatic Pain Tablets
(Booker)
'Heath & Heather'

Dose: 1 tablet 3 times a day with water.
Product licence: No. P/L1713/5046R.
Constituents: bogbean (*Menyanthes trifoliata*) 330 mg, celery seed (*Apium graveolens*) 200 mg, guaiacum resin 70 mg, microcrystalline cellulose, dicalcium phosphate, sodium starch glycolate, stearic acid, magnesium stearate; coating hypromellose, polyethylene glycol, iron oxide, titanium dioxide.
Uses: to relieve the symptoms of backache, lumbago, fibrositis, rheumatic pain.
Special notes: vegan, yeast free.
Caution: not recommended for children. Not to be used in pregnancy without practitioner supervision. Susceptible individuals may experience some gastro-intestinal disturbance.

Rheumatic Pain Tablets
(Potters)

Dose: 2 tablets 3 times a day.
Product licence: 0250/5162R
Constituents: bogbean (*Menyanthes trifoliata*), yarrow (*Achillea millefolium*), burdock root (*Arctium lappa*), guaiacum resin, nutmeg (*Myristica fragrans*), excipients.
Uses: relief of aches and pains of rheumatism.
Special notes:
Caution: not recommended for children or during pregnancy or breastfeeding.

Rhus toxicodendron (Rhus tox.)
(Weleda 6c 30c; Nelsons, 6c)

Prepared from leaves of *Rhus toxicodendron* plant (oakleaf poison ivy) gathered at sunset just before flowering.

Uses: strains, sprains, overexertion, strains of muscles and tendons, pain in ligaments, rheumatism, stiffness, arthritis, sciatica, shooting pains, cold sores, herpes, eczema, tickling cough, restlessness.
Symptoms better for: continued movement, heat, hot bathing, rubbing, stretching, warm dry weather.
Symptoms worse for: first movement, cold, wet, drafts, before storms.
Low time: after midnight.

Rhus Tox. Ointment
(Weleda)

Dose: apply directly to the affected part or on a dry dressing.
Product licence: No. PL0298/6374.
Constituents: per 100 g: oakleaf poison ivy (*Rhus toxicodendron*) tincture (1:2) 10 ml, base containing lanolin, beeswax, and vegetable oils.
Uses: to ease rheumatic pain.
Caution: some individuals may be sensitive to lanolin.

Rite-Diet gluten-free
(Nutricia)

Gluten-free preparation supplied as high-fibre crackers, biscuits, pasta, flour mix, baking mix, white bread mix, brown bread mix, white loaf, high-fibre loaf, brown bread, canned white loaf and used for patients suffering coeliac disease or other digestive disorders where sensitivity to gluten occurs.

Caution: unsuitable for low-protein diets, phenylketonuria, galactosaemia (except pasta, low-protein flour mix, and canned white bread.

Rite-Diet low protein
(Nutricia)

Low-phenylalanine, low-electrolyte, gluten- and lactose-free preparation supplied as flour mix, baking mix, canned bread, white bread, flavoured wafers, biscuits, and pasta for patients suffering from phenylketonuria and other conditions where there is intolerance to amino acids, kidney and liver failure, cirrhosis of the liver, and digestive disorders where there is sensitivity to gluten.

Caution: biscuits and wafers are not suitable for gluten-sensitive digestive disorders.

Rite-Diet low-sodium bread
(Nutricia)

Bread containing carbohydrate, minerals, vitamins, and trace elements and used for patients needing low-sodium diets.

Roccal
(Winthrop)

A solution used as a disinfectant for cleansing and disinfecting the skin before surgery.

Dose: dilute the solution and use as needed.
Side effects:
Caution:
Not to be used for:
Not to be used with:

Contains: benzalkonium chloride.
Other preparations:

Rose Bengal
(SNP)

Drops used as a dye to stain the eye for finding degenerated cells in dry eye syndrome.

Dose: 1-2 drops in the eye as needed.
Side effects: severe smarting
Caution:
Not to be used for: children.
Not to be used with:
Contains: rose Bengal.
Other preparations:

Roter
(Roterpharma)

A pink tablet used as an antacid and antibulking agent to treat peptic ulcer, gastritis.

Dose: 1-2 tablets 3 times a day.
Side effects: constipation, nerve damage.
Caution:
Not to be used for: infants.
Not to be used with: tetracycline antibiotics.
Contains: magnesium carbonate, bismuth subnitrate, sodium bicarbonate, frangula.
Other preparations:

Rotersept
(Roterpharma)

An aerosol used as a disinfectant for the prevention of mastitis, and to treat cracked nipples.

Dose: spray on to the breast before and after feeding.
Side effects:
Caution:
Not to be used for: children.
Not to be used with:
Contains: chlorhexidine gluconate.
Other preparations:

Rowatinex
(Tillotts)

Volatile oils used to treat urinary stones, kidney disorders, prevention of urinary stones.

Dose: 3-5 drops 4-5 times a day before food.
Side effects:
Caution:
Not to be used for: children.
Not to be used with:
Contains: pinene, camphene, anethol, fenchone, cineole, olive oil.
Other preparations:

Ruta graveolens (Ruta grav.)
(Weleda 6c, 30c; Nelson 6c)

Prepared from entire *Ruta graveolens* plant (rue).

Uses: bruised bones, injuries to periosteum (membrane covering the bone), strains and sprains where Rhus tox. is ineffective, bruised sore aching with restlessness, synovitis, rheumatism, tennis elbow, eye strain.
Symptoms better for: warmth, movement, rubbing.

Symptoms worse for: overexertion, cold, menstruation.
Low time: evening.

Ruta Ointment
(Weleda)

Dose: apply directly to the affected part or on a dry dressing.
Product licence: No. PL0298/6393.
Constituents: rue (*Ruta graveolens*) tincture (1:3) 15 %, base.
Uses: to ease and aid healing of strains and sprains
Caution:

Rynacrom Spray
(Fisons)

A spray used as an anti-allergy treatment for allergic rhinitis.

Dose: 1 spray into each nostril 4-6 times a day.
Side effects: temporary itching nose, rarely bronchial spasm.
Caution:
Not to be used for:
Not to be used with:
Contains: sodium cromoglycate.
Other preparations: Rynacrom Nasal Drops, Rynacrom Cartridges, Rynacrom Compound.

Salactol
(Dermal)

A paint used as a skin softener to treat warts.

Dose: apply to the wart once a day and rub down with a pumice stone.
Side effects:
Caution: do not apply to healthy skin.

Not to be used for: warts on the face or anal and genital areas.
Not to be used with:
Contains: salicyclic acid, lactic acid.
Other preparations:

Salonair
(Salonpas)

An aerosol used as an analgesic rub to relieve muscular and rheumatic pain.

Dose: spray on to the affected area 1-2 times a day.
Side effects: may be irritant.
Caution:
Not to be used for: areas near the eyes, broken or inflamed skin, or on membranes (such as the mouth).
Not to be used with:
Contains: glycol salicylate, menthol, camphor, squalane, benzyl nicotinate.
Other preparations:

Salzone
(Wallace)

A syrup supplied at a strength of 120 mg/5 ml teaspoonful and used as an analgesic to relieve pain and reduce fever.

Dose: children ½-2 5 ml teaspoonsful every 4 hours according to age.
Side effects:
Caution: in children suffering from liver or kidney disease.
Not to be used for:
Not to be used with:
Contains: paracetamol.
Other preparations:

Sandocal
(Sandoz)

An orange effervescent tablet used as a calcium supplement in additional treatment for osteoporosis, osteomalacia, rickets, pregnancy, lactation, undernourishment, and after gastric surgery when absorption is poor.

Dose: adults 3-4 tablets a day dissolved in water; children 1-2 tablets a day dissolved in water.
Side effects: diarrhoea, nausea, flushes.
Caution: in patients suffering from kidney disease, unbalanced electrolyte levels, congestive heart failure. Your doctor may advise that calcium levels should be checked regularly.
Not to be used for: patients suffering from raised calcium levels in the blood or urine, severe kidney failure, kidney stones, galactosaemia.
Not to be used with: thiazides, tetracyclines.
Contains: calcium lactate gluconate, sodium bicarbonate, potassium bicarbonate.
Other preparations: Calcium Sandoz Syrup, Calcium Sandoz Injection.

Sando-K
(Sandoz)

A white effervescent tablet used as a potassium supplement to treat potassium deficiency.

Dose: 2-4 tablets a day dissolved in water.
Side effects: stomach upset
Caution: in patients suffering from kidney disease.
Not to be used for: children.
Not to be used with:
Contains: potassium bicarbonate, potassium chloride.
Other preparations: Kloref-S.

Savloclens
(ICI)

A solution in a sachet used as a disinfectant for cleansing and disinfecting wounds and burns.

Dose: use neat as needed.
Side effects:
Caution:
Not to be used for:
Not to be used with:
Contains: chlorhexidine gluconate, cetrimide.
Other preparations:

Savlodil
(ICI)

A solution in a sachet used as a disinfectant for cleansing and disinfecting wounds and burns.

Dose: use neat as needed.
Side effects:
Caution:
Not to be used for:
Not to be used with:
Contains: chlorhexidine gluconate, cetrimide.
Other preparations:

Savlon
(Ciba)

Savlon contains chlorhexidine and cetrimide and is available as a cream, liquid, barrier cream, nappy rash cream, sachets, and spray (containing povidine iodine). It is a useful antiseptic cream suitable for all age groups.

Savlon Hospital Concentrate
(ICI)

A solution used as a disinfectant and general antiseptic.

Dose: adequate amounts.
Side effects:
Caution:
Not to be used for:
Not to be used with:
Contains: chlorhexidine gluconate, cetrimide.
Other preparations:

Sciargo
(Potters)

Dose: 2 tablets 3 times a day.
Product licence: 0250/5229R.
Constituents: shepherd's purse (*Capsella bursa-pastoris*), wild carrot (Daucus carota), clivers (*Galium aparine*), uva ursi (*Arctostaphylos uva-ursi*), juniper berry (*Juniperus communis*) oil, excipients.
Uses: diuretic, anti-inflammatory, for the relief of sciatica.
Special notes:
Caution: not recommended during pregnancy.

Selora
(Winthrop)

Fine white grabules used as a common salt substitute for patients on low-sodium diets.

Dose: normal salt use.
Side effects:
Caution:
Not to be used for: patients suffering from kidney disease.

Not to be used with:
Contains: potassium chloride.
Other preparations:

Selsun
(Abbott)

A suspension used as an anti-dandruff treatment for dandruff, tinea versicolor (a scalp condition).

Dose: shampoo twice a week for 2 weeks, then once a week for 2 weeks, or apply to lesions and leave overnight.
Side effects:
Caution: keep out of the eyes or broken skin; do not use within 48 hours of using waving or colouring substances.
Not to be used for:
Not to be used with:
Contains: selenium sulphide.
Other preparations:

---

senna tablets

A tablet supplied at a strength of 7.5 mg and used as a stimulant laxative to treat constipation.

Dose: adults 2-4 tablets at bedtime; children 6-12 years half adult dose.
Side effects:
Caution:
Not to be used for: pregnant women, children under 6 years.
Not to be used with:
Contains: sennosides.
Other preparations:

Senna Tablets
(Potters)

Dose: 2 tablets at bedtime when required; children over 8 years: 1 tablet in the morning when required.
Product licence: 0250/5181R.
Constituents: senna Alexandrian (*Cassia senna*), excipients.
Uses: the relief of occasional constipation.
Special notes:
Caution: senna is not to be used in colitis or spastic colon. May cause harmless coloration of urine or stools. Not to be used for children under 8 years or during pregnancy or breastfeeding without practitioner supervision.

Senokot
(Reckitt & Colman)

A brown tablet supplied at a strength of 7.5 mg and used as a stimulant to treat constipation.

Dose: adults 2-4 tablets at bedtime; children 2-6 years 2.5-5 ml syrup (see below) in morning; children over 6 years half adult dose in morning.
Side effects:
Caution:
Not to be used for: infants under 2 years.
Not to be used with:
Contains: Sennoside B.
Other preparations: Senokot granules, Sennokott syrup.

Sepia
(Weleda 6c, 30c; Nelsons 6c)

Prepared from the ink of *Sepia officinalis* (common cuttlefish).
Uses: depression, indifference to loved ones, menopause, hot

flushes, hot sweats, hair loss, irregular periods, premenstrual tension, uterine pain with bearing down sensation, loss of sex drive, headache comes in shocks, sluggish irregular circulation, sudden tiredness.

Suited to: those who become depressed easily and lose interest in work, pleasure, loved ones, and sex.

Symptoms better for: exercise, dancing, hot applications.

Symptoms worse for: cold air, rest.

Low time: afternoon, evening.

Seravit Paediatric
(S.H.S.)

Low-sodium and potassium powder used as a source of carbohydrate, minerals, vitamins, and trace elements for infants and children where supplements are needed in special diets.

Setlers

Setlers contain calcium carbonate, magnesium carbonate and hydroxide, and aluminium hydroxide. Setlers Tums contain calcium carbonate only. Various strength and flavours are available and there are liquid and tablet preparations.

Shock and Distress Relief
(Nelsons)

Combination of Arnica 6c, Hypericum 6c, Rhus tox. 6c, Ruta grav. 6c, Symphytum 6c.

Uses: to relieve the effects of physical shock and trauma.

Silica
(Weleda 6c, 30c; New Era 6x; Nelsons 6c)

Prepared from flint.

Uses: abcesses, boils, expulsion of foreign bodies, acne, fungal infections, athlete's foot, tendency to suppurate, whitlow, offensive sweats particularly of the feet, persistent colds, hayfever, chilliness, swollen glands, migraine, poor assimilation of nutrients, brittle unhealthy nails, white spots on nails, constipation.
Suited to: delicate, pale, fair-haired people who are both timid and obstinate.
Symptoms better for: warmth, summer, humidity.
Symptoms worse for: cold, drafts, noise, touch, alcohol.
Low time: morning.

Sinotar
(Modern Health)

Dose: 2 tablets to be taken 3 times a day before meals; children 5-12 years tablet 3 times a day before meals.
Product licence: No. 1146/5011R.
Constituents: elderflower (*Sambucus*) 50 mg, marshmallow root (*Althaea officinalis*) 80 mg, coneflower (*Echinacea*) 75 mg, excipients.
Uses: sinusitis, catarrh, expectorant, soothes and lubricates nasal passages, antiseptic, increases resistance to infection.
Special notes: not tested on animals.
Caution: not recommended for children under 5 years or during pregnancy or breastfeeding unless prescribed.

Skin Cleanser
(Larkhall)
'Cantassium'

Dose: 1-2 tablets to be taken after meals with plenty of water.
Product licence: No. PL0912/7197R.
Constituents: senna extract 125 mg, burdock extract (*Arctium lappa*) 10 mg, fumitory (*Fumaria officinalis*) extract 10 mg, clivers extract (*Galium aparine*) 8 mg, buckbean extract (*Menyanthes trifoliata*), gum acacia, sago starch, magnesium trisilicate, vegetable fatty acid.
Uses: to cleanse the body to help clear skin blemishes.
Special notes: vegan, yeast free, hypoallergenic.
Caution: senna is not to be used in spastic colon or colitis. Large doses of senna cause nausea, griping pain, and red coloration of urine. Not recommended for children or during pregnancy or breastfeeding.

Skin Clear Ointment
(Potters)

Dose: apply to the affected parts morning and night.
Product licence: No. PL0250/5133R.
Constituents: starch, sublimed sulphur, zinc oxide, ti tree oil, yellow soft paraffin.
Uses: antiseptic, astringent, for mild acne, mild dry eczema, mild dermatitis.
Caution: not to be used on children under 5 years. Jewellery should be removed.

Skin Clear Tablets
(Potters)

Dose: 2 tablets 3 times a day.
Product licence: No. 0250/5208R.
Constituents: coneflower (*Echinacea*) root, excipients.
Uses: minor skin conditions, blemishes.
Special notes:
Caution: not recommended during pregnancy or lactation.

Skin Eruptions Mixture
(Potters)

Dose: 1 5 ml teaspoonful 3 times a day.
Product licence: No. PL0250/5002R.
Constituents: blue flag (*Iris versicolor*) extract, burdock root (*Arctium lappa*), yellow dock (*Rumex crispus*), sarsaparilla (*Smilax*), cascara (*Rhamnus purshiana*), buchu leaf (*Barosma betulina*), excipients.
Uses: symptomatic relief of mild eczema, psoriasis, and other skin diseases. These herbs aid elimination by diureses (buchu) and by gentle purging (cascara and yellow dock).
Special notes:
Caution: not recommended for children or in pregnancy or breastfeeding.

Skin Tablets
(Booker)
'Heath & Heather'

Dose: 2 tablets 3 times a day with water.
Product licence: No. P/L1713/5047R.
Constituents: burdock root (*Arctium lappa*) 500 mg, wild pansy (*Viola tricolor*) 375 mg, microcrystalline cellulose, stearic acid, magnesium stearate; coating hypromellose, polyethylene glycol, glycerin, iron oxide, titanium dioxide.
Uses: to help clear spots, skin blemishes, dry eczema.
Special notes: vegan, yeast free.
Caution: not recommended for children. Not to be taken in pregnancy without practitioner supervision. Susceptible individuals may experience gastro-intestinal upset.

SLIPPERY ELM PREPARATIONS

Dose: see product pack.
Constituents: slippery elm bark (*Ulmus rubra*).

Uses: soothes the gastro-intestinal mucosa, eases constipation. May help gastritis, diverticulitis, spastic colon, ulcerative colitis.

Caution: not recommended for children under 12 years. Not to be used in pregnancy without practitioner supervision. The (Potters) preparation may antidote any homoeopathic remedies you are taking.

Slippery Elm 400 mg Tablets
(Gerard House)

Slippery elm bark, gum myrrh 15 mg, malto-dextrin 265 mg, talc 16 mg, magnesium stearate 4mg.
Product licence: No. 1661/5025R.

Slippery Elm Stomach Tablets
(Potters)

Slippery elm bark, cinnamon oil, clove oil, peppermint oil.
Product licence: No. 0250/5209R.

Slow-Fe
(Ciba)

An off-white tablet supplied at a strength of 160 mg and used as an iron supplement to treat iron-deficiency anaemia.

Dose: adults 1-2 tablets a day; children 6-12 years 1 tablet a day.
Side effects: nausea, constipation.
Caution:
Not to be used for: children under 6 years.
Not to be used with: tetracyclines.
Contains: ferrous sulphate.
Other preparations:

Slow-K
(Ciba)

An orange tablet supplied at a strength of 600 mg and used as a potassium supplement to treat potassium deficiency.

Dose: adults 2-6 tablets a day or every other day after food; children as advised by a physician.
Side effects: blocked or ulcerated small bowel.
Caution: in patients suffering from kidney disease or peptic ulcer.
Not to be used for: patients suffering from advanced kidney disease.
Not to be used with:
Contains: potassium chloride.
Other preparations:

Slow Sodium
(Ciba)

A white tablet supplied at a strength of 600 mg and used as a salt supplement to treat salt deficiency.

Dose: adults 4-20 tablets times a day; children in proportion to dose for 70 kg adult.
Side effects:
Caution:
Not to be used for: patients suffering from fluid retention, heart disease, heart failure.
Not to be used with: diuretics, lithium.
Contains: sodium chloride.
Other preparations:

Sno Tears
(SNP)

Drops used to lubricate the eyes.

Dose: 1 or more drops into the eye as needed.
Side effects:
Caution:
Not to be used for: patients who wear soft contact lenses.
Not to be used with:
Contains: polyvinyl alcohol.
Other preparations:

Soliwax
(Martindale)

A red capsule used as a wax softener to soften and remove
hardened ear wax and to clean the canal.

Dose: insert the contents of 1 capsule into the ear, plug, and
leave overnight, then syringing if necessary.
Side effects:
Caution:
Not to be used for: patients suffering from perforated eardrum.
Not to be used with:
Contains: sodium docusate.
Other preparations:

Solpadeine
(Sterling Research Laboratories)

A white, effervescent tablet used as an analgesic to relieve
rheumatic, muscle, bone pain, headache, sinusitis, influenza.

Dose: adults 2 tablets in water 3-4 times a day; children 7-12½-
1 tablet 3-4 times a day.
Side effects: constipation.
Caution: in patients suffering from liver or kidney disease, or
who have a restricted salt consumption.

Not to be used for: children under 7 years.
Not to be used with:
Contains: paracetamol, codeine phosphate, caffeine.
Other preparations:

Solprin
(Reckitt & Colman)

A white, soluble tablet supplied at a strength of 300 mg used as an analgesic to relieve pain and to treat rheumatic conditions.

Dose: 1-3 tablets in water every 4 hours to a maximum of 12 tablets in 24 hours; higher doses for rheumatoid arthritis.
Side effects:
Caution:
Not to be used for: children.
Not to be used with:
Contains: aspirin.
Other preparations: Solprin 75 mg.

Solvazinc
(Thames)

An off-white effervescent tablet supplied at a strength of 200 mg and used as a zinc supplement to treat zinc deficiency.

Dose: adults and children over 30 kg body weight 1 tablet dissolved in water 1-3 times a day after food; children under 10 kg body weight ½ tablet in water once a day after food, 10-30 kg half adult dose.
Side effects: stomach upset.
Caution: in patients suffering from kidney failure.
Not to be used for:
Not to be used with: tetracyclines.
Contains: zinc sulphate.
Other preparations:

Sorbitrate
(Stuart)

A yellow, oval, scored tablet or a blue, oval, scored tablet according to strengths of 10 mg, 20 mg and used as a nitrate for the prevention of angina.

Dose: 10-40 mg 3-4 times a day.
Side effects: headache, flushes, dizziness.
Caution:
Not to be used for: children.
Not to be used with:
Contains: isosorbide dinitrate.
Other preparations:

Spanish Tummy Mixture
(Potters)

Dose: 1 5 ml teaspoonful every hour.
Product licence: No. PL0250/5088R.
Constituents: American blackberry root (*Rubus villosus*) extract, catechu (*Uncaria gambier*) tincture.
Uses: the treatment of non-persistent diarrhoea.
Special notes:
Caution: shake bottle before use.

Spasmonal
(Norgine)

A blue/grey capsule supplied at a strength of 60 mg and used as an anti-spasmodic treatment for irritable bowel syndrome.

Dose: 1-2 capsules 1-3 times a day.
Side effects: blurred vision, confusion, dry mouth.
Caution:
Not to be used for: children or for patients suffering from

glaucoma, inflammatory bowel disease, intestinal obstruction, enlarged prostate.
Not to be used with:
Contains: alverine citrate.
Other preparations:

Ster-Zac DC
(Hough, Hoseason)

A cream used as a disinfectant for cleansing and disinfecting the hands before surgery.

Dose: use as a liquid soap.
Side effects:
Caution: in children under 2 years.
Not to be used for:
Not to be used with:
Contains: hexachlorophane.
Other preparations:

Ster-Zac Powder
(Hough, Hoseason)

A powder used as a disinfectant for the prevention of infections in newborn infants, and to treat recurring skin infections.

Dose: adults apply to the affected area once a day; infants dust the affected area at each change of nappy.
Side effects:
Caution: in patients where the skin is broken.
Not to be used for:
Not to be used with:
Contains: hexachlorophane.
Other preparations:

Stomach Mixture
(Potters)

Dose: 1 5 ml teaspoonful 3 times a day.
Product licence: No. PL0250/5016R.
Constituents: dandelion root (*Taraxacum officinale*) extract, gentian (*Gentiana lutea*) root extract, compound rhubarb tincture, buchu (*Agathosma betulina*), bismuth ammonium citrate solution.
Uses: to relieve stomach ache and stomach upsets.
Special notes:
Caution: not recommended for children nor during pregnancy or breastfeeding. Shake bottle before use.

Strength Tablets
(Potters)

Dose: 2 tablets 3 times a day.
Product licence: 0250/5193R.
Constituents: kola (*Cola acuminata*), damiana (*Turnera diffusa*), saw palmetto (*Serenoa repens*), excipients.
Uses: contains the stimulants caffeine and theobromine, for short-term fatigue or times when extra energy is called for.
Special notes:
Caution: use of stimulants such as caffeine may tire the body in prolonged use.

Stugeron
(Janssen)

A white, scored tablet supplied at a strength of 15 mg and used as an antihistamine treatment for vestibular disorders, travel sickness.

Dose: vestibular disorders adults 2 tablets 3 times a day; travel sickness 1 tablet 2 hours before journey, then 1 every 8 hours

during the journey. Children 5-12 years half adult dose.
Side effects: drowsiness, reduced reactions, rarely skin erup-
tions.
Caution: in patients suffering from liver or kidney disease.
Not to be used for: children under 5 years.
Not to be used with: MAOIs, sedatives, alcohol.
Contains: cinnarizine.
Other preparations:

Sudafed
(Calmic)

A red tablet supplied at a strength of 60 mg and used as a
sympathomimetic treatment to relieve congestion of the nose,
sinuses, and upper respiratory tract.

Dose: adults1 tablet 3 times a day; children use elixir.
Side effects: anxiety, tremor, rapid or abnormal heart rate, dry
mouth, brain stimulation.
Caution: in patients suffering from diabetes.
Not to be used for: patients suffering from cardiovascular
disorders, overactive thyroid.
Not to be used with: MAOIs, tricyclics.
Contains: pseudoephedrine.
Other preparations: Sudafed Elixir, Sudafed SA, Sudafed-Co,
Sudafed Expectorant.

Sudafed Plus
(Calmic)

A white, scored tablet used as an antihistamine,
sympathomimetic treatment for allergic rhinitis.

Dose: adults1 tablet 3 times a day; children over 2 years use
Syrup.
Side effects: drowsiness, rash, disturbed sleep, rarely halluci-

nations.
Caution: in patients suffering from raised eye pressure, enlarged prostate.
Not to be used for: infants under 2 years, or for patients suffering from severe high blood pressure, coronary artery disease, overactive thyroid.
Not to be used with: MAOIs, sympathomimetics, furazolidone alcohol.
Contains: triprolidine hydrochloride, pseudoephedrine hydrochloride.
Other preparations: Sudafed Plus Syrup.

Suleo-C
(International)

A lotion used as a pediculicide to treat head lice.

Dose: rub into the scalp as directed.
Side effects:
Caution: keep out of the eyes.
Not to be used for:
Not to be used with:
Contains: carbaryl.
Other preparations: Suleo-C Shampoo.

Suleo-M
(International)

A lotion used as a pediculicide to treat head lice.

Dose: rub into the scalp as directed.
Side effects:
Caution: keep out of the eyes.
Not to be used for:
Not to be used with:
Contains: malathion.

Other preparations:

Sulphur
(New Era 6c, 30c; Nelsons 6c)

Prepared from sublimated sulphur.

Uses: skin eruptions which are hot and burning, redness, eczema, acne, burning pains, excoriating discharges, itching, mid-morning hunger, early morning diarrhoea, unrefreshing sleep, flushes of heat, burning soles of feet, burning itching haemorrhoids, insomnia.
Suited to: intellectual, self-absorbed, and untidy people.
Symptoms better for: open air, walking, movement.
Symptoms worse for: bathing, becoming overheated, standing, eating sweets, atmospheric changes.
Low time: late morning

Summer Catarrh Tablets
(Larkhall)
'Cantassium'

Dose: 1-2 tablets 3 times a day with water, preferably after a meal.
Product licence: PL/0912/6107R.
Constituents: lobelia (*Lobelia inflata*) 22.5 mg, vervain (*Verbena officinalis*) extract 17 mg, sage (*Salvia*) extract 17 mg, yarrow (*Achillea millefolium*) extract 17 mg, horehound extract (*Marrubium vulgare*) 7.5 mg, boneset (*Eupatorium perfoliatum*) 50 mg, capsicum powder 22.5 mg, calcium phosphate tribasic 234.5 mg, vegetable fatty acid.
Uses: to relieve catarrh in the upper respiratory tract during the hayfever season.
Special notes: vegan, yeast free, hypoallergenic.
Caution: not to be used in pregnancy or breastfeeding nor for children. Do not exceed the stated dose. Large doses of *Lobelia*

may cause nausea and vomiting.

Sunerven
(Modern Health)

Dose: 2 tablets to be taken after meals and 2 tablets before going to bed.
Product licence: No. PL/2452/5000R.
Constituents: valerian extract 90 mg, passionflower (*Passiflora*) extract 45 mg, motherwort (*Leonorus cardica*) 45 mg, vervain (*Verbena officinalis*) extract 90 mg, excipients.
Uses: anxiety, irritability, fatigue, insomnia.
Special notes: not tested on animals.
Caution: not recommended for children under 14 years nor in pregnancy or breastfeeding unless prescribed. Valerian should not be taken in large doses for an extended period of time. *Passiflora* may induce drowsiness in high doses.

Surbex T
(Abbott)

An orange, oval tablet used as a multivitamin treatment for vitamin B and vitamin C deficiencies.

Dose: adults 1 or more tablets a day; children 6-12 years 1 tablet a day.
Side effects:
Caution:
Not to be used for: children under 6 years.
Not to be used with: levodopa.
Contains: thiamine, riboflavine, nicotinamide, pyridoxine, ascorbic acid.
Other preparations:

Suscard Buccal
(Pharmax)

A white tablet supplied at strengths of 1 mg, 2 mg, 3 mg, 5 mg and used as a nitrate to treat angina, acute heart failure, congestive heart failure.

Dose: 5 mg 3 times a day at first or repeated until symptoms are relieved, allowing tablet to dissolve between upper lip and gum. For angina 1 mg as required or 1 mg 3 times a day increasing strength and frequency as needed.
Side effects: headache, flushes.
Caution:
Not to be used for: children.
Not to be used with:
Contains: glyceryl trinitrate.
Other preparations:

Symphytum
(Weleda 6c)

Prepared from *Symphytum officinale* plant (comfrey).

Uses: facilitates union of fractured bones (do not take unless you know the bones are in good alignment), pricking stitching pains, cartilage injuries, painful old injuries, blows to the eye from blunt objects.
Symptoms worse for: touch.
Symptoms better for:
Low time:

Syndol
(Merrell Dow)

A yellow, scored tablet used as an analgesic, antihistamine treatment for tension headache after dental or other surgery.

Dose: 1-2 tablets every 4-6 hours up to a maximum of 8 tablets in 24 hours.
Side effects: drowsiness, constipation.
Caution: in patients suffering from liver or kidney disease.
Not to be used for: children.
Not to be used with: alcohol, sedatives.
Contains: paracetamol, codeine phosphate, doxylamine succinate, caffeine.
Other preparations:

Synogist
(Townendale)

A shampoo used as an antifungal, antibacterial treatment for seborrhoea of the scalp.

Dose: shampoo twice a week for 4 weeks, then once a week.
Side effects:
Caution: keep out of the eyes.
Not to be used for:
Not to be used with:
Contains: sodium sulphosuccinated undecyclenic monoalkylolamide.
Other preparations:

Sytron
(Parke-Davis)

An elixir used as an iron supplement to treat iron-deficiency anaemia.

Dose: adults 1 5 ml teaspoonful 3 times a day at first increasing gradually to 2 teaspoonsful 3 times a day; children 0-1 year ½ teaspoonful twice a day, 1-5 years ½ teaspoonful 3 times a day, 6-12 years 1 teaspoonful 3 times a day.
Side effects: nausea, diarrhoea.

Caution:
Not to be used for:
Not to be used with: tetracyclines.
Contains: sodium iron edetate.
Other preparations:

Tabritis
(Potters)

Dose: 2 tablets 3 times a day. Needs to be taken for at least 6 weeks for maximum effect.
Product licence: 0250/5179R.
Constituents: elder flowers (*Sambucus*), prickly ash bark (*Zanthoxylum americanum*), yarrow (*Achillea millefolium*), burdock (*Arctium lappa*), clivers (*Galium aparine*), poplar bark, uva ursi (*Arctostaphylos uva-ursi*), senna (*Cassia senna*).
Uses: anti-inflammatory, analgesic, helps detoxify the body, for the relief of rheumatic and arthritic pain and stiffness.
Special notes:
Caution: not recommended during pregnancy or breastfeeding nor for children.

Tachyrol
(Duphar)

A white, scored tablet supplied at a strength of 0.2 mg and used as a source of vitamin D to treat rickets, osteomalacia, underactive parathyroid gland, kidney osteodystrophy (bone problems due to kidney disease).

Dose: adults 1 tablet a day at first, adjusted as needed; children as advised by a physician.
Side effects: raised blood or urine clacium levels.
Caution: in patients suffering from kidney disease. Blood calcium should be checked regularly.
Not to be used for:

Not to be used with: barbiturates, anticonvulsant drugs.
Contains: dihydrotachysterol.
Other preparations:

Tavegil
(Sandoz)

A white, scored tablet supplied at a strength of 1 mg and used as an antihistamine treatment for allergic rhinitis, dermatoses, urticaria, allergy to other drugs.

Dose: adults 1 tablet night and morning; children ½-1 tablet night and morning.
Side effects: drowsiness, reduced reactions, rarely dizziness, dry mouth, palpitations, gastro-intestinal disturbances.
Caution:
Not to be used for:
Not to be used with: MAOIs, sedatives, alcohol.
Contains: clemastine.
Other preparations: Tavegil Elixir.

TCP

TCP contains phenol and salicylate and is available as an antiseptic and lotion and ointment and throat pastilles containing blackcurrant, honey, and menthol or lemon. TCP is an efficient antiseptic which should be diluted with water to avoid too strong an astringent effect.

Tears Naturale
(Alcon)

Drops used to lubricate dry eyes.

Dose: use as needed.

Side effects:
Caution:
Not to be used for: patients who wear soft contact lenses.
Not to be used with:
Contains: dextran, hypromellose.
Other preparations:

Teejel
(Napp Consumer)

A gel used as an antiseptic, analgesic treatment for mouth ulcers, stomatitis, gingivitis, glossitis, teething, uncomfortable dentures.

Dose: rub gently into the affected area every 3-4 hours.
Side effects:
Caution:
Not to be used for: infants under 4 months.
Not to be used with:
Contains: choline salicylate, cetalkonium chloride.
Other preparations:

Tercoda
(Sinclair)

A syrup used as an opiate, expectorant, antussive, sputum softener to treat bronchitis.

Dose: 1-2 5 ml teaspoonsful 3 times a day.
Side effects: constipation.
Caution: in patients suffering from asthma.
Not to be used for: children, or for patients suffering from liver disease.
Not to be used with: MAOIs.
Contains: codeine phosphate, terpin hydrate, cineole, menthol, peppermint oil, pumilio pine oil.

Other preparations:

Terpoin
(Hough, Hoseason)

An elixir used as an opiate treatment for dry cough.

Dose: 1 5 ml teaspoonful every 3 hours.
Side effects: constipation.
Caution: in patients suffering from asthma.
Not to be used for: children under 5 years, or for patients suffering from liver disease.
Not to be used with: MAOIs.
Contains: codeine phosphate, cineole, menthol.
Other preparations:

Tetmosol
(ICI)

A solution used as a scabicide to treat scabies.

Dose: dilute and apply to the body as directed.
Side effects:
Caution: keep out of the eyes.
Not to be used for:
Not to be used with: alcohol.
Contains: monosulfiram.
Other preparations: Tetmosol Soap.

T Gel
(Neutrogena)

A shampoo used as an antipsoriatic treatment for dandruff, seborrhoea, and psoriasis of the scalp.

Dose: shampoo 1-2 times a week.
Side effects: irritation.
Caution:
Not to be used for: patients suffering from acute psoriasis.
Not to be used with:
Contains: coal tar extract.
Other preparations:

Theodrox
(3M Riker)

A white tablet used as a bronchodilator to treat bronchial spasm brought on by asthma, chronic bronchitis.

Dose: 1 tablet 4 times a day including 1 tablet at night.
Side effects: rapid heart rate, stomach upset, headache, sleeplessness, abnormal heart rhythms.
Caution: in the elderly, pregnant women, nursing mothers, and in patients suffering from heart or liver disease or peptic ulcer.
Not to be used for: children.
Not to be used with: cimetidine, erythromycin, ciprofloxacin, interferon.
Contains: aminophylline, aluminium hydroxide gel.
Other preparations:

Thephorin
(Sinclair)

A white tablet supplied at a strength of 25 mg and used as an antihistamine to treat allergies.

Dose: 1-2 tablets 3 times a day before 4.00 in the afternoon.
Side effects: dry mouth, stomach upset, rarely drowsiness.
Caution:
Not to be used for: children.
Not to be used with: MAOIs, sedatives, alcohol,

anticholinergics.
Contains: phenindamine tartrate.
Other preparations:

Theraderm
(Westwood)

A gel used as an antibacterial skin softener to treat acne.

Dose: wash and dry the affected area, then apply 1-2 times a day.
Side effects: irritation, peeling.
Caution: keep out of the eyes, nose, mouth.
Not to be used for:
Not to be used with:
Contains: benzoyl peroxide.
Other preparations:

Thuja
(Weleda 6c, 30c; Nelsons 6c)

Prepared from fresh green twigs of *Thuja occidentalis* tree (American arbor vitae, northern white cedar).

Uses: warts, catarrh, stabbing headaches, migraine, vertigo when closing the eyes, tooth decay at roots, ear inflammations, cystitis, insomnia, rumbling and flatulence in abdomen.
Suited to: dark-haired, dark-skinned, reserved and perhaps inflexible people.
Symptoms better for: warmth, movement, sneezing, rubbing.
Symptoms worse for: cold, damp, menstruation, tea, coffee, sweets, onions, bright light, sun.
Low time: mid-afternoon, night.

Thyme Formula
(Bio-Strath: imported by Cedar Health Ltd)

Dose: 20 drops (0.6 ml) in a little water every 2 hours.
Product licence: No. PL04210/0002.
Constituents: thyme leaf (*Thymus vulgaris*) extract 45 %, primula root (*Primula officinalis*) extract 5 %, *Torula utilis* yeast plasmolysate 50 %, (ethanol content 35.5 % v/v approx.).
Uses: antiseptic, for the temporary relief of coughs.
Special notes:
Caution: not recommended during pregnancy.

Timoped
(Reckitt & Colman)

A cream used as an antifungal treatment for athlete's foot and similar skin infections.

Dose: rub gently into the affected area and allow to dry.
Side effects:
Caution:
Not to be used for:
Not to be used with:
Contains: tolnaftate, triclosan.
Other preparations:

Tineafax
(Wellcome)

An ointment used as an antifungal treatment for athlete's foot and similar skin infections.

Dose: apply to the affected area twice a day at first, then once a day.
Side effects:
Caution:

Not to be used for:
Not to be used with:
Contains: zinc undecenoate, zinc naphthenate.
Other preparations: Tineafax Powder.

Tisept
(Seaton-Prebbles)

A solution in a sachet used as a disinfectant for cleansing and disinfecting wounds and burns, changing dressing, obstetrics.

Dose: use neat as needed.
Side effects:
Caution:
Not to be used for:
Not to be used with:
Contains: chlorhexidine gluconate, cetrimide.
Other preparations:

Titralac
(3M Riker)

A white tablet used as a calcium supplement.

Dose: to be adjusted for individuals.
Side effects:
Caution:
Not to be used for:
Not to be used with:
Contains: calcium carbonate, glycine.
Other preparations: Kloref-S.

Tonivitan
(Medo)

A brown capsule used as a multivitamin treatment for vitamin deficiencies.

Dose: 1-3 capsules 3 times a day.
Side effects:
Caution:
Not to be used for:
Not to be used with:
Contains: vitamin A, thiamine, nicotinic acid, ascorbic acid, calciferol, dried yeast.
Other preparations:

Tonivitan A & D
(Medo)

A syrup used as a source of vitamins A and D and minerals, and used as a tonic.

Dose: adults and children over 10 years 2 5 ml teaspoonsful 3 times a day; infants under 1 year ½ teaspoonful 3 times a day, 1-10 years 1 teaspoonful 3 times a day.
Side effects:
Caution:
Not to be used for:
Not to be used with:
Contains: vitamin A, thiamine, calciferol, ferric ammonium citrate, calcium glycerophosphate, manganese glycerophosphate, copper sulphate.
Other preparations:

Tonivitan B
(Medo)

A syrup used as a source of vitamin B and minerals, and used as a tonic.

Dose: adults 1-2 5 ml teaspoonsful 3 times a day; children as advised by a physician.
Side effects:
Caution:
Not to be used for:
Not to be used with: levodopa.
Contains: thiamine hydrochloride, riboflavine, pyridoxine hydrochloride, nicotinamide, calcium glycerophosphate, manganese glycerophosphate.
Other preparations:

Topal
(ICI)

A cream tablet used as an antacid to treat oesophagitis, heartburn, gastritis.

Dose: adults 1-3 tablets 3-4 times a day between meals and at bedtime; children half adult dose.
Side effects: occasionally constipation.
Caution:
Not to be used for: infants.
Not to be used with: tetracycline antibiotics.
Contains: aluminium hydroxide, magnesium carbonate, alginic acid.
Other preparations:

Topiclens
(S & N)

A solution in a sachet used to wash out the eyes, wounds, or burns.

Dose: use as needed.
Side effects:
Caution: throw away any remaining solution.
Not to be used for:
Not to be used with:
Contains: sodium chloride.
Other preparations:

Torbetol
(Torbet Laboratories)

A lotion used as an antibacterial treatment for acne.

Dose: apply to the affected area 3 times a day.
Side effects:
Caution:
Not to be used for:
Not to be used with:
Contains: cetrimide, benzalkonium chloride, hexachlorophane.
Other preparations:

Transiderm-Nitro
(Ciba)

Patches supplied at strengths of 5 mg, 10 mg and used as a nitrate for the prevention of angina..

Dose: apply a patch to a hairless part of the chest every 24 hours on a different place each time.
Side effects: headache, rash, dizziness.
Caution: the treatment should be reduced gradually and re-placed with decreasing doses of oral nitrate.
Not to be used for: children.
Not to be used with:
Contains: glyceryl trinitrate.
Other preparations:

Transvasin
(Lloyds)

A cream used as an analgesic rub for the relief of rheumatic and muscular pain.

Dose: massage into the affected area at least twice a day.
Side effects:
Caution:
Not to be used for:
Not to be used with:
Contains: thurfyl salicylate, ethyl nicotinate, n-hexyl nicotinate, benzocaine.
Other preparations:

Travasept 100
(Baxter)

A solution used as an aminoglycocide antibiotic, antibacterial preparation for disinfecting wounds and burns.

Dose: use neat as needed.
Side effects:
Caution:
Not to be used for:
Not to be used with:
Contains: chlorhexidine acetate, cetrimide.
Other preparations:

Travel Sickness
(Nelsons)

Combination of *Apomorphium* 6c, *Staphisagria* 6c, *Cocculus indicus* 6c, Nux vom. 6c, petroleum 6c, *Tabacum* 6c, *Theridion* 6c.

Uses: the relief of travel sickness.

Travel Sickness Naturtabs
(Larkhall)
'Cantassium'

Dose: 3 tablets with water ½ hour before meals or ½ hour before beginning a journey; children 6-12 years 1-2 tablets as above.
Product licence: No. PL0912/7219R.
Constituents: ginger (*Zingiber officinale*) 250 mg, calcium phosphate tribasic 0.18 g, calcium sulphate dihydrate 88 mg, potato starch 20 mg, vegetable fatty acid 2 mg, isopropyl alcohol 83ul.
Uses: the relief of travel sickness and nausea.
Special notes: vegan, yeast free.
Caution:

Triclosept
(Hough, Hoseason)

A cream used as a disinfectant for cleansing and disinfecting the hands and skin.

Dose: rub vigorously into the affected area until the cream has been absorbed.
Side effects:
Caution:
Not to be used for:
Not to be used with:
Contains: triclosan.
Other preparations:

Triludan
(Merrell Dow)

A white, scored tablet supplied at a strength of 60 mg and used as an antihistamine treatment for allergies including hay fever and rhinitis.

Dose: adults 1 tablet twice a day or 2 tablets once a day; children 6-12 years ½ tablet twice a day.
Side effects: rash, sweating, headache, mild stomach disturbances.
Caution:
Not to be used for: children under 6 years.
Not to be used with:
Contains: terfenadine.
Other preparations: Triludan Forte, Triludan Suspension.

Triosorbon
(Merck)

Gluten-, sucrose-, fructose-, and galactose-free, low-lactose powder used as a source of protein, carbohydrate, fat, vitamins, and minerals for patients suffering from short bowel syndrome, intractable poor absorption, dysphagia, inflammatory bowel disease, cachexia, anorexia nervosa, or for undernourished patients before surgery or after complete gastrectomy.

Caution: unsuitable as the only source of nutrition for children under 5 years.
Not to be used for: infants under 1 year.

Tritamyl
(Procea)

Gluten- and lactose-free, starch-based self-raising flour used for patients suffering from coeliac disease, dermatitis herpetiformes, and digestive disorders sensitive to gluten.

Other preparations: Tritamyl PK

Trufree
(Cantassium)

Various gluten-free flours used for patients suffering from digestive disorders sensitive to gluten.

Tyrozets
(MSD)

A pink lozenge used as an antibiotic and local anaesthetic to treat mild mouth and throat disorders.

Dose: allow 1 lozenge to dissolve in the mouth every 3 hours to a maximum of 8 lozenges in 24 hours.
Side effects: additional infection, blackening or soreness of mouth and tongue.
Caution:
Not to be used for:
Not to be used with:
Contains: tyrothricin, benzocaine.
Other preparations:

Uniflu & Gregovite C
(Unigreg)

A red, oblong tablet and a yellow tablet used as an analgesic, opiate, antussive, xanthine, antihistamine treatment for cold and flu symptoms.

Dose: 1 each of the tablets every 4 hours up to a maximum of 6 of each tablets in 24 hours.
Side effects: constipation, drowsiness, reduced reactions, anxiety, hands shaking, irregular or rapid heart rate, dry mouth, excitement, rarely skin eruptions.
Caution: in patients suffering from asthma, kidney disease, diabetes.

Not to be used for: children, or for patients suffering from liver disease, heart or thyroid disorders.
Not to be used with: MAOIs, sedatives, alcohol, tricyclics.
Contains: paracetamol, codeine phosphate, caffeine, diphenhydramine hydrochloride, phenylphrine hydrochloride, ascorbic acid.
Other preparations:

Unisept
(Seton-Prebbles)

A solution used as a disinfectant and general antiseptic.

Dose: use neat as needed.
Side effects:
Caution:
Not to be used for:
Not to be used with:
Contains: chlorhexidine gluconate.
Other preparations:

Urisal
(Sterling Research Laboratories)

Orange-flavoured granules in sachets of 4 g used as an alkalizing agent to relieve the pain of cystitis.

Dose: the contents of 1 sachet dissolved in water 3 times a day for 3 days.
Side effects:
Caution: in patients suffereing from kidney disease.
Not to be used for: children, pregnant women, or for patients suffering from heart disease, high blood pressure, or with a history of kidney disease.
Not to be used with:
Contains: sodium citrate.

Other preparations:

Urtica Urens
(Weleda 6c)

Prepared from the flowering *Urtica urens* plant
(nettle).

Uses: skin rashes and irritations especially from heat or allergy,
stinging and burning pains, urticaria, itchy red raised blotches,
minor burns which do not blister, sunburn, insufficient breast
milk, gout.
Symptoms better for:
Symptoms worse for: cool bathing, cool moist air, touch.
Low time:

Valerian Compound
(Gerard House)

Dose: 2 tablets to be taken in the early evening and 2 tablets
immediately before bedtime.
Product licence: 1661/5029R.
Constituents: hops (*Humulus lupulus*)50 mg, passionflower
(*Passiflora*) 50 mg, valerian (*Valeriana officinalis*) extract 18
mg, wild lettuce (*Lactuca virosa*) extract 9 mg, Jamaican
dogwood (*Piscidia erythrina*) extract 11 mg, scullcap (*Scutellaria*)
45 mg, malto-dextrin 58 mg, sodium starch glycollate 1.26 mg,
magnesium stearate 0.75 mg, talc 13 mg, lactose 13 mg;
coating iron oxide, titanium dioxide, and syrup.
Uses: to relieve restlessness and aid sleep.
Special notes: vegan, yeast free.
Caution: not recommended for children under 12 years. Not to
be used in pregnancy or breastfeeding. Sedative action may
cause drowsiness if taken during the day.

Valerian Formula
(Bio-Strath: imported by Cedar Health Ltd)

Dose: 20 drops (0.6 ml) in a little water 3 times a day before meals and ½ hour before going to bed.
Product licence: No. PL04210/0005.
Constituents: valerian root (*Valeriana officinalis*) extract 22.5 %, passionflower leaf (*Passiflora incarnata*) extract 22.5 %, peppermint leaf (*Mentha piperita*) extract 5 %, *Torula utilis* yeast plasmolysate 50 %, (ethanol content 40 % v/v approx.).
Uses: to calm and relieve nervousness and irritability.
Special notes:
Caution: shake bottle before use. Not recommended in pregnancy or breastfeeding nor for children. May antidote any homoeopathic remedies you are taking. May cause drowsiness.

Varicose Ointment
(Potters)

Dose: apply to the affected parts morning and evening.
Product licence: No. PL0250/5136R.
Constituents: cade oil, witch hazel (*Hamamelis*) water, zinc oxide, base.
Uses: to relieve skin conditions of the lower limbs where there is much irritation due to varicosity.
Caution:

Vegetable Cough Remover
(Potters)

Dose: 2 5 ml teaspoonsful 3-4 times a day; children over 8 years 1 5 ml teaspoonful 3 times a day; children 5-7 years 1 5 ml teaspoonful every 12 hours.
Product licence: No. 0250/5090R.
Constituents: black cohosh (*Cimicifuga racemosa*),

ipecacuanha (*Cephalis ipecacuanha*), lobelia (*Lobelia inflata*), pleurisy root (*Asclepias tuberosa*), scullcap (*Scutellaria*), elecampane (*Inula helenium*) extract, horehound (*Marrubium vulgare*) extract, hyssop (*Hyssopus officinalis*) extract, liquorice (*Glycyrrhiza glabra*), anise oil (*Pimpinella anisum*) syrup.
Uses: the symptomatic relief of coughs.
Special notes:
Caution: not to be used in pregnancy or breastfeeding nor for children under 5 years. Do not exceed the stated dose. Shake bottle before use.

Vegetex
(Modern Health)

Dose: 3 tablets 3 times a day before meals.
Product licence: No. 1146/5000R.
Constituents: celery (*Apium graveolens*) 87 mg, buckbean (*Menyanthes trifoliata*) 37.5 mg, black cohosh (*Cimicifuga racemosa*) 37.5 mg, horseradish (*Armoracia rusticana*), excipients.
Uses: rheumatic pain, fibrositis, sciatica. It is formulated to reduce body acids and thereby relieve symptoms.
Special notes: not tested on animals.
Caution: not recommended for children under 12 years. Black cohosh is not to be used in pregnancy. Large doses of buckbean may cause vomiting and diarrhoea. Large doses of horseradish may cause skin or gastro-intestinal irritation in some patients.

Veracur
(Typharm)

A gel used as a skin softener to treat warts.

Dose: apply to the wart twice a day and cover, rubbing down with a pumic stone between treatments.
Side effects:

Caution: do not apply to healthy skin.
Not to be used for: warts on the face or anal and genital areas.
Not to be used with:
Contains: formaldehyde.
Other preparations:

Verdiviton
(Squibb)

A liquid used as a source of vitamin B complex for maintaining vitamin B complex levels.

Dose: 3 5 ml teaspoonsful 3 times a day before food.
Side effects:
Caution:
Not to be used for: children, or for patients suffering from hepatitis, alcoholism
Not to be used with: levodopa
Contains: glycerophosphates of calcium, sodium, potassium, manganese, cyanocobalamin, d-panthenol, nicotinamide, pyridoxine, riboflavine, thiamine, alcohol.
Other preparations:

Verrugon
(Pickles)

An ointment with corn rings and plasters used as a skin softener to treat warts.

Dose: protect healthy skin, apply the ointment to the wart, and cover with a plaster, rubbing down with pumice stone between treatments.
Side effects:
Caution: do not apply to healthy skin
Not to be used for: warts on the face or anal and genital regions.

Not to be used with:
Contains: salicyclic acid.
Other preparations:

Verucasep
(Galen)

A gel used as a virucidal, anhidrotic treatment for viral warts.

Dose: apply twice a day, paring down any hard skin around the wart.
Side effects: stains the skin.
Caution: do not apply to healthy skin.
Not to be used for: warts on the face or anal and genital regions.
Not to be used with:
Contains: glutaraldehyde.
Other preparations:

Vick

Vicks preparations contain basic ingredients similar to Day Nurse. In addition, there is an expectorant which contains guaiphenesin and citrate, and a Medinite preparation which has ephedrine, doxylamine, and alcohol. Vicks Sinex spray contains oxymetalozine, menthol, camphor and eucalyptol. Vicks throat spray and vapour rub are also available. The side effects of these preparations depend upon the main ingredients but they should be treated similarly to Actifed.

Videne Powder
(3M Riker)

A powder used as an antiseptic treatment for infections in wounds and burns.

Dose: dust the affected area lightly with the powder.
Side effects:
Caution:
Not to be used for:
Not to be used with:
Contains: povidone-iodine.
Other preparations: Videne Solution, Videne Tincture, Videne Surgical

---

Visclair
(Sinclair)

A yellow tablet supplied at a strength of 100 mg and used as a mucus softener to treat bronchitis, phlegm.

Dose: adults 2 tablets 3-4 times a day for 6 weeks then 2 tablets twice a day; children over 5 years 1 tablet 3 times a day.
Side effects: stomach upset.
Caution:
Not to be used for: children under 5 years.
Not to be used with:
Contains: methylcysteine hydrochloride.
Other preparations:

Vita-E
(Bioglan)

An ointment used as an anti-oxidant to treat wounds, bed sores, burns, skin ulcers.

Dose: apply to the affected area as needed.
Side effects:
Caution:
Not to be used for: patients suffering from overactive thyroid gland.
Not to be used with: fish liver oils, digitalis, insulin.

Contains: d-alpha-tocopheryl acetate.
Other preparations:

Waterlex
(Gerard House)

Dose: 1-2 tablets 3 times a day.
Product licence: 0770/5116R.
Constituents: dandelion (*Taraxacum officinale*) 90 mg, horsetail (*Equisetum arvense*) extract 10 mg, uva ursi (*Arctostaphylos uva-ursi*) extract 75 mg, starch 1500 12.25 mg, sugar 37.50 mg, talc 3.75 mg, magnesium stearate 1.5 mg; titanium dioxide and syrup as coating.
Uses: diuretic, antiseptic, helpful for fluid retention and pre-menstrual tension.
Special notes: vegan, yeast free.
Caution: not recommended for children under 12 years. Not to be used in pregnancy without practitioner supervision.

Water Naturtabs
(Larkhall)
'Cantassium'

Dose: 1-2 tablets 3 times a day.
Product licence: No. PL0912/7199R.
Constituents: bladderwrack (*Fucus vesiculosus*) extract 50 mg, burdock (*Arctium lappa*) extract 25 mg, ground ivy (*Glechoma hederacea*) extract 25 mg, clivers (*Galium aparine*) extract 25 mg, calcium phosphate tribasic 100 mg, sago flour 20 mg, magnesium trisilicate 4 mg, vegetable fatty acid 1 mg.
Uses: to relieve fluid retention and premenstrual tension.
Special notes: vegan, yeast free.
Caution: not to be used for children nor in pregnancy or breastfeeding without practitioner supervision.

Water Relief
(Booker)
'Heath & Heather'

Dose: 1-2 tablets 3 times a day for up to 7 days before expected onset of menstruation.
Product licence: No. P/L1713/5023R.
Constituents: bladderwrack (*Fucus vesiculosus*) 200 mg, clivers (*Galium aparine*) 200 mg, ground ivy (*Glechoma hederacea*) 200 mg, burdock root (*Arctium lappa*) 100 mg, dicalcium phosphate, microcrystalline cellulose, stearic acid, magnesium stearate; coating hypromellose, polyethylene glycol, titanium dioxide.
Uses: diuretic, to provide relief from premenstrual tension.
Special notes: vegan, yeast free.
Caution: not recommended for children. Not to be taken in pregnancy.

Waxsol
(Norgine)

Drops used as a wax softener to remove wax from the ears.

Dose: fill the ear with the solution for 2 nights before they are to be syringed.
Side effects: temporary irritation.
Caution:
Not to be used for: patients suffering from inflammation of the ear or perforated eardrum.
Not to be used with:
Contains: sodium docusate.
Other preparations:

WCS Dusting Powder
(Weleda)

Dose: dust the affected area liberally and cover with a dry dressing. Change the dressing twice a day.
Product licence: No. PL0298/5565.
Constituents: per 100 g: arnica (*Arnica montana*) 1 g, marigold (*Calendula*) 1.65 g, purple coneflower (*Echinacea angustifolia*) 0.5 g, silica 0.1 g, Stibium Metallicum Praep. 0.1 g, purified talc.
Uses: for the treatment of minor burns and wounds which need to be kept dry.
Caution:
Not to be used for: patients where a deep infection is present because *Calendula* promotes surface healing and may seal in sepsis.
Availability: pharmacies only.

Wellwoman Tablets
(Potters)

Dose: 2 tablets 3 times a day.
Product licence: No. PL0250/5207R.
Constituents: yarrow (*Achillea millefolium*), motherwort (*Leonorus cardiaca*), lime flowers (*Tilia platyphylla*), scullcap (*Scutellaria*), valerian (*Valeriana officinalis*).
Uses: to relieve menopausal symptoms.
Special notes:
Caution: not recommended in pregnancy or breastfeeding.

Willow Formula
(Bio-Strath: imported by Cedar Health Ltd)

Dose: 50 drops (1.5 ml) in a little water 3 times a day before meals.
Product licence: No. PL04210/0003.
Constituents: willow bark (*Salix purpurea*) extract 35 %, primula

root (*Primula officinalis*) extract 15 %, *Torula utilis* yeast plasmolysate 50 %, (ethanol content 39 % v/v approx.).

Uses: analgesic, anti-inflammatory, to relieve backache, lumbago, sciatica, fibrositis, and muscular pain. Willow contains salicin and salicylic acid and is considered to be the natural form and origin of modern aspirin.

Special notes:
Caution: not recommended for children or during pregnancy or breastfeeding.

---

witch hazel (see also **Optrex**)

witch hazel is a solution which is useful in reducing the reddening and soreness of skin inflammations.

Wysoy
(Wyeth)

Gluten-, milk protein-, and lactose-free powder used as a source of protein, carbohydrate, fat, vitamins, minerals, and trace elements for patients suffering from galactosaemia, low galactokinase, intolerance to milk or lactose.

Xylocaine

Xylocaine gel, ointment, and spray contain a local anaesthetic which can be used to suppress pain from local mouth disorders. It only masks the pain, however, and should not be used for more than a few days.

Yomesan
(Bayer)

A yellow tablet supplied at a strength of 500 mg used to treat tapeworm.

Dose: as advised by the physician.
Side effects: stomach upset, lightheadedness, itch.
Caution:
Not to be used for:
Not to be used with: alcohol.
Contains: niclosamide.
Other preparations:

Zeif
(New Era)

Combination of Ferr. Phos. 6x, Nat. Phos. 6x, Nat. Sulph. 6x, Silica 6x.

Uses: rheumatic pain and allied conditions.

Z Span Spansule
(S K & F)

A blue/clear capsule used as a zinc supplement for the prevention and treatment of zinc deficiency.

Dose: adults and children over 1 year 1 capsule 1-3 times a day.
Side effects: stomach upset.
Caution: in patients suffering from kidney failure.
Not to be used for: infants under 1 year.
Not to be used with: tetracyclines.
Contains: zinc sulphate monohydrate.
Other preparations:

Glossary

adrenal glands
the adrenal glands are organs situated above the kidneys which produce hormones, including steroids.

anticholinergic
a drug which blocks the action of acetyl choline, a nerve transmitter. Anticholinergics are used to reduce muscle spasm. The effects include dry mouth, difficulty passing urine, and possibly confusion.

beta-blocker (ß-blocker)
a drug which blocks some of the effects of adrenaline in the body. Beta-blockers are used to treat angina, high blood pressure, and other conditions.

MAOI (mono-amine oxidase inhibitor)
an antidepressant agent which may interact with some foods and other drugs.

nitrate
a drug used to treat poor blood supply to the heart muscle (angina). Nitrates reduce the work which the heart has to do.

tricyclic antidepressant
a drug used to treat depression but which may cause sedation and dryness of the mouth.

INDEX

If you look up a condition from which you may be suffering, you will be referred to the name of one or more medicines which may be used to treat the condition. You can refer directly to each of these medicines in Part 3: Alphabetical Listing. In addition, you will see a page number. This is the number of the page in Parts 1 and 2 of the book and, in Part 1, you will also find the other medicines in that section used to treat related disorders.

A

B

C

D

E

H

I

N

O

P

T

Magnesia Phosphorica 354

Z

zinc deficiency

Notes

Notes

Notes